Pediatric Head and Neck Imaging

Editor

WILLIAM T. O'BRIEN SR

NEUROIMAGING CLINICS OF NORTH AMERICA

www.neuroimaging.theclinics.com

Consulting Editor
SURESH K. MUKHERJI

November 2023 • Volume 33 • Number 4

ELSEVIER

1600 John F. Kennedy Boulevard • Suite 1800 • Philadelphia, Pennsylvania, 19103-2899

http://www.neuroimaging.theclinics.com

NEUROIMAGING CLINICS OF NORTH AMERICA Volume 33, Number 4
November 2023 ISSN 1052-5149, ISBN 13: 978-0-323-93901-0

Editor: John Vassallo (j.vassallo@elsevier.com)
Developmental Editor: Saswoti Nath

Neuroimaging Clinics of North America (ISSN 1052-5149) is published quarterly by Elsevier Inc., 360 Park Avenue South, New York, NY 10010-1710. Months of issue are February, May, August, and November. Business and editorial offices: 1600 John F. Kennedy Blvd., Suite 1800, Philadelphia, PA 19103-2899. Business and editorial offices: 6277 Sea Harbor Drive, Orlando, FL 32887-4800. Periodicals postage paid at New York, NY, and additional mailing offices. Subscription prices are USD 413 per year for US individuals, USD 745 per year for US institutions, USD 100 per year for US students and residents, USD 483 per year for Canadian individuals, USD 949 per year for Canadian institutions, USD 562 per year for international individuals, USD 949 per year for international institutions, USD 100 per year for Canadian students and residents and USD 260 per year for foreign students and residents. To receive student/resident rate, orders must be accompanied by name of affiliated institution, date of term, and the *signature* of program/residency coordinator on institution letterhead. Orders will be billed at individual rate until proof of status is received. Foreign air speed delivery is included in all *Clinics* subscription prices. All prices are subject to change without notice. POSTMASTER: Send address changes to *Neuroimaging Clinics of North America*, Elsevier Health Sciences Division, Subscription **Customer Service, 3251 Riverport Lane, Maryland Heights, MO 63043. Telephone: 1-800-654-2452 (U.S. and Canada); 314-447-8871 (outside U.S. and Canada). Fax: 314-447-8029. E-mail: journalscustomerservice-usa@elsevier.com (for print support); journals onlinesupport-usa@elsevier.com (for online support)**.

Reprints. For copies of 100 or more of articles in this publication, please contact the Commercial Reprints Department, Elsevier Inc., 360 Park Avenue South, New York, NY 10010-1710. Tel.: 212-633-3874; Fax: 212-633-3820; E-mail: reprints@elsevier.com.

Neuroimaging Clinics of North America is covered by *Excerpta Medical/EMBASE,* the RSNA Index of Imaging Literature, *MEDLINE/PubMed (Index Medicus),* MEDLINE/MEDLARS, SciSearch, Research Alert, and Neuroscience Citation Index.

PROGRAM OBJECTIVE

The goal of *Neuroimaging Clinics of North America* is to keep practicing radiologists and radiology residents up to date with current clinical practice in radiology by providing timely articles reviewing the state of the art in patient care.

TARGET AUDIENCE

Practicing radiologists, radiology residents, and other healthcare professionals who utilize neuroimaging findings to provide patient care.

LEARNING OBJECTIVES

Upon completion of this activity, participants will be able to:

1. Review characteristic imaging features of some of the more common congenital, acquired, and neoplastic head and neck masses in children.
2. Discuss salient imaging features, important complications, and pertinent clinical and surgical considerations for various pediatric head and neck infections.
3. Recognize both strengths and limitations radiologists face when utilizing various imaging modalities available to pediatric patients.

ACCREDITATION

The Elsevier Office of Continuing Medical Education (EOCME) is accredited by the Accreditation Council for Continuing Medical Education (ACCME) to provide continuing medical education for physicians.

The EOCME designates this journal-based CME activity for a maximum of 11 *AMA PRA Category 1 Credit*(s)™. Physicians should claim only the credit commensurate with the extent of their participation in the activity.

All other healthcare professionals requesting continuing education credit for this enduring material will be issued a certificate of participation.

DISCLOSURE OF CONFLICTS OF INTEREST

The EOCME assesses conflict of interest with its instructors, faculty, planners, and other individuals who are in a position to control the content of CME activities. All relevant conflicts of interest that are identified are thoroughly vetted by EOCME for fair balance, scientific objectivity, and patient care recommendations. EOCME is committed to providing its learners with CME activities that promote improvements or quality in healthcare and not a specific proprietary business or a commercial interest.

The planning committee, staff, authors, and editors listed below have identified no financial relationships or relationships to products or devices they or their spouse/life partner have with commercial interest related to the content of this CME activity:
Berna Aygun, MBBS, MRes, FRCR; Asthik Biswas, MBBS, DNB; Timothy N. Booth, MD; Michael C. Brodsky, MD; Rebekah Clarke, MD; Felice D'Arco, MD; Sri Gore, MBBS, FRCOphth; Julie B. Guerin, MD; Kothainayaki Kulanthaivelu, BCA, MBA; Martin Lewis, MD; Michelle Littlejohn; Mark D. Mamlouk, MD; Kshitij Mankad, MD, FRCR; William T. O'Brien, Sr., DO; Caroline D. Robson, MBChB; V. Michelle Silvera, MD; Ajay Taranath, MD, FRANZCR; Jennifer A. Vaughn, MD; Oi Yean Wong, MBBS, FRCR; Harun Yildiz, MD

UNAPPROVED/OFF-LABEL USE DISCLOSURE

The EOCME requires CME faculty to disclose to the participants:

1. When products or procedures being discussed are off-label, unlabelled, experimental, and/or investigational (not US Food and Drug Administration [FDA] approved); and
2. Any limitations on the information presented, such as data that are preliminary or that represent ongoing research, interim analyses, and/or unsupported opinions. Faculty may discuss information about pharmaceutical agents that is outside of FDA-approved labelling. This information is intended solely for CME and is not intended to promote off-label use of these medications. If you have any questions, contact the medical affairs department of the manufacturer for the most recent prescribing information.

TO ENROLL

To enroll in the *Neuroimaging Clinics of North America* Continuing Medical Education program, call customer service at 1-800-654-2452 or sign up online at http://www.theclinics.com/home/cme. The CME program is available to subscribers for an additional annual fee of USD 359.00.

METHOD OF PARTICIPATION

In order to claim credit, participants must complete the following:

1. Complete enrolment as indicated above.
2. Read the activity.
3. Complete the CME Test and Evaluation. Participants must achieve a score of 70% on the test. All CME Tests and Evaluations must be completed online.

CME INQUIRIES/SPECIAL NEEDS

For all CME inquiries or special needs, please contact elsevierCME@elsevier.com.

NEUROIMAGING CLINICS OF NORTH AMERICA

FORTHCOMING ISSUES

February 2024
Vasculitis
Mahmud Mossa-Basha, Carlos A. Zamora, and
Mauricio Castillo, *Editors*

May 2024
**Advanced Imaging in Ischemic and
Hemorrhagic Stroke**
Joseph J. Gemmete and Zachary M. Wilseck,
Editors

August 2024
**Multiple Sclerosis and Associated
Demyelinating Disorders**
Frederik Barkhof and Yaou Liu, *Editors*

RECENT ISSUES

August 2023
Spinal Tumors
Carlos H. Torres, *Editor*

May 2023
MRI and Traumatic Brain Injury
Pejman Jabehdar Maralani and Sean Symons,
Editors

February 2023
Central Nervous System Infections
Tchoyoson Lim Choie Cheio, *Editor*

SERIES OF RELATED INTEREST

Advances in Clinical Radiology
Available at: https://www.advancesinclinicalradiology.com/
MRI Clinics of North America
Available at: https://www.mri.theclinics.com/
PET Clinics
Available at: https://www.pet.theclinics.com/
Radiologic Clinics of North America
Available at: https://www.radiologic.theclinics.com/

THE CLINICS ARE AVAILABLE ONLINE!
Access your subscription at:
www.theclinics.com

Contributors

CONSULTING EDITOR

SURESH K. MUKHERJI, MD, MBA, FACR
Professor of Radiology, University of Louisville, Louisville, Kentucky, USA; Professor of Radiology, University of Illinois, Peoria, Illinois, USA; Professor of Radiation Oncology, Robert Wood Johnson Medical School, Rutgers University, New Brunswick, New Jersey, USA; Faculty, Otolaryngology–Head Neck Surgery, Michigan State University, Farmington Hills, Michigan, USA; National Director of Head and Neck Radiology, Marian University, Head and Neck Radiology, ProScan Imaging, Carmel, Indiana, USA

EDITOR

WILLIAM T. O'BRIEN SR. DO, FAOCR
Chief, Pediatric Neuroradiology, Orlando Health - Arnold Palmer Hospital for Children, Orlando, Florida, USA

AUTHORS

BERNA AYGUN, MBBS, MRES, FRCR
Department of Neuroradiology, Neuroradiologist, King's College Hospital NHS Foundation Trust, Department of Neuroradiology, Neuroradiologist, Great Ormond Street Hospital for Children NHS Foundation Trust, London, United Kingdom

ASTHIK BISWAS, MBBS, DNB
Department of Neuroradiology, Neuroradiologist, Great Ormond Street Hospital for Children NHS Foundation Trust, London, United Kingdom

TIMOTHY N. BOOTH, MD
Professor of Radiology and Otolaryngology, University of Texas Southwestern, Children's Health of Texas, Dallas, Texas, USA

MICHAEL C. BRODSKY, MD
Professor of Ophthalmology and Neurology, Department of Ophthalmology, Mayo Clinic, Rochester, Minnesota, USA

REBEKAH CLARKE, MD
Assistant Professor, Department of Pediatric Radiology, University of Texas Southwestern, Children's Health Dallas, Dallas, Texas, USA

FELICE D'ARCO, MD
Pediatric Neuroradiologist, Department of Radiology, Great Ormond Street Hospital for Children NHS Foundation Trust, London, United Kingdom

SRI GORE, MBBS, BSC FRCOPHTH, PGDIP ED
Department of Ophthalmology, Consultant Ophthalmologist and Lead Oculoplastic Surgeon, Great Ormond Street Hospital for Children NHS Foundation Trust, London, United Kingdom

JULIE B. GUERIN, MD
Assistant Professor, Department of Radiology, Mayo Clinic, Rochester, Minnesota, USA

MARTIN LEWIS, MD
Department of Radiology, Great Ormond Street Hospital for Children NHS Foundation Trust, London, United Kingdom

MARK D. MAMLOUK, MD
Regional Neuroradiology Lead, Department of
Radiology, The Permanente Medical Group,
Kaiser Permanente Medical Center, Santa
Clara, California, USA; Assistant Clinical
Professor of Neuroradiology - Volunteer,
Department of Radiology and Biomedical
Imaging, University of California, San
Francisco, San Francisco, California, USA

KSHITIJ MANKAD, MBBS, FRCR
Department of Neuroradiology,
Neuroradiologist, Great Ormond Street
Hospital for Children NHS Foundation Trust,
London, United Kingdom; Associate Professor,
UCL GOS Institute of Child Health, London,
United Kingdom

WILLIAM T. O'BRIEN SR. DO, FAOCR
Chief, Pediatric Neuroradiology, Orlando
Health - Arnold Palmer Hospital for Children,
Orlando, Florida, USA

CAROLINE D. ROBSON, MB, ChB
Neuroradiology Division Chief, Department of
Radiology, Boston Children's Hospital,
Associate Professor in Radiology, Harvard
Medical School, Boston, Massachusetts, USA

V. MICHELLE SILVERA, MD
Associate Professor, Department of Radiology,
Mayo Clinic, Rochester, Minnesota, USA

AJAY TARANATH, MBBS, MD, FRANZCR
Department of Medical Imaging,
Neuroradiologist, Women's and Children's
Hospital, South Australia Medical Imaging,
University of Adelaide, South Australia,
Australia

JENNIFER A. VAUGHN, MD
Department of Radiology, Phoenix Children's
Hospital, Clinical Assistant Professor,
Radiology, University of Arizona College of
Medicine, Clinical Assistant Professor,
Radiology, Creighton University School of
Medicine, Barrows Neurological Institute,
Phoenix, Arizona, USA

OI YEAN WONG, MBBS, FRCR
Department of Neuroradiology, Fellow, Great
Ormond Street Hospital for Children NHS
Foundation Trust, London, United Kingdom

HARUN YILDIZ, MD
Department of Radiology, Radiologist, Bursa
Dortcelik Children's Hospital, Bursa, Turkey

Contents

limitations of the various imaging modalities available to image pediatric patients presenting with cervical adenopathy, provide guidance on when to image, and highlight the imaging appearance of both common and uncommon disorders affecting the cervical nodes in children to aid the radiologist in their clinical practice.

Congenital cystic masses are commonly encountered when imaging a patient presenting with a neck mass. Congenital cysts are present at birth; however, these cysts may not present until later in life with some growing slowly and others rapidly increasing in size due to hemorrhage or infection. A neonatal presentation is rare but when present may allow a narrower differential diagnosis. Imaging plays a significant role in defining a lesion as cystic, assessing location, and directing the next step in evaluation and/or intervention.

Neck masses are frequent in the pediatric population and are usually divided into congenital, inflammatory, and neoplastic. Many of these lesions are cystic and are often benign. Solid masses and vascular lesions are relatively less common, and the imaging appearances can be similar. This article reviews the clinical presentation and imaging patterns of pediatric solid and vascular neck masses.

In this article, we will discuss the essential MR imaging protocol required for the assessment of ocular abnormalities including malignancies. Then we will describe relevant anatomy, ocular embryogenesis, and genetics to establish a profound understanding of pathophysiology of the congenital ocular malformations. Finally, we will discuss pediatric ocular malignancies, benign mimics, and the most common congenital ocular malformations with case examples and illustrations and give tips on how to distinguish these entities on neuroimaging.

In this article, we will describe relevant anatomy and imaging findings of extraocular and orbital rim pathologic conditions. We will highlight important clinical and imaging pearls that help in differentiating these lesions from one another, and provide a few practical tips for challenging cases.

Neck infections are common in children, though the clinical presentation is often vague and nonspecific. Therefore, imaging plays a key role in identifying the site and extent of infections, evaluating for potentially drainable collections, and assessing for airway and vascular complications. This review focuses on imaging features associated with common and characteristic neck infections in children to include tonsillar, retropharyngeal, and otomastoid infections; suppurative adenopathy; superimposed inflammation or infection of congenital cystic lesions; and Lemierre syndrome.

Odontogenic and sinogenic infections are frequently encountered in the pediatric population. Although the diagnosis is often suspected clinically, imaging can play a significant role in localizing the site of infection, assessing for involvement of deep neck spaces, detection of abscess and other potentially life-threatening complications, and providing valuable information to help with treatment planning. This article reviews the general imaging considerations and anatomy relevant to odontogenic and paranasal sinus infections and describes the salient clinical and imaging features of infectious diseases of the dentition and sinuss.

Most primary orbital pathology in children is due to bacterial infection. Radiologists typically encounter these cases to evaluate for clinically suspected postseptal orbital involvement. Contrast-enhanced cross-sectional imaging is important for the detection and early management of orbital infection and associated subperiosteal/orbital abscess, venous thrombosis, and intracranial spread of infection. Benign mass-like inflammatory processes involving the pediatric orbit are rare, have overlapping imaging features, and must be distinguished from orbital malignancies.

Foreword
Pediatric Head and Neck Imaging

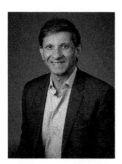

Suresh K. Mukherji, MD, MBA, FACR
Consulting Editor

Children are NOT little adults! This adage succinctly summarizes why we decided to have an issue for *Neuroimaging Clinics* devoted to pediatric head and neck. I often joke that head and neck studies are frequently left for those radiologists who are on an exotic vacation or a lavish meeting…and it is even more true for pediatric head studies, which require a unique understanding of embryology, developing anatomy, and unique pathologic conditions.

Dr William O'Brien has masterfully created an issue that is both practical and state-of-the-art and covers a variety of pathologic conditions encountered in clinical practice. The articles are clinically oriented and provide comprehensive reviews of congenital, inflammatory, and neoplastic lesions in children who present with neck masses, hearing loss, sinonasal disorders, and vision loss. The article authors are an international "Who's Who" in pediatric head and neck radiology. The content is superb, and the articles are beautifully illustrated.

I would like to thank Dr O'Brien for accepting this difficult task and all of the authors for their outstanding contributions. Pediatric head and neck is always a challenging topic, and I always lamented about the lack of a concise book that I could reference when I had that challenging case. Well…thanks to Dr O'Brien and his wonderful team…now we do!

Suresh K. Mukherji, MD, MBA, FACR
University of Louisville & Proscan Imaing
ProScan Imaging
1185 West Carmel Drive, Suite D D1
Carmel, IN 46032, USA

E-mail address:
sureshmukherji@hotmail.com

Neuroimag Clin N Am 33 (2023) xiii
https://doi.org/10.1016/j.nic.2023.07.012
1052-5149/23/© 2023 Published by Elsevier Inc.

Preface

Pediatric Head and Neck Imaging: Understanding the Nuances and Complexities

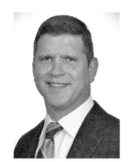

William T. O'Brien Sr, DO, FAOCR
Editor

Perhaps the only thing that imparts more fear and dread than opening a complex head and neck case on a worklist is opening a complex *pediatric head and neck* case on a worklist. If this pertains to you, then you are in good company, since even the most experienced pediatric head and neck radiologists not only began feeling that way but also continue to experience those feelings from time to time.

One issue cannot encompass all that is the wonderful world of pediatric head and neck imaging, so for this issue, we focused on covering a mix of common and more complex topics that are frequently encountered in clinical practice. For the common topics, such as cervical lymphadenopathy and a variety of head and neck infections, the charge for the authors was to emphasize the important, "bread-and-butter" imaging manifestations and to highlight important findings or complications that may impact clinical or surgical management. For the more complex topics, such as those covering various types of hearing loss, with a focus on congenital causes—this is a pediatric issue after all—and a wide range of head and neck masses, the expert authors were given carte blanche as to their approach to the topics, in terms of both content and format. As a result, there is truly something for everyone in this issue, whether you are in training or early in your career or if you are an experienced head and neck radiologist looking for a refresher of common or a deeper dive into complex pediatric head and neck topics.

I am deeply indebted to the world-class, international group of authors who came together for this issue. They devoted their time, expertise, and teaching cases, so that we may learn the intricacies associated with pediatric head and neck imaging and better care for the children and families behind all of our imaging studies. After all, when you truly think about it, that is what it is all about.

William T. O'Brien Sr, DO, FAOCR
Division of Pediatric Neuroradiology
Orlando Health –
Arnold Palmer Hospital for Children
92 West Miller Street
Orlando, FL 32806, USA

E-mail address:
william.obrien@orlandohealth.com

https://doi.org/10.1016/j.nic.2023.07.011
1052-5149/23/© 2023 Published by Elsevier Inc.

neuroimaging.theclinics.com

Non-Syndromic Sensorineural Hearing Loss in Children

Caroline D. Robson, MB, ChB[a,*], Martin Lewis, MD[b], Felice D'Arco, MD[b]

KEYWORDS

- Hearing loss • Sensorineural hearing loss • Non-syndromic hearing loss • Temporal bone
- Inner ear malformation • Enlarged vestibular aqueduct • Cytomegalovirus infection • Labyrinthitis

KEY POINTS

- Computerized tomography and MR provide complimentary information in the evaluation of non-syndromic hearing loss.
- Protocols require high-definition, thin-section, detailed images.
- Interpretation requires an advanced knowledge of normal temporal bone anatomy.
- Imaging may provide clues as the etiology and prognostic implications of hearing loss.
- Imaging provides information that is critical in the preoperative evaluation of potential surgical candidates including demonstration of potential surgical hazards.

INTRODUCTION

Bilateral severe-to-profound hearing loss (HL) is present in 1 to 2/1000 live births with a prevalence that increases with every decade.[1] Although universal newborn hearing screening has been mandated at the state level in the United States, it is possible for a neonate with congenital HL to pass newborn hearing screening, so if HL is suspected then a more compete diagnostic audiometric examination should be obtained.[2] Moreover, not all childhood HL is present at birth, so hearing screening is recommended throughout childhood and adolescence to identify later onset HL. Subsequent evaluation helps identify the type, severity, and etiology of HL to provide comprehensive support of language, communication, social and emotional development, and academic advancement. Radiological evaluation helps establish the cause of HL in some cases, is used to determine suitability for surgery if indicated, and provides useful anatomic information

that helps identify potential risk factors for surgery sometimes guiding the type of procedure performed. It is estimated that a definite or probable cause of HL is established in about 50% to 60% of cases.[1] Interestingly, some cases of "congenital" HL are acquired in utero, whereas some congenital malformations may manifest apparently as acquired HL.

HL is categorized as syndromic or non-syndromic and described in terms of age of onset, type of HL (sensorineural, conductive, or mixed), stability, laterality and degree of HL, and audiometric configuration. Ototoxic agents that can cause permanent HL include aminoglycosides, antineoplastic agents (especially cisplatin), and loop diuretics; potentially reversible HL can be caused by salicylates and macrolides such as azithromycin.[3] Multifactorial etiologies are exemplified by prematurity and neonatal intensive care-related HL with hyperbilirubinemia, hypoxia, subarachnoid hemorrhage, neonatal bacterial meningitis, ototoxic medication, prolonged ventilation,

[a] Department of Radiology, Boston Children's Hospital, Harvard Medical School, 300 Longwood Avenue, Boston, MA, USA; [b] Department of Radiology, Great Ormond Street Hospital for Children, Great Ormond Street, London, WC1N 3JH, UK
* Corresponding author. Division of Neuroradiology, Department of Radiology, Boston Children's Hospital, 300 Longwood Avenue, Boston, MA 02115.
E-mail address: caroline.robson@childrens.harvard.edu

Neuroimag Clin N Am 33 (2023) 531–542
https://doi.org/10.1016/j.nic.2023.05.005

and extracorporeal membrane oxygenation all playing a role in the development of sensorineural HL (SNHL).[4]

For the purposes of this review, following a description of various inner ear malformations, etiologies will be divided into non-syndromic malformations and genetic causes, infectious and inflammatory disorders, trauma, and benign masses and tumors. Entities that can occur in children but are more typically seen in adults such as otospongiosis will not be covered in this review.

CLINICAL EVALUATION

The approach to imaging depends on whether HL is congenital or acquired, whether there is pure SNHL or mixed HL, and whether the patient is a potential candidate for surgery. Computerized tomography (CT) and MR imaging provide complementary information that is critical for planned cochlear implantation and helps guide the surgical approach, implantation method, type of electrode, timing of surgery, and potential surgical pitfalls.

High-resolution CT (HRCT), flat panel, or cone-beam CT examinations with submillimeter bone algorithm axial images of the temporal bones are ideally reformatted in a plane parallel to that of the horizontal semicircular canal (SCC), which is also parallel to the plane of the hard palate. Coronal reformatted images should be created perpendicular to the plane of the hard palate. Short axis reformats (45° oblique or Pöschl plane) are parallel to the plane of the superior SCC (across the short axis of the petrous bone), and long axis reformats are at right angles to the plane of the superior SCC, along the long axis of the petrous bone.

CT depicts the osseous anatomy of the inner ear structures (Fig. 1) to diagnose inner ear malformations, fractures in post-traumatic SNHL, and labyrinthine ossification. Critical information includes the identification of findings that pose potential surgical hazards, such as oval window and facial nerve canal (FNC) anomalies (with or without oval window stenosis/atresia), and malformations, fractures, or erosive lesions associated with perilymph fistula (PLF), cerebrospinal fluid (CSF) gusher and potential risk of meningitis. The size and position of the posterior recesses and round window should also be assessed for potential cochlear implant candidates. CT also provides information that helps determine feasibility of cochlear implantation, side selection, and type of device to be implanted.[5]

MR depicts the anatomy of the fluid-containing spaces of the inner ear, demonstrates the size and course of each facial nerve (FN), vestibulocochlear nerve (VCN) and cochlear nerve (CN) (Fig. 2), and provides detailed assessment of the brain. MR is the examination of choice for evaluation of tumors associated with SNHL and for detecting enhancement in acute and subacute labyrinthitis and loss of fluid signal in labyrinthine fibrosis or ossification. The protocol for MR includes routine brain sequences and high-resolution submillimeter slice thickness 3D axial T2-weighted (eg, sampling perfection with application-optimized contrasts using different flip angle evolution or "SPACE" sequence).[6] The normal CN should be the same size or larger than a normal facial nerve (FN) in cross-section (see Fig. 2C). High-resolution thin-section axial T1-weighted images and contrast-enhanced fat-suppressed (FS) axial and coronal T1-weighted images are reserved for acquired SNHL in the absence of other explanation usually to assess for the presence of labyrinthine enhancement due to labyrinthitis.

CLASSIFICATION OF MALFORMATIONS

Approximately 80% of patients with congenital SNHL have radiologically occult abnormality affecting the membranous labyrinth, whereas a minority of patients have a variety of radiologically demonstrable inner ear malformations, for which the morphological classification provided by Sennaroglu and Bajin, as summarized below, is widely used.[7]

1. Labyrinthine aplasia: Absent cochlea, vestibule, and SCCs (Fig. 3A); variable petrous bone and otic capsule hypoplasia/aplasia; FNC may be present.
2. Rudimentary otocyst: Small cyst representing the membranous labyrinth; absent internal auditory canal (IAC) (Fig. 3B).
3. Cochlear aplasia: Absent cochlea, vestibule, and SCC normal or malformed with dilated vestibule ± malformed SCCs. The vestibule is along the posterior aspect of the IAC fundus (Fig. 3C).
4. Common cavity: Single, ovoid or rounded structure representing cochlea and vestibule, with central entrance of IAC, variable SCC malformation (Fig. 3D, E). May have single VCN with variable percentage of CN fibers.
5. Cochlear hypoplasia: Small cochlea often with reduced number of turns. Spectrum of severity from pronounced reduction in size and number of turns to mildly flattened upper turns (Fig. 4A).
6. Cochlear incomplete partition (IP) anomalies:
   a. Type 1 (IP-I): Includes cystic cochleovestibular anomaly; featureless cochlea, normal to

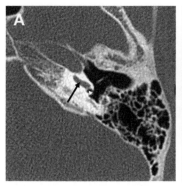
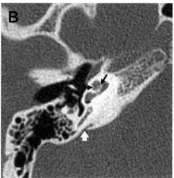
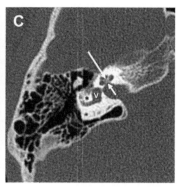

Fig. 1. Axial CT images depicting normal inner ear anatomy. The normal cochlea consists of 2$\frac{1}{2}$ to 2$\frac{3}{4}$ turns. (*A*) Inferior image at the level of the cochlear basal turn shows the round window (*white arrowhead*) and the faintly visualized osseous spiral lamina within the center of the basal turn (*long black arrow*), with uniform diameter of the turn. (*B*) A more cephalad image showing the interscalar septum (*short black arrows*) which becomes progressively thinner as it separates the upper cochlear turns. The posterior semicircular canal (SCC) (*white asterisk*) is shown as is a normal-sized vestibular aqueduct (*short, thick white arrow*). (*C*) The box or bowtie-shaped modiolus (*long, thin white arrow*) is well seen at the level of the cochlear aperture (*short white arrow*). The vestibule (*V*) and horizontal SCC (white *asterisk*) are also shown with the intervening bone island (*black asterisk*).

large in size, without internal structure (Fig. 4B), and variably malformed vestibule sometimes forming common cavity with horizontal SCC, with or without partially formed SCC.

b. Type II (IP-II): Normal basal turn, deficient interscalar septum between upper cochlear turns with variably malformed, deficient or absent modiolus (Fig. 4C, D).

c. Type III (IP-III): Deficient internal structure with corkscrew like external morphology.

Misshapen cochlea, partially formed interscalar septa, absent modiolus, bulbous IAC, and abnormal vestibule.[8]

7. Enlarged vestibular aqueduct (EVA): Midpoint measurement ≥ 1 mm transverse (TR), optimally measured on oblique short axis reformat[9-11], opercular measurement ≥ 2 mm TR.[11] Usually associated with variable cochlear malformation ranging from mild modiolar malformation to IP-II (see Fig. 4C, D). Atypical EVA also described, for example,

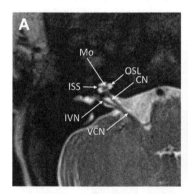
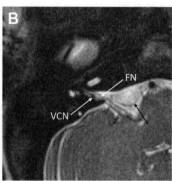
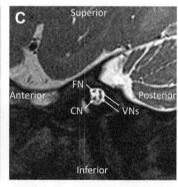

Fig. 2. (*A, B*) Axial and sagittal oblique (*C*) T2-sampling perfection with application-optimized contrasts using different flip angle evolution (SPACE) MR images depicting normal inner ear anatomy. (*A*) The fluid-filled cochlear turns are shown separated by the interscalar septum (*arrow* ISS). The osseous spiral lamina (*arrow* OSL) is faintly seen as a thin hypointense structure in the center of each turn. The modiolus (*arrow* Mo) is at the level of the cochlear aperture. The vestibulocochlear nerve (*arrow* VCN) cisternal segment divides within the internal auditory canal (IAC) into the anterior inferior cochlear nerve (*arrow* CN) and the posteroinferior inferior vestibular nerve (*arrow* IVN). Note the diverging course of the CN and IVN. (*B*) A more cephalad image shows the facial nerve (*arrow* FN) coursing anterior and parallel to the superior vestibular nerve (*arrow* SVN). A loop of the anterior inferior cerebellar artery (*black arrow*) courses ventral to the FN. (*C*) Cross-section of the IAC with orientation as depicted demonstrates four nerves: the anteroinferior cochlear nerve (*arrow* CN) is similar to slightly larger in cross-section when compared with the anterosuperior facial nerve (*arrow* FN). The diverging vestibular nerves (*arrow* VNs) course posteriorly.

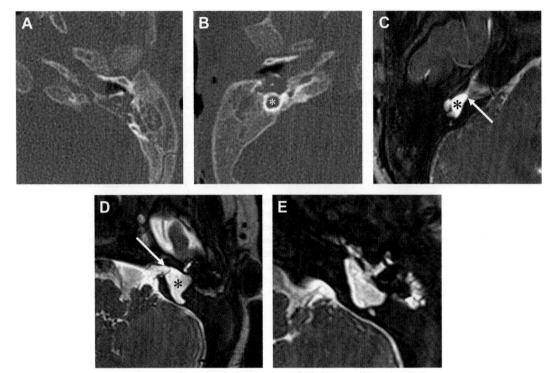

Fig. 3. Inner ear malformations. Axial CT (*A* and *B*) and axial T2 SPACE MR images (*C–E*). (*A*) Complete labyrinthine aplasia. The petrous apex is diminutive and the otic capsule bone and inner ear structures are absent. (*B*) Rudimentary otocyst. There is a small, fluid-filled round structure (*white asterisk*) and all other inner ear structures are absent. A small amount of dense otic capsule bone is present and the petrous apex is hypoplastic. (*C*) Cochlear aplasia with dilated vestibule (*black asterisk*) and malformed SCC. Note that the vestibule connects with the posterolateral aspect of the fundus of the IAC (*long white arrow*). (*D*) Common cavity. Although similar in appearance to (*C*), there is a single common cavity (*black asterisk*) representing vestibule, cochlea, and the horizontal SCC that connects centrally with the fundus of the IAC (*long white arrow*). The posterior SCC is also malformed protruding dorsally off the common cavity. (*E*) The same patient as (*D*). A more inferior image shows continuity of fluid within the labyrinth with fluid in the middle ear space consistent with a perilymph fistula.

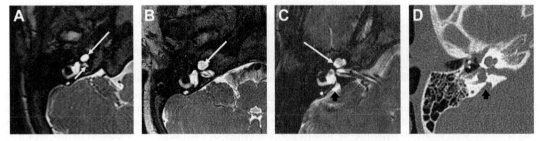

Fig. 4. Cochlear malformations. Axial T2 SPACE MR images (*A–C*) and axial CT (*D*). (*A*) Cochlear hypoplasia type I. There is a single cochlear turn without internal structure (*long white arrow*). The cochlear aperture is absent and the IAC is markedly narrowed (*short white arrow*). (*B*) Incomplete partition type I (IP-I). The cochlear turns are mildly enlarged and the internal structure is absent (*white arrow*). The vestibule and SCC are mildly enlarged. (*C, D*) IP-II with enlarged endolymphatic sac and duct and EVA. The interscalar septum between the mildly enlarged upper cochlear turns is absent, resulting in mild flattening of the posterolateral aspect of the cochlea (*white arrow*). The modiolus is also absent. Note the enlarged endolymphatic sac in (*C*) and vestibular aqueduct in (*D*) (*black arrows*).

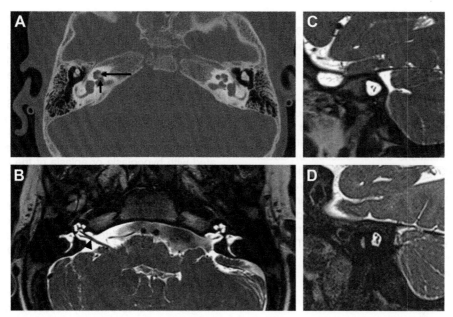

Fig. 5. Cochlear aperture stenosis and CN aplasia (*A–C*) and hypoplasia (*D*). (*A*) Axial CT and (*B*) axial T2 SPACE MR and sagittal oblique (*C*, *D*) T2 SPACE MR. (*A*) CT demonstrates the thickened, more densely ossified left modiolus compared with the normal right modiolus (*long black arrow*). There is left cochlear aperture stenosis which is significantly narrower than the normal right side (*short black arrow*). (*B*) MR shows that the left cochlear nerve is absent, whereas the right VCN (*arrowhead*) splits into a normal cochlear nerve ventrally and vestibular nerve posteriorly. (*C*) The left CN is absent with visualization of the FN anterosuperiorly and dividing vestibular nerves posteriorly (compare with normal anatomy in Fig. 2C). (*D*) A different patient with a very faintly visualized, hypoplastic CN.

with borderline measurements on CT, focal prominence, or large extra-osseous endolymphatic sac on MR.[12]

8. Cochlear aperture (CN canal or fossette) abnormalities:
   a. Atresia: Associated with absent CN; IAC normal or narrowed; thickened modiolus.
   b. Stenosis: Diameter less than 1.4 mm TR.[13] Associated with CN hypoplasia/aplasia; IAC normal or narrowed (<2.5 mm midpoint width); ± thickened modiolus (Fig. 5A).
   c. Widened: Diameter greater than 3.0 mm ± associated with absent modiolus and risk of CSF gusher[13]; IAC normal or bulbous.
9. CN abnormalities (± narrowed cochlear aperture) (Fig. 5B, C).
   a. Absent CN
   b. Hypoplastic CN (smaller in cross-section than normal FN)
   c. Absent VCN
   d. Hypoplastic VCN

Not included in the classification scheme above.

10. Isolated cochlear modiolar malformation: Asymmetric, misshapen, too small or too thick.

11. Congenital PLF: Small communication at the oval or round windows between perilymph containing inner ear structures and the middle ear space. Typically in association with inner ear malformation (eg, common cavity and IP-I), CSF enters the perilymph space and leaks via the fistula into the middle ear space (otogenic CSF fistula) (see Fig. 3E).[14]

NON-SYNDROMIC MALFORMATIONS AND GENETIC CAUSES

HL that occurs as an isolated finding without abnormality affecting other organ systems is considered non-syndromic in nature. Etiologies include genetic mutations and teratogenic insults. In developed countries, it is estimated that at least 60% of educationally significant congenital and early-onset HL is attributable to genetic factors that can be classified by mode of inheritance and whether the HL is syndromic or non-syndromic in nature.[2] HL genes are transmissible with associated disorders that are designated with "deafness neurosensory" (DFN) acronyms to reflect their pattern of inheritance as autosomal recessive (DFNB), autosomal dominant, X-linked, or mitochondrial patterns of inheritance with numeric designations for specific disorders.[2] Non-syndromic HL accounts for 70% to 75% of hereditary HL.[15] Over 100 genes are associated with non-syndromic genetic HL.[2]

DFNB1

Non-syndromic HL is most often inherited in an autosomal recessive pattern and is most frequently due to DFNB1 with gap junction beta (GJB) 2 mutations and/or deletion of GJB6.[2,16] GJB2 and GJB6 encode the gap junction proteins connexin 26 and connexin 30. Temporal bone imaging in DFNB1 is more likely to be normal than in non-DFNB1-related HL patients and detection of the often subtle, nonspecific abnormalities requires determination of absolute CT measurements for inner ear structures rather than visual inspection alone.[16–18]

Non-Syndromic Enlarged Vestibular Aqueduct

One of the most commonly detected inner ear malformations in HL of genetic origin is EVA. The gross anatomic features of this entity were originally described by Mondini in association with a minimally dilated vestibule and shortened or deficient cochlear interscalar septum between the upper cochlear turns.[19] EVA is either non-syndromic (only the temporal bone is involved) or syndromic in nature (see subsequent chapter). Non-syndromic autosomal recessive EVA (DFNB4) has been linked to a variety of genetic mutations with approximately 50% of cases linked to biallelic SLC26A4 mutations.[15] Clinical manifestations include SNHL with or without vestibular symptoms.

CT reveals EVA and frequently variable cochlear malformation, ranging from minimal modiolar malformation to IP-II anomaly with more pronounced malformation, deficiency or absence of the modiolus and slightly plump cochlear turns (see Fig. 4C, D). The deficient interscalar septum that characterizes IP-II results in flattening of the notch between the upper cochlear turns such that the cochlea resembles a baseball cap. MR reveals enlargement of the endolymphatic sac and duct. Measurements of the size of the cochlear scalar chambers and the angle between the upper cochlear turns for detection of IP II on MR have been well described in the literature.[20,21] Modiolar deficiency sometimes causes CSF oozing and gusher at the cochleostomy site during cochlear implant surgery.[7]

COCHLEAR NERVE HYPOPLASIA/APLASIA

The cochlear aperture (CN canal or fossette) is the space between the base of the modiolus and the fundus of the IAC that transmits the CN. The cochlear aperture is measured in the axial plane at the level of the modiolus on CT and is considered abnormally narrowed if less than 1.4 mm and abnormally widened if greater than 3 mm.[13] Pronounced narrowing or atresia of the cochlear aperture is usually associated with an abnormally thickened modiolus. Patients with SNHL are more likely to have narrower cochlear apertures than patients with normal hearing, and a significantly narrowed cochlear aperture is often associated with hypoplasia or aplasia of the CN.[22] The most common etiology of unilateral congenital SNHL, accounting for at least 25% of cases, is CN hypoplasia or aplasia.[23] This anomaly often occurs as an isolated finding in children with non-syndromic unilateral SNHL but is also seen in association with other inner ear anomalies in patients with syndromic SNHL.

The width of the cochlear aperture is readily measured on either axial CT or MR images. The images should be carefully assessed for associated modiolar thickening which almost invariably predicts CN aplasia or severe hypoplasia (see Fig. 5). MR is required for optimal assessment of CN diameter. High-resolution, direct sagittal oblique, heavily T2-weighted submillimeter images (eg, T2 SPACE or equivalent) are ideal for determining the presence and cross-sectional size of the CN (see Figs. 2C and 5C, D).

INFECTION AND INFLAMMATION
Congenital Cytomegalovirus Infection

Congenital cytomegalovirus (cCMV) infection is the most common cause of nongenetic pediatric SNHL and is estimated to affect 0.2% to 2.5% of all live born neonates worldwide, with an incidence of 1% to 5% in developing countries.[24] Up to 50% of symptomatic and 15% of asymptomatic infants with cCMV present with SNHL either at birth or subsequently.[25] Approximately 15% of neonatal SNHL is attributable to cCMV infection with progressive HL in about 20% of cases.[24] SHNL caused by cCMV is often initially unilateral in neonates, especially with otherwise asymptomatic infection, but can progress to bilateral HL.[26] Based on experimental evidence in murine models, it has been extrapolated that human CMV infection results in damage to the stria vascularis and the physiological consequences of this may contribute to HL.[27] Other congenital infections such as zika virus, syphilis, and rubella can also cause HL.[3]

cCMV infection does not produce radiological abnormality within the temporal bones but produces a typical constellation of findings on fetal or postnatal brain imaging (Fig. 6). Although cranial sonography demonstrates some of these

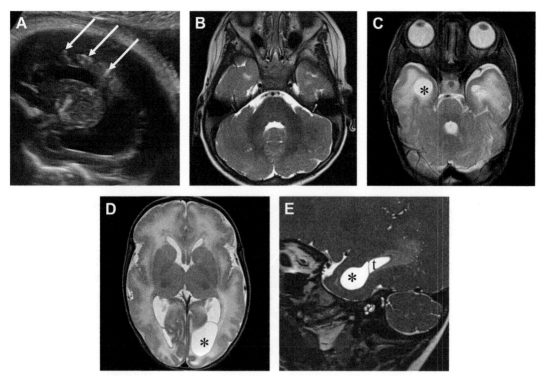

Fig. 6. Congenital CMV infection. (*A*) Fetal MR demonstrates ventriculomegaly in the setting of microcephaly. There are multiple hyperechoic, mineralized foci in the periventricular white matter (*arrows*). (*B* -*D*) Axial T2-weighted MR images of the brain showing bilateral cerebellar malformation, extensive polymicrogyria, abnormal T2 prolongation in the anterior temporal and occipital subcortical white matter and bilateral subependymal cysts (*asterisks*). (*E*) Sagittal oblique T2 SPACE MR image demonstrating a typical anterior temporal lobe subependymal cyst (*asterisks*) ventral to the temporal horn (t).

findings, MR is the examination of choice. Findings include microcephaly, ventriculomegaly (primarily ex vacuo), polymicrogyria that is usually asymmetric (usually due to early gestational cCMV), decreased parenchymal volume, asymmetric, patchy, non-confluent white matter T2 prolongation (associated with late gestational cCMV), white matter mineralization, cerebellar malformation, and subependymal cysts.[28,29] In particular, subependymal cysts ventral to the temporal horns of the lateral ventricles are a typical finding resulting from cCMV infection (see Fig. 6C, E).

The current recommendation for diagnosis is polymerase chain reaction assay in blood, urine, and saliva in neonates with suspected cCMV infection. Symptomatic cCMV is treated with IV ganciclovir transitioning to oral valganciclovir or with valganciclovir alone. Treatment is typically started during the first month of life with modest efficacy for hearing and long-term outcomes.[30,31]

Labyrinthitis and Labyrinthitis Ossificans

Labyrinthitis is usually infectious in nature (eg, viral, bacterial, or fungal) or due to noninfectious inflammatory causes such as autoimmune disorders, sarcoidosis, or ischemic insults. Infectious labyrinthitis occurs via hematogenous, meningeal, or tympanogenic routes of spread. Bacterial meningitis is one of the most common causes of acquired pediatric SNHL with a rapid onset of progressive SNHL. Predisposing events include bacterial meningitis alone or in association with congenital anomalies, otic capsule violating (OCV) trauma, otomastoiditis (eg, tympanogenic spread), and foreign bodies such as cochlear implant devices. Causative bacterial pathogens associated with post-meningitic labyrinthitis are usually *Streptococcus pneumoniae* and *Hemophilus influenzae* with labyrinthine ossification (LO) more frequently seen with the meningogenic route of spread and *S. pneumoniae* infection.[32] Following acute inflammation labyrinthine fibrosis typically ensues and ultimately LO with pathologic neo-ossification of the membranous labyrinth (Fig. 7). Multiorganism infection can complicate cochlear implantation, sometimes with otic capsule erosion and PLF (Fig. 8). LO has also been described in association with sickle cell disease.[33]

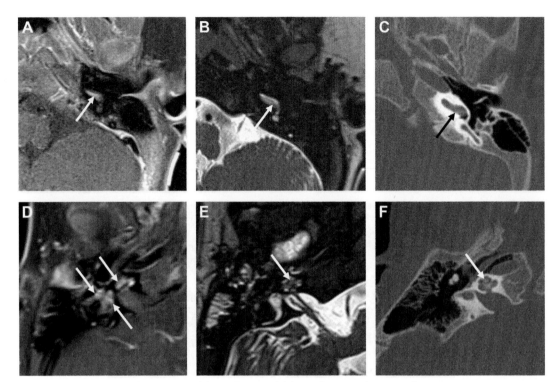

Fig. 7. Post-pneumococcal meningitic labyrinthitis and labyrinthine ossification of varying severity in two patients (*A–C* and *D–F*). (*A* and *D*) Axial gadolinium-enhanced, fat-suppressed (FS) T1-weighted MR images a few weeks after admission show enhancement within (*A*) the scala tympani of the cochlear basal turn, and (*D*) within the cochlea, vestibule and horizontal SCC (*white arrows*). (*B, E*) Same day axial T2 SPACE MR images show corresponding loss of fluid signal (*B*) in the scala tympani due to fibrosis (no visible ossification on CT a day later), and (*E*) throughout the cochlea due fibrosis and/or ossification (*white arrows*). (*C, F*) Axial CT of the temporal bone (*C*) 2 months later shows slight hazy ossification in the scala tympani consistent with cochlear ossification (*black arrow*), and (*F*) 7 weeks later in the second patient shows extensive cochlear ossification (*white arrow*).

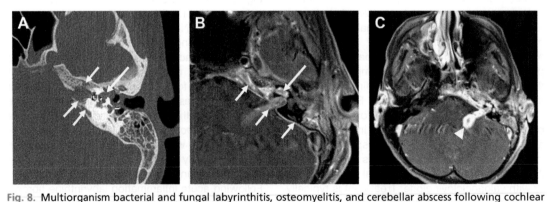

Fig. 8. Multiorganism bacterial and fungal labyrinthitis, osteomyelitis, and cerebellar abscess following cochlear implantation. (*A*) Axial CT shows the cochlear implant device in situ. There is erosion of otic capsule bone around the cochlear apical turn (*long arrow*) resulting in perilymph fistula that was confirmed at surgery and erosion of the petrous apex (*short arrows*). Mastoid air cells and the middle ear space are opacified. The infected device was removed. (*B, C*) Gadolinium-enhanced, FS T1-weighted MR images show enhancement of the cochlea (*long arrow*), IAC, petrous apex, clivus, and adjacent dura (*short arrows*). A ring-enhancing abscess is present in the left middle cerebellar peduncle (*arrowhead*). Enhancement and fluid are present within the middle ear space and mastoid air cells. Culture of mastoid bone cement grew Zygomycetes and coagulase-negative staphylococci.

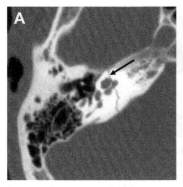 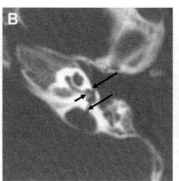 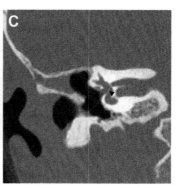

Fig. 9. Temporal bone trauma. (A) SNHL following occipital trauma. Axial CT image demonstrates a transverse otic capsule violating fracture that traverses the right cochlea (*long black arrow*). (B) Remote history of temporal bone trauma complicated by persistent CSF leak and recurrent meningitis. Axial CT shows a non-united left otic capsule violating fracture that traverses the cochlear basal turn, inferior aspect of the vestibule, and jugular foramen (*long black arrows*). There is ossification of the cochlear basal turn (*short black arrow*). Evidence of prior left tympanomastoidectomy and middle ear space obliteration. (C) Sudden onset of SNHL and vestibular symptoms concerning for labyrinthine violation following mastoidectomy for cholesteatoma. Coronal reformatted CT image shows that the stapedial footplate has subluxed into the vestibule (*black arrowhead*).

LO is associated with bilateral HL in over 80% of patients and is attributable to meningitis in approximately 80% cases.[34] Pathologic evidence of labyrinthine fibrosis has been identified as early as 1.5 weeks after meningitic labyrinthitis with subsequent LO that commences within the scala tympani at the round window and extends along the basal turn, with variable involvement of the scala vestibuli.[32] Profound SNHL meriting cochlear implantation may present a challenge depending on the extent and severity of LO.

A diagnosis of labyrinthitis should be considered in any child with acute bacterial meningitis and labyrinthitis and/or LO should also be a consideration in any child presenting with otherwise unexplained acquired SNHL. MR is the examination of choice for diagnosing early manifestations of labyrinthitis and subsequent labyrinthine fibrosis/ossification. HRCT is used to detect ossification which typically appears months following infection. For those patients with profound SNHL requiring cochlear implantation, the presence of florid ossification requiring drill out may preclude successful implantation; therefore, early diagnosis before this stage is imperative.[35]

There are three phases of infectious labyrinthitis depicted on high-resolution temporal bone imaging:

Acute phase
Labyrinthine enhancement on contrast-enhanced T1-weighted MR (see Fig. 7A, D).

Subacute phase
Decreased enhancement, loss of labyrinthine fluid signal on T2 weighted MR due to fibrosis (see Fig. 7B, E).

Chronic phase
Loss of labyrinthine fluid signal on T2-weighted MR with ossification on CT (see Fig. 7C, F).

Other findings
Bacterial, fungal, and granulomatous infection can also result in mass-like enhancement within the IAC with associated dural enhancement that gradually resolves with effective treatment.

Other infectious causes of SNHL include measles, mumps, and varicella zoster with potentially treatable HL from Lyme disease.[3] Autoimmune causes of HL include disorders primarily localized to the inner ear or systemic disorders such as Cogan syndrome (interstitial keratitis, progressive HL, and vestibular dysfunction), Takayasu arteritis, and granulomatosis with polyangiitis among other entities.[36]

TRAUMA

Temporal bone trauma can result in fracture or concussive injury without fracture. The consequences of trauma to the temporal bone include HL (SNHL, conductive HL, or mixed HL), vestibular symptoms, temporary or permanent FN paralysis, CSF leak, and meningitis. Etiologies of post-traumatic SHNL include trauma to the cochlea, CN, post-traumatic PLF, or intracranial injury. Temporal bone fractures were originally classified according to the direction of the fracture with respect to the long axis of the petrous bone and described as longitudinal, transverse, oblique, or mixed. However, a more predictive classification is whether or not the fracture disrupts the otic capsule. These fractures are known as OCV or

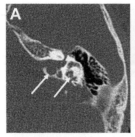
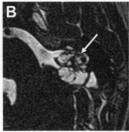
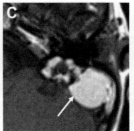
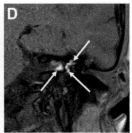

Fig. 10. Cholesterol granuloma with perilymph fistula resulting in profound SNHL. (*A*) Axial CT shows an erosive lesion involving the left petrous bone with destruction of the posterior wall of the IAC, posterior aspect of the vestibule and SCCs (*arrows*). (*B*) Axial T2 SPACE MR image shows the petrous bone and IAC lesion and heterogeneous signal intensity with loss of fluid signal within the vestibule and horizontal SCC (*arrow*). (*C*) Axial T1-weighted MR image shows that the lesion is predominantly hyperintense on T1 (*arrow*). (*D*) High-resolution fat-suppressed T1-weighted MR image shows cholesterol granuloma within the IAC, proximal cochlear basal turn, vestibule, and SCCs (*arrows*). This case highlights the complementary roles of CT (extent of bone erosion) and MR (cholesterol granuloma within the cochlea, vestibule, and SCCs).

sparing fractures. OCV fractures are rarely associated with longitudinal fractures and are typically attributable to transverse or mixed fractures.[37] Sudden, permanent SNHL has been reported to occur in approximately 22% pediatric OCV fractures compared with 100% incidence in adults, possibly related to different mechanisms of trauma and anatomic differences.[38] FN injury has been reported to occur in approximately 45% of OCV fractures.[39] Temporary or permanent SHNL can also result from traumatic brain injury without temporal bone or skull fracture.[40]

Temporal bone CT is the examination of choice for the evaluation of temporal bone trauma in the acute setting. CT demonstrates the fracture trajectory and whether or not there is evidence of OCV fracture (Fig. 9). Pneumolabyrinth is also sometimes present. The images should also be carefully assessed for fracture of the FNC, carotid canal, jugular foramen, and ossicular chain disruption. Long-term radiological complications include OCV fracture nonunion (sometimes resulting in prolonged or persistent PLF/CSF leak) and LO (see Fig. 9B). Trauma can also result from penetrating foreign bodies or surgery resulting in subluxation of stapes into the vestibule resulting in very subtle ossific density within the vestibule (see Fig. 9C).

BENIGN MASSES AND TUMORS

A variety of non-syndromic benign lesions, benign tumors, and malignant primary and metastatic tumors can result in SNHL. Tumor locations include the petrous apex with otic capsule and/or IAC erosion or within the IAC involving the CN, VCN, or multiple nerves, the VCN cisternal segment or VCN or the adjacent brainstem. Benign lesions include aggressive cholesteatoma and cholesterol

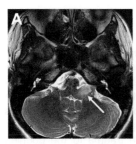
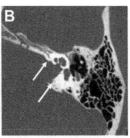
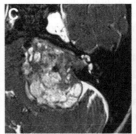
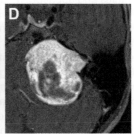

Fig. 11. Tumors. (*A*) Axial T2 MR image showing a relatively hyperintense tumor (*arrow*) involving the dorsolateral medulla, cerebellum, inferior, and middle cerebellar peduncles, and the root entry zone and cisternal segment of the left VCN. Histopathology showed low-grade glioma. (*B*) Different patient. Axial CT, (*B*) T2 SPACE MR and (*C*) gadolinium-enhanced FS T1-weighted MR image showing a large tumor centered in the cerebellopontine angle cistern with mass effect on the cerebellum and a widened left IAC. Notice the well-defined margins of the remodeled IAC on CT (*arrow*). The tumor is heterogeneous with hypointense solid components on T2 which enhance avidly with contrast. Histopathology confirmed a schwannoma. The patient had a history of leukemia but no evidence of neurofibromatosis type 2 on DNA extraction and next-generation sequencing from blood lymphocytes.

granuloma both of which can erode otic capsule bone resulting in PLF and/or CSF leak, SNHL, and vestibular symptoms (Fig. 10). Benign and malignant tumor types include Langerhans cell histiocytosis, sporadic schwannoma, rhabdomyosarcoma, atypical teratoid rhabdoid tumor, metastatic neuroblastoma, or leukemia. CT and MR provide complimentary information regarding the extent of disease, presence and pattern of osseous destruction (CT), and tumor type (MR) (Fig. 11).

SUMMARY

Childhood HL is common and imaging plays an essential role in helping determine the cause of HL, providing invaluable information that helps assess prognosis and determine therapeutic options and highlights potential risks of surgery. Many of the conditions described in this review have characteristic imaging findings, as exemplified by cCMV, various inner ear malformations, and a variety of inflammatory, neoplastic, and traumatic entities.

CLINICS CARE POINTS

- CT and MR provide complementary information that is critical for planned cochlear implantation and helps guide the surgical approach, implantation method, type of electrode, timing of surgery, and potential surgical pitfalls.
- CT is used to help diagnose inner ear malformations, otic capsule violating fractures in trauma and labyrinthine ossification that may complicate bacterial meningitis.
- Potential surgical hazards include facial nerve canal aberrancy.
- MR demonstrates the fluid containing membranous labyrinth, cranial nerves and brain parenchyma and is used for the assessment of acute inflammatory disorders, tumors and for preoperative assessment of inner ear anatomy and the presence and size of the cochlear nerves.
- Cochlear aperture stenosis or atresia is associated with absence or hypoplasia of the cochlear nerve.
- Deficient internal structure of the cochlea with enlarged cochlear turns suggests perilymph hydrops with potential for CSF leak at the time of cochleostomy.
- Congenital CMV is a common cause of SNHL and does not produce inner ear malformations. The diagnosis is readily suggested by

findings such as anterior temporal lobe and other subependymal cysts, asymmetric polymicrogyia, patchy white matter abnormality and parenchymal mineralization.

- Bacterial meningitis is one of the most common causes of acquired pediatric SNHL, with potential rapid progression to labyrinthine fibrosis and ossification.
- Otic capsule violating fractures are associated with sudden, permanent SNHL, facial nerve injury and sometimes CSF leak with subsequent meningitis.

DISCLOSURE

The authors have nothing to disclose.

REFERENCES

1. Kenna MA. Acquired Hearing Loss in Children. Otolaryngol Clin 2015;48(6):933–53.
2. Li MM, Tayoun AA, DiStefano M, et al. Clinical evaluation and etiologic diagnosis of hearing loss: A clinical practice resource of the American College of Medical Genetics and Genomics (ACMG). Genet Med 2022;24(7):1392–406.
3. Lieu JEC, Kenna M, Anne S, et al. Hearing Loss in Children: A Review. JAMA 2020;324(21):2195–205.
4. Korver AM, Smith RJ, Van Camp G, et al. Congenital hearing loss. Nat Rev Dis Prim 2017;3:16094.
5. Young JY, Ryan ME, Young NM. Preoperative imaging of sensorineural hearing loss in pediatric candidates for cochlear implantation. Radiographics 2014;34(5):E133–49.
6. D'Arco F, Mertiri L, de Graaf P, et al. Guidelines for magnetic resonance imaging in pediatric head and neck pathologies: a multicentre international consensus paper. Neuroradiology 2022;64(6):1081–100.
7. Sennaroglu L, Bajin MD. Classification and Current Management of Inner Ear Malformations. Balkan Med J 2017;34(5):397–411.
8. Phelps PD, Reardon W, Pembrey M, et al. X-linked deafness, stapes gushers and a distinctive defect of the inner ear. Neuroradiology 1991;33(4):326–30.
9. Bouhadjer K, Tissera K, Farris CW, et al. Retrospective Review of Midpoint Vestibular Aqueduct Size in the 45 degrees Oblique (Poschl) Plane and Correlation with Hearing Loss in Patients with Enlarged Vestibular Aqueduct. AJNR Am J Neuroradiol 2021;42(12):2215–21.
10. Juliano AF, Ting EY, Mingkwansook V, et al. Vestibular Aqueduct Measurements in the 45 degrees Oblique (Poschl) Plane. AJNR Am J Neuroradiol 2016; 37(7):1331–7.
11. Vijayasekaran S, Halsted MJ, Boston M, et al. When is the vestibular aqueduct enlarged? A statistical

analysis of the normative distribution of vestibular aqueduct size. AJNR Am J Neuroradiol 2007;28(6): 1133–8.

12. Wang L, Qin Y, Zhu L, et al. Auditory and imaging markers of atypical enlarged vestibular aqueduct. Eur Arch Oto-Rhino-Laryngol 2022;279(2):695–702.

13. Stjernholm C, Muren C. Dimensions of the cochlear nerve canal: a radioanatomic investigation. Acta Otolaryngol 2002;122(1):43–8.

14. Ng MMY, D'Arco F, Chorbachi R, et al. Oval window perilymph fistula in child with recurrent meningitis and unilateral hearing loss. BMJ Case Rep 2020;(7): 13. https://doi.org/10.1136/bcr-2020-234744.

15. Roesch S, Rasp G, Sarikas A, et al. Genetic Determinants of Non-Syndromic Enlarged Vestibular Aqueduct: A Review. Audiol Res 2021;11(3):423–42.

16. Oonk AM, Beynon AJ, Peters TA, et al. Vestibular function and temporal bone imaging in DFNB1. Hear Res 2015;327:227–34.

17. Kenna MA, Rehm HL, Frangulov A, et al. Temporal bone abnormalities in children with GJB2 mutations. Laryngoscope 2011;121(3):630–5.

18. Kochhar A, Angeli SI, Dave SP, et al. Imaging correlation of children with DFNB1 vs non-DFNB1 hearing loss. Otolaryngol Head Neck Surg 2009;140(5): 665–9.

19. Mondini C. Minor works of Carlo Mondini: the anatomical section of a boy born deaf. Am J Otol 1997;18(3):288–93.

20. Reinshagen KL, Curtin HD, Quesnel AM, et al. Measurement for Detection of Incomplete Partition Type II Anomalies on MR Imaging. AJNR Am J Neuroradiol 2017;38(10):2003–7.

21. Booth TN, Wick C, Clarke R, et al. Evaluation of the Normal Cochlear Second Interscalar Ridge Angle and Depth on 3D T2-Weighted Images: A Tool for the Diagnosis of Scala Communis and Incomplete Partition Type II. AJNR Am J Neuroradiol 2018; 39(5):923–7.

22. Wilkins A, Prabhu SP, Huang L, et al. Frequent association of cochlear nerve canal stenosis with pediatric sensorineural hearing loss. Arch Otolaryngol Head Neck Surg 2012;138(4):383–8.

23. Dewyer NA, Smith S, Herrmann B, et al. Pediatric Single-Sided Deafness: A Review of Prevalence, Radiologic Findings, and Cochlear Implant Candidacy. Ann Otol Rhinol Laryngol 2022;131(3):233–8.

24. Goderis J, De Leenheer E, Smets K, et al. Hearing loss and congenital CMV infection: a systematic review. Pediatrics 2014;134(5):972–82.

25. Boppana SB, Ross SA, Fowler KB. Congenital cytomegalovirus infection: clinical outcome. Clin Infect Dis 2013;57(Suppl 4):S178–81.

26. Tissera KA, Williams A, Perry J, et al. Hearing Stability in Patients With Unilateral Hearing Loss Due to Congenital CMV. Otolaryngol Head Neck Surg 2022;167(4):739–44.

27. Yu Y, Shi K, Nielson C, et al. Hearing loss caused by CMV infection is correlated with reduced endocochlear potentials caused by strial damage in murine models. Hear Res 2022;417:108454.

28. Hranilovich JA, Park AH, Knackstedt ED, et al. Brain Magnetic Resonance Imaging in Congenital Cytomegalovirus With Failed Newborn Hearing Screen. Pediatr Neurol 2020;110:55–8.

29. Manara R, Balao L, Baracchini C, et al. Brain magnetic resonance findings in symptomatic congenital cytomegalovirus infection. Pediatr Radiol 2011; 41(8):962–70.

30. Lanzieri TM, Pesch MH, Grosse SD. Considering Antiviral Treatment to Preserve Hearing in Congenital CMV. Pediatrics 2023;(2):151.

31. Leung J, Grosse SD, Yockey B, et al. Ganciclovir and Valganciclovir Use Among Infants With Congenital Cytomegalovirus: Data From a Multicenter Electronic Health Record Dataset in the United States. J Pediatric Infect Dis Soc 2022;11(8):379–82.

32. Trakimas DR, Knoll RM, Castillo-Bustamante M, et al. Otopathologic Analysis of Patterns of Postmeningitis Labyrinthitis Ossificans. Otolaryngol Head Neck Surg 2021;164(1):175–81.

33. Liu BP, Saito N, Wang JJ, et al. Labyrinthitis ossificans in a child with sickle cell disease: CT and MRI findings. Pediatr Radiol 2009;39(9):999–1001.

34. Booth TN, Roland P, Kutz JW Jr, et al. High-resolution 3-D T2-weighted imaging in the diagnosis of labyrinthitis ossificans: emphasis on subtle cochlear involvement. Pediatr Radiol 2013;43(12):1584–90.

35. Durisin M, Buchner A, Lesinski-Schiedat A, et al. Cochlear implantation in children with bacterial meningitic deafness: The influence of the degree of ossification and obliteration on impedance and charge of the implant. Cochlear Implants Int 2015; 16(3):147–58.

36. Espinoza GM, Wheeler J, Temprano KK, et al. Cogan's Syndrome: Clinical Presentations and Update on Treatment. Curr Allergy Asthma Rep 2020;20(9): 46.

37. Wexler S, Poletto E, Chennupati SK. Pediatric Temporal Bone Fractures: A 10-Year Experience. Pediatr Emerg Care 2017;33(11):745–7.

38. Bhindi A, Carpineta L, Al Qassabi B, et al. Hearing loss in pediatric temporal bone fractures: Evaluating two radiographic classification systems as prognosticators. Int J Pediatr Otorhinolaryngol 2018;109: 158–63.

39. Brodie HA, Thompson TC. Management of complications from 820 temporal bone fractures. Am J Otol 1997;18(2):188–97.

40. Chen JX, Lindeborg M, Herman SD, et al. Systematic review of hearing loss after traumatic brain injury without associated temporal bone fracture. Am J Otolaryngol 2018;39(3):338–44.

Conductive Hearing Loss in Children

Caroline D. Robson, MB, ChB

KEYWORDS

- Pediatric hearing loss • Conductive hearing loss • Temporal bone • Ossicles
- Craniofacial microsomia • Cholesteatoma • Cholesterol granuloma

KEY POINTS

- Computerized tomography is the imaging modality of choice for the assessment of pediatric conductive hearing loss.
- Familiarity with normal anatomy of the temporal bone is required in order to diagnose the various congenital and acquired abnormalities implicated in pediatric conductive hearing loss.

INTRODUCTION

Pediatric conductive hearing loss (CHL) is prevalent and usually results from abnormal mechanical transmission of sound from the external and middle ear to the oval window and ultimately the cochlea. Under normal circumstances, sound is transmitted mechanically by the tympanic membrane (TM) and ossicles resulting in movement of the stapedial footplate-oval window complex. This is accompanied by a compensatory opposite phase motion of the round window membrane, with the generation of fluid oscillations in the cochlea. These mechanical signals are then converted by cochlear sensory hair cells into chemical signals that activate innervating cochlear nerves to generate electrical impulses that are centrally transmitted to the brain stem.[1] Abnormalities resulting in CHL can be located anywhere from the pinna and external auditory canal (EAC) to the stapedial footplate and also include so-called third window lesions. Multifactorial causes frequently coexist and mixed hearing loss (MHL), which is a combination of CHL and sensorineural hearing loss (SNHL), is sometimes present.

CHL is characterized by an air bone gap on audiogram, which is a difference between air conduction and bone conduction audiometric thresholds.[2] Bone conduction thresholds should be normal with pure CHL but air conduction thresholds indicate hearing loss. Common causes such as cerumen impaction, TM perforation, and acute and chronic otitis media will not be considered here. Coalescent mastoiditis is discussed in a subsequent article. For the purposes of this review, causes will be divided into congenital malformations of the external and middle ear, isolated congenital ossicular anomalies, syndromes, chronic inflammatory disorders, tumors, vascular lesions, third window lesions, and trauma. Entities that can occur in children but are more typically seen in adults will not be discussed in this article.

Radiological Evaluation

CHL is primarily evaluated with computerized tomography (CT) of the temporal bones with thin section, high-resolution CT (HRCT), flat panel, or cone beam CT protocol as outlined in the earlier article on non-syndromic sensorineural hearing loss. Indications in addition to CHL include congenital malformation, as suggested by anomalies of the external ear, craniofacial region or an underlying syndrome, trauma, suspected coalescent mastoiditis, or the presence of a mass. CT depicts the presence, size, position and morphology of the EAC, tympanic plate, TM, middle ear space (MES), ossicles, adjacent vascular structures, and inner ear. Familiarity with normal anatomy is essential (Fig. 1). Assessment of surrounding structures such as the size of the oval window and course

Department of Radiology, Boston Children's Hospital, Harvard Medical School, 300 Longwood Avenue, Boston, MA 02115, USA
E-mail address: Caroline.robson@childrens.harvard.edu

Neuroimag Clin N Am 33 (2023) 543–562
https://doi.org/10.1016/j.nic.2023.05.006
1052-5149/23/© 2023 Elsevier Inc. All rights reserved.

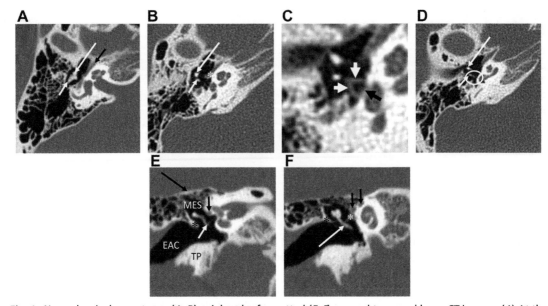

Fig. 1. Normal ossicular anatomy. (*A–D*) axial and reformatted (*E–F*) coronal temporal bone CT images. (*A*) At the level of the epitympanum the incudomalleal joint is shown as a faint lucency between the head of the malleus (*long thin white arrow*) and the articular facet on the body of the incus. The short process of the incus is directed posteriorly (*short thin white arrow*) and connected by a short ligament to the fossa incudis. The ossicles resemble an ice cream cone. The tympanic segment of the FNC is also shown (*short thin black arrow*). (*B*) A more caudal image shows the malleus anteriorly (*long thin white arrow*) and the incus posteriorly (*short thin white arrow*). The semicanal housing the tensor tympani courses over the cochlear promontory (*white asterisk*). (*C*) A magnified, slightly more caudal axial image shows the anterior and posterior stapedial crura (*short thick white arrows*). Connecting the crura is the foot plate of the stapes. The footplate, annular ligament, and oval window membrane form a thin linear density (*short wide black arrow*) overlying the vestibule, nestled inferior to the FNC. The obturator foramen is the space between the crura and footplate. (*D*) The ossicles seem as 2 parallel dashes with the anterior malleus (*long thin white arrow*) and the posterior incus (*short thin white arrow*). There is a faint lucency representing the IS articulation between the lenticular process of the incus and the stapedial capitulum (enclosed in the oval). (*E*) The body of the incus tapers to form the long process which then makes a 90° bend at the junction with the lenticular process (*short thin white arrow*). The tympanic segment of the FNC (*short thin black arrow*) courses immediately cephalad to the incus. The scutum is also seen (black *asterisk*). Note the normal morphology of the EAC and subjacent tympanic plate (TP). The tegmen tympani (long thin *black arrow*) forms the roof of the MES. (*F*) A more anterior image shows the malleus with the manubrium attached to the TM at the umbo (long thin *white arrow*). The labyrinthine and tympanic segments of the FNC are seen (*short thin black arrows*) cephalad to the tensor tympani tendon (*white asterisk*) and cochlea. Prussak space is located between the scutum (*black asterisk*), the malleus and the lateral suspensory ligament of the malleus.

and integrity of the facial nerve canal (FNC), carotid canal and jugular foramen is imperative in order to detect anomalies that may pose a hazard at the time of surgery. Contrast is reserved for specific clinical indications such as suspected coalescent mastoiditis, vascular lesions or tumors, in order to characterize the nature and extent of the abnormality and to detect associated complications.

MR imaging is reserved for the assessment of MHL, and/or for entities such as coalescent mastoiditis with complications, suspected cephalocele, cholesteatoma (residual or recurrence), cholesterol granuloma, and tumors. MR provides complimentary information to that provided by CT. The protocol for temporal bone MR depends on

the clinical indication and may include high-resolution, <1 mm slice thickness 3D axial T2-weighted (eg, Sampling Perfection with Application optimized Contrasts using different flip angle Evolution or "SPACE" sequence) images; axial and coronal thin section, high-resolution fat-suppressed (FS) T2-weighted images; axial thin section, high-resolution T1-weighted images; and nonechoplanar or multishot echoplanar diffusion-weighted imaging (DWI). High-resolution, thin-section, contrast-enhanced FS axial and coronal T1-weighted images are reserved for infectious and neoplastic causes. Magnetic resonance venography, magnetic resonance angiography (MRA), and contrast-enhanced gradient echo T1-weighted sequences of the brain are acquired as needed.

Congenital External and Middle Ear Malformation

The external ear, MES, and contents are derived primarily from the first and second pharyngeal apparatus with contributions from neural crest cells.[3,4] This development is distinct from the otocyst-derived inner ear structures other than the labyrinthine aspect of the stapedial footplate, which originates from the mesenchyme of the otic capsule.[4] As a result, external ear anomalies such as EAC atresia (also known as congenital aural atresia) and stenosis are also associated with malformations involving the size and shape of the MES together with variable deficiency, malformation, rotation, and sometimes ankylosis of the ossicles.[5]

Clinical presentation depends on whether the anomaly is nonsyndromic or syndromic in nature. Nonsyndromic or "isolated" congenital external and middle ear malformation (CEMEM) is usually unilateral, associated with CHL and physical clues such as anotia, microtia, a misshapen pinna (Fig. 2A), polyotia, and atresia or stenosis of the EAC. More than 80% of patients with microtia have congenital EAC stenosis or atresia, and isolated microtia has a right ear predominance.[6]

Syndromic CEMEM may be unilateral or bilateral and symmetric or asymmetric in nature. Physical signs include those associated with nonsyndromic CEMEM, other craniofacial findings (such as micrognathia), pharyngeal apparatus remnants (preauricular skin tags, sinuses, fistulae, cysts, and/or squamous remnants) and other organ system abnormalities such as cardiac, renal, and/or vertebral anomalies. Micrognathia may be unilateral or bilateral, symmetric or asymmetric, and typically associated with a low set pinna or pinnae.

Environmental causes of CEMEM include isoretinion embryopathy, prenatal alcohol syndrome and maternal diabetic embryopathy.[7–9] Syndromic causes include multifactorial or uncertain cause, for example, craniofacial microsomia, chromosomal abnormalities (eg, trisomy 13, 18, 22), and single gene mutations (eg, Treacher Collins syndrome [TCS]).[6]

CT helps distinguish between EAC atresia and stenosis. The tympanic plate and TM are absent in EAC atresia (see Fig. 2). As assessed on coronal images, EAC atresia is characterized as bony (thick vs thin atresia plate), part bony and part membranous, or membranous in nature. EAC stenosis is characterized by a narrow EAC with variable hypoplasia of the tympanic plate (Fig. 3).

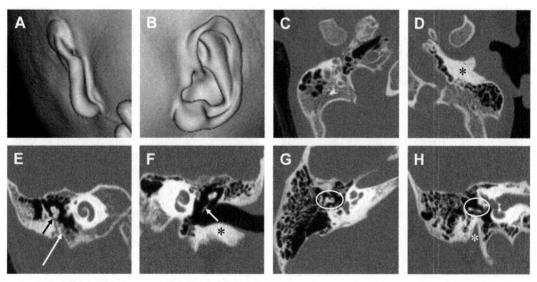

Fig. 2. EAC atresia right ear; normal left ear. (A and B) CT 3D surface rendered images demonstrate (A) microtia and (B) a normal pinna. (C and D) Axial CT images show (C) Right EAC atresia. The right EAC and TP are absent. The absent TP corroborates that this is atresia rather than a stenotic, completely opacified EAC. (D) Normal TP (black *asterisk*) on the left. (E and F) Reconstructed coronal CT images. (E) Absent EAC with a complete osseous atresia plate on the right (*long white arrow*). The manubrium of the malleus is absent, and the malleus is rotated and ankylosed to the atresia plate (*short black arrow*). There is mild hypoplasia of the MES. (F) Note the normal EAC, tympanic plate (black *asterisk*), TM, scutum, and malleus with the manubrium attached at the umbo to the TM (*short white arrow*). (G) Axial CT at the level of the attic shows that the misshapen and rotated incus has a "boomerang" shape (enclosed in white oval). (H) Reconstructed coronal CT shows the flattened, misshapen, horizontally inclined incus (enclosed in white oval) with a very obtuse angle between the long and lenticular processes of the incus. The descending FNC is ventrally positioned (*white asterisk*).

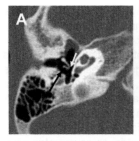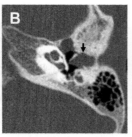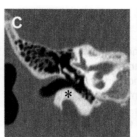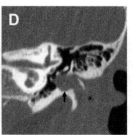

Fig. 3. Bilateral EAC stenosis with ossicular anomaly and left EAC cholesteatoma. (*A* and *B*) Axial and (*C* and *D*) reformatted coronal CT images. (*A*) The stenotic EACs are partially visualized. (*A*) The manubrium of the malleus is dorsally angulated and abuts the lenticular process of the incus (short *white arrow*). There is opacification of the anterior MES. The facial recess is hypoplastic (*long black arrow*). (*B*) Left side at the same level showing an opacity that remodels the anterior aspect of the stenotic EAC (*short black arrow*). There is partial opacification of the anterior MES. Although the incus is not seen on this image, there was no evidence of ossicular erosion at surgery. (*C* and *D*) Mildly stenotic EACs. Contrast the normal upward convexity of the right TP (*black asterisk,* *C*) with the well-defined erosion of the left EAC (*short black arrow, D*). At surgery, keratin debris and an EAC cholesteatoma was removed from the stenotic left EAC.

The stenotic canal is at risk for trapped debris (keratosis obturans) and EAC cholesteatoma. Both of these entities manifest as opacification of the EAC with paradoxic widening due to bone remodeling (see Figs. 3B and D).

The MES is sometimes absent or severely hypoplastic with absent or rudimentary ossicles and mastoid underpneumatization, as is typical of some syndromes described in the ensuing sections. With milder MES hypoplasia or near normal MES size, the posterior recesses may be variably shallow or misshapen (see Fig. 3A). When the ossicles are present, there is frequently truncation or deficiency of the neck, manubrium and umbo of the malleus, shortened length of the incus long process, and a relatively obtuse incudostapedial (IS) angle (as measured between the incus long process and lenticular process/stapes on coronal CT) (see Fig. 2).[10] The ossicles are also sometimes ankylosed laterally to the atresia plate (see Fig. 2E). The observation of a misshapen incus fused to a rudimentary hypoplastic malleus head with absence/hypoplasia of the stapedial capitulum, ossicular discontinuity and fibrous attachment of the incus to the tympanic segment of the FNC has been described as a "boomerang."[5] This refers to visualization of the malleus head and entirety of the incus on a single axial image (see Fig. 2G). The correlate for the "boomerang" morphology on coronal images is the obtuse angle between the shortened long and lenticular process of the incus (see Fig. 2H).

For those anomalies that affect primarily first pharyngeal arch derivatives, the oval window is normal in size. Oval window stenosis or atresia implicates involvement of second pharyngeal arch derivatives and/or neural crest cells, and in this situation, the stapes may be misshapen or malpositioned together with aberrancy and sometimes dehiscence of the tympanic segment of the FNC. With EAC atresia, the descending FNC is invariably ventrally positioned (see Fig. 2H) because the intervening tympanic plate is absent, and the stylomastoid foramen is sometimes in close to the posterior aspect of the temporomandibular joint (TMJ).

Surgical repair of EAC atresia or stenosis is complicated to perform and is undertaken in an attempt to restore the normal sound conduction mechanism of the ear.[11] Surgical candidacy is based on audiometric findings and temporal bone anatomy as shown on HRCT, for which the Jahrsdoerfer 10-point grading scale is widely used.[11,12] In order to be considered a surgical candidate and graded, cochlear function has to be present and the inner ear structure should be normal on imaging.[12] Scores regarding presence or absence of structures are assigned as follows with 1 point for every structure (other than stapes which is assigned 2 points): Stapes present, oval window "open," MES, facial nerve, malleus-incus complex, mastoid pneumatization, incus-stapes connection, round window, external ear.[12] Patients with a score of 7 or greater have significantly better hearing postoperatively.[11,12]

Isolated Congenital Ossicular Anomalies

When pediatric CHL occurs without evidence of otitis media, with a normal TM and an aerated tympanic cavity, the differential diagnoses includes juvenile otosclerosis, congenital stapes ankylosis, anomalies of the ossicular chain, osteogenesis imperfecta, and atresia of the round window.[13] Congenital ossicular anomalies are however a rare cause of CHL, with an incidence of 0.5% to 1.2%.[14,15] Ossicular anomalies are associated with an underlying syndrome in approximately 25% of cases.[16] Conversely, diagnosis of a specific genetic syndrome may prompt the assessment for certain types of ossicular anomalies. Ossicular malformation can also be simulated by inflammatory, ischemic, or posttraumatic insult to the ossicles.

Congenital stapes footplate fixation has been reported to be the most prevalent ossicular anomaly and is attributed to maldevelopment of the annular ligament of the oval window with or without other ossicular or FNC abnormalities.[17] Congenital stapes footplate fixation is distinguished clinically from juvenile onset otosclerosis by lifelong, nonprogressive CHL while otosclerosis is suggested by age usually greater than 6 years, progressive CHL, and a positive family history.[13] In isolated stapes fixation, CT is typically normal or near normal, whereas otosclerosis is characterized by otic capsule demineralization. For suspected stapes footplate fixation, CT is however indicated to avoid performing stapedotomy on children at high risk for cerebrospinal fluid (CSF) gusher and resultant SNHL.[17]

The 2 most recent operative classifications of congenital ossicular anomalies are based on the Cremers classification[18,19]:

Class I: Isolated stapes footplate fixation.

Class II: Stapes fixation with another congenital ossicular chain anomaly.

a. Ossicular discontinuity
b. Epitympanic fixation
c. Tympanic fixation

Class III Ossicular chain anomaly but mobile stapes footplate.

a. Ossicular discontinuity
b. Epitympanic fixation
c. Tympanic fixation

Class IV Congenital aplasia/malformation of the oval window or round window

a. Aplasia
b. Dysplasia
  b1. Abnormal facial nerve
  b2. Persistent stapedial artery (PSA)

Temporal bone CT evaluation assists with the above classification. Stapedial anomalies that can be diagnosed on CT include absent stapedial superstructure, monopod or columellar stapes, abnormal and/or asymmetric height, thickness or positioning of the anterior and posterior crura, thickening of the crura at the junction with the oval window and deficiency of the capitulum or IS joint (Fig. 4). Abnormal ossification of the stapedius muscle/tendon is also occasionally seen.

Oval window stenosis/atresia is also associated with variable malformation or abnormal positioning of the stapes and tympanic segment of the FNC (see Figs. 4B and C).[20] In this situation, the FNC sometimes courses over the oval window, promontory or even across the floor of the MES, and is sometimes dehiscent. Anomalies of the malleus and incus include abnormalities in size, shape and orientation, ankylosis to each other or to the MES, and ossified ligaments or disconnected ossicles (see Figs. 4E and F). A deficient incus longlenticular process can be congenital or acquired (eg, tympanosclerosis, posttraumatic). Recent reports suggest that ossicular chain anomaly with a mobile stapes footplate is more common than isolated stapes footplate fixation.[21]

Syndromes

There are several genes involved in a variety of cellular processes that are required for the normal development of the ear and mandible.[22]

- Transcription factors involved in neural crest cell migration and patterning: *SIX1*, *SIX5*, *EYA1*, *HOXA10*, *HOXA2*, *SALL1*; for example, Branchio-oto-renal (BOR) syndrome, Townes-Brocks syndrome
- Chromatin modifiers: *CHD7*, *KMT2D*, *KDM6A*; for example, CHARGE syndrome, Kabuki syndrome
- Growth factors and their receptors: *GDF6*, *FGF3*, *FGF10*, *FGFR2*, *FGFR3*
- DNA prereplication complexes: *ORC1*, *ORC4*, *ORC6*, *CDC6*, *CDT1*
- Ribosome assembly: *TCOF1*, *POL1RC*, *POL1RD*; for example, Treacher-Collins syndrome
- Spliceosome: *EFTUD2*, *TXNL4A*, *SF3B4*; for example, Craniofacial microsomia, Nager syndrome

Craniofacial Microsomia

Craniofacial microsomia (CFM) represents the second most common congenital craniofacial defect after cleft lip and palate, occurring in 1 in 3000 to 5000 live births.[23] CFM is characterized by unilateral or bilateral underdevelopment of facial structures derived from the first and second pharyngeal arches and encompasses a wide variety of phenotypes that range from mild to severe.[24,25] CFM has been previously termed first and second branchial arch syndrome, otomandibular dysostosis, oculo-auriculo-vertebral syndrome, hemifacial microsomia, and Goldenhar syndrome.

The most common clinical presentation is auricular malformation and underdevelopment of the

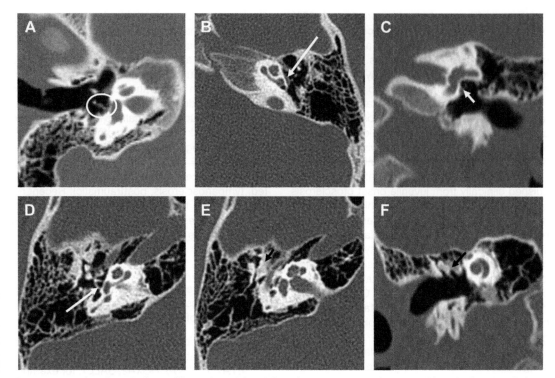

Fig. 4. Nonsyndromic ossicular malformations (*A*) Axial CT shows a monopod stapes with a single stapedial crus directed toward the middle third of the oval window (enclosed in oval). (*B*) Axial CT and (*C*) reformatted coronal CT images show opacification between abnormally short stapedial crura (*long white arrow, B*). The tympanic segment of the FNC (short *white arrow, C*) is aberrant and dehiscent, coursing over the cochlear promontory, through the stapedial obturator foramen. (*D and E*) Axial and (*F*) reformatted coronal CT images. (*D*) The stapedial crura are abnormally thickened (*long white arrow*). (*E and F*) There is hypoplasia of the attic, fusion of the incudomalleal joint and ankylosis of the ossicles to the walls of the attic (*short black arrows*). A similar appearance can be seen in tympanosclerosis; however, this patient had congenital CHL.

mandible on one or both sides.[26] Microtia, preauricular tags, EAC atresia, ossicular anomalies, oval window anomalies, and sometimes cochlear and semicircular canal (SCC) anomalies are the most frequently reported external, middle, and inner ear findings. Hearing loss, usually CHL, is reported in 29% to 100% of patients.[27] Other affected structures include the muscles of mastication, maxilla, palate, zygomatic arch, orbit, parotid gland, and facial nerve. CFM can be also be associated with lateral oral clefts, epibulbar dermoids, and anomalies of the nervous system, kidneys, spine, limbs, and heart.[23,25,26] There are several other syndromes that have overlapping clinical features of micrognathia and microtia, notably Townes-Brocks, Treacher Collins, and CHARGE syndromes.

CFM has been reported in association with a variety of maternal risk factors (eg, diabetes, smoking, vasoactive medications, and assisted reproductive technology) and may result from a range of causes such as vascular injury, teratogenic exposure, or genetic mutations.[24] Although most cases are sporadic, associated genetic mutations include loss of function variants of SF3B2 with autosomal dominant inheritance.[26] More recently, damaging variants in *FOXI3* have been reported to be the second most common genetic cause of CFM associated with approximately 1% of cases, particularly in the setting of bilateral microtia with a positive family history.[28] Putative mechanisms for CFM include bleeding around the stapedial artery leading to insufficient blood supply to the first and second pharyngeal arches, abnormal development of Meckel cartilage and abnormal neural crest cell formation, migration, or differentiation.[23]

CT demonstrates unilateral or bilateral asymmetric micrognathia with hypoplasia of the mandibular ramus, hypoplasia or absence of the condyle, and a small, abnormally positioned or absent TMJ (**Figs. 5**A–C). The zygomatic arch is frequently cleft or deficient with only a small anterior component present. There is variable midface hypoplasia and sometimes cleft palate. Temporal bone anomalies include unilateral EAC atresia or stenosis (see **Figs. 5**B and C) with the contralateral

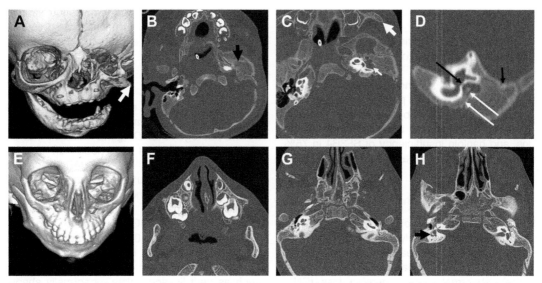

Fig. 5. (*A–D*) CFM. (*A*) CT 3D model shows asymmetric micrognathia with absence of the left mandibular ramus and condyle. The patient also has ipsilateral midface hypoplasia and a small deformed orbit. (*A* and *C*) Note the hypoplastic, cleft zygomatic arch (short thick *white arrow*). (*B* and *C*) Axial CT images show left EAC atresia and absent left mastoid pneumatization. Note the sphenosquamosal suture, which is rotated 90° into a transverse orientation (short thick *black arrow*, B). (*C*) Axial and (*D*) reformatted coronal images revealing the small, opacified left MES (short thin *white arrow*, C). The ossicles are not visualized. (*D*) There is oval window atresia (long thin *black arrow*) and aberrancy of the FNC (long thin *white arrows*) which courses over the floor of the MES and descends ventrally. Note the low position of the middle cranial fossa (short thin *black arrow*) related to absent mastoid pneumatization. (*E–H*) TCS. (*E*) CT 3D model shows symmetric micrognathia with midface hypoplasia and down slanting orbits. (*F*) Axial CT image shows posteriorly slanted maxillae. (*G* and *H*) Axial CT images demonstrate bilateral EAC atresia, severely hypoplastic MESs, mastoid non-pneumatization, absent ossicles, and absent zygomatic arches. (*H*) There is a malformed right horizontal SCC with small bone island (short thick *black arrow*).

EAC appearing normal or mildly stenotic, associated ossicular anomalies, MES hypoplasia, oval window atresia or stenosis (see Fig. 5D), anomalies of the FNC and sometimes inner ear anomalies. The OMENS-Plus(+) acronym and classification of CFM uses a 0 to 3 scoring system for each of the 5 major manifestations of CFM: O for orbital distortion; M for mandibular hypoplasia; E for ear anomaly; N for nerve involvement; S for soft tissue deficiency; and Plus for extracraniofacial anomalies.[29,30] Extracraniofacial anomalies occur in approximately 55% of patients particularly those with higher OMENS scores.[29]

A CFM-like phenotype associated with auricular, anal, hand, and thumb anomalies is characteristic of Townes-Brocks syndrome. It is important to distinguish between CFM and Townes-Brocks syndrome because the latter is caused by heritable autosomal dominant *SALL1* transcription factor mutations.[31]

Treacher Collins Syndrome

TCS, also known as mandibulofacial dysostosis, is a rare craniofacial disorder with an incidence of approximately 1 in 50,000 live births.[32–34] A family history of TCS is present in approximately 40% and de novo mutations in 60% of affected individuals.[32] Clinical features include micrognathia, microtia, CHL, down-slanting palpebral fissures, eyelid coloboma, and midface hypoplasia sometimes with nasal cavity stenosis. There are at least 4 subtypes of TCS with different associated genetic mutations and predominantly autosomal dominant inheritance: TCS1: *TCOF1*; TCS2: *POLR1D*; TCS3: *POLR1C*; and TCS4: *POLR1B*.[32–34] TCS is considered a ribosomopathy and neurocristopathy with facial features attributed to abnormal neural crest cell migration.[34]

CT shows bilateral micrognathia, sometimes resulting in glossoptosis, U-shaped cleft palate and Robin sequence. There is also variable deficiency of the mandibular rami, condyles, TMJs, and zygomatic arches with malar hypoplasia with posteriorly slanted malar eminences (see Figs. 5E and F). Temporal bone findings include bilateral, symmetric or asymmetric microtia, EAC atresia or stenosis, MES hypoplasia, ossicular anomaly including rudimentary, fused ossicles or even absent ossicles, poor or absent mastoid pneumatization, oval window atresia, and aberrancy of the FNCs (see Figs. 5G and H).[35,36] Inner ear anomalies are sometimes seen and include malformation of the horizontal SCC with a small bone island (see Fig. 5H).

In the differential diagnosis for TCS is Nager syndrome, also known as preaxial acrofacial dysostosis, characterized by hypoplastic neural crest-derived craniofacial bones, limb malformations, and haploin insufficiency of SF3B4 in 75% of cases.[37–39] Imaging features overlap those of TCS.

Branchio-Oto-Renal Syndrome

BOR is a craniofacial disorder with an estimated frequency of approximately 1 in 40,000.[40] Clinical features include pharyngeal apparatus anomalies (cysts, sinus tracts, preauricular tags or pits, fistulae), abnormal pinnae, hearing loss (CHL, MHL, or SNHL), facial asymmetry, and renal anomalies.[41] Approximately 40% of patients with BOR have autosomal dominant EYA1 gene mutations and a significantly smaller percentage have SIX5 or SIX1 mutations.[41–44] When renal anomalies are absent, the disorder is referred to as branchio-otic syndrome.

CT demonstrates variable EAC stenosis or normal EACs. The MES is misshapen and the ossicles are usually malformed, abnormally positioned, and/or ankylosed (Fig. 6).[1] Shortening and calcification of the superior malleal ligament is also considered a feature of BOR.[45] A characteristic finding of BOR is marked dilatation and sometimes anomalous course of the Eustachian tubes (see Fig. 6C). The EYA1–BOR phenotype has a characteristic "unwound" appearance of the cochlea such that the basal turn is tapered while the upper turns are hypoplastic and anteriorly offset (see Fig. 6B).[46–48] Additional features include funnel-shaped enlargement of the vestibular aqueducts, enlarged vestibules, malformed posterior SCCs, funnel-shaped internal auditory canals (IACs) and anomalous course of the FNCs.[45,48]

CHARGE Syndrome

CHARGE syndrome is an uncommon autosomal dominant syndrome that most commonly results from a pathogenic CHD7 gene mutation that encodes ATP-dependent chromodomain helicase DNA-binding protein 7.[49,50] The CHARGE acronym refers to coloboma, heart defects, atresia choanae, retardation of growth and/or development, genitourinary abnormalities, and ear abnormalities and deafness. CHARGE syndrome occurs in approximately 1 in 10,000 births worldwide, and phenotypic expression is variable.[49] Clinical presentation also includes craniofacial abnormalities such as cleft lip and palate, abnormally shaped ears, anosmia, facial palsy, hearing loss (SNHL or MHL), and tracheo-esophageal anomaly.[51]

CT demonstrates the inner ear anomalies characteristic of CHARGE syndrome including variable cochlear malformation, cochlear aperture stenosis, hypoplastic vestibules, rudimentary or absent SCCs, and sometimes funnel-shaped enlarged vestibular aqueducts (Fig. 7A).[52] Ossicular anomalies include malformation, abnormally positioned or absent stapes, malformation and abnormal orientation of the malleus and incus, and ossicular ankyloses (see Fig 7). If cochlear implantation is being considered, it is important to detect associated large emissary veins, mastoid under pneumatization, oval and round window stenosis and aberrancy of the FNC, for example, coursing over the atretic oval window, or inferiorly over the cochlear promontory, sometimes with dehiscence (see Fig. 7).[53,54] Additional findings on CT include hypoplasia and/or clefting of the basiocciput, a small deep set pituitary fossa, choanal atresia,

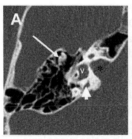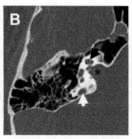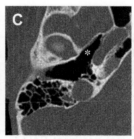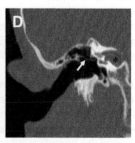

Fig. 6. BOR syndrome. (A–C) Axial and (D) reformatted coronal CT images. (A) The body of the incus is broadened (long thin *white arrow*) with possible ankylosis of the medial aspect of the incudomalleal joint. Note the widened vestibule (*V*). (B and D) The long and lenticular process of the incus is deficient with only a thin, abnormal, obtusely angled vestige seen on the coronal reformatted image (*short thin white arrow*, D). (A–D) Note the widened, flared IAC (black *asterisks*), bulbous, enlarged vestibular aqueduct (*short thick white arrows*), "unwound" appearance of the malformed cochlea with offset, hypoplastic upper turns (*short thick black arrow*) and dilated Eustachian tube (*white asterisk*). (D) The EAC is angled upward.

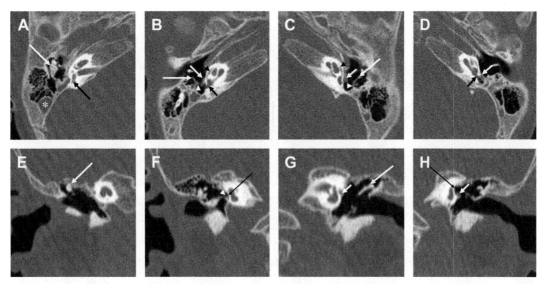

Fig. 7. CHARGE syndrome. (*A* and *B* right side, *C* and *D* left side) Axial CT images and (E and F right side, G and H left side) reformatted coronal CT images. (*A*) The body and short process of the incus are mildly broadened (*long white arrow*). Inner ear anomalies typical of CHARGE syndrome including a small vestibule (*long black arrow*), absent SCCs and absent cochlear apical turn with atretic cochlear aperture are also shown. Note the large mastoid emissary vein (*asterisk*). (*B–D*) The lenticular process of the incus is directed posteriorly (*long white arrows*) with a rudimentary small stapes (*arrowheads*) abutting the pyramidal eminence. The tympanic segment of the FNC is abnormally low, coursing over the cochlear promontory (*short white arrows*). The round window is stenotic and opacified (*short black arrows*). The cochlear turns and modioli are misshapen. Normal developmental cartilaginous cochlear clefts are seen (*black arrowheads*). (*E*) The head of the malleus is ankylosed to the tegmen tympani (*arrow*). Notice the shallow height of the epitympanum. (*F–H*) The malformed and likely ankylosed stapes abuts the FNC (*arrowhead*). Note the abnormally shaped incus (*long white arrow*), which has an abnormally obtuse angle at the junction of the long and lenticular processes. A myringotomy tube is in place. There is oval window atresia (*thin black arrows*) and the FNC courses over the atretic oval window then inferiorly along the cochlear promontory (*short white arrows*).

ocular colobomata, parotid hypoplasia, cleft palate, and vertebral anomalies.[55]

In the differential diagnosis for CHARGE syndrome are 22q11.2 deletion syndrome, Kabuki syndrome, CFM, and TCS. However, the temporal bone findings of CHARGE syndrome are usually distinctive and differ from these entities.

22q11.2 deletion syndrome

Chromosome 22q11.2 deletion syndrome, also known as velocardiofacial or DiGeorge syndrome, is the most common human microdeletion syndrome affecting between 1:3000 and 1:6000 live births.[56–59] This autosomal dominant syndrome has considerable variation in penetrance and severity, with clinical features including congenital heart disease, renal insufficiency, hypoparathyroidism, thymic hypoplasia with immunodeficiency, autoimmunity, neurocognitive disorders, characteristic facial features, micrognathia, cleft palate (associated with the Robin sequence), and velopharyngeal insufficiency.[57,59] The chromosomal microdeletion results in haploin sufficiency of approximately 106 genes (notably including the

Tbx1 gene), which affect the development of the pharyngeal arches, pouches, and arteries.[57] Hearing impairment affects close to 40% of patients with CHL being most common.[58] Causes for hearing impairment include middle and inner ear malformation, Eustachian tube dysfunction, and otitis media.[60]

Temporal bone CT findings in 22q11.2 deletion syndrome include stenotic or occasionally atretic EACs, variably small MES, dense manubrium of the malleus (sometimes with fixation), abnormal thinning of the long process of the incus with horizontal orientation, IS disconnection, dense stapedial superstructure with variable abnormality in orientation, elongated cochlear basal turn, slightly deficient cochlear interscalar septum and a widened vestibule and malformed horizontal SCC with either a small or absent bone island, and occasionally malformation affecting the posterior SCC (**Fig. 8**).[60,61] An important finding that should not be overlooked is a lateralized course (see **Fig. 8**A) and sometimes dehiscence of the petrous carotid canal accompanied by pulsatile tinnitus.[60] The dense stapedial superstructure in conjunction

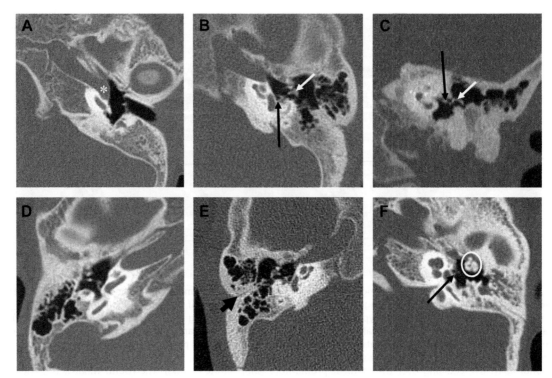

Fig. 8. (*A–C*) 22q11.2 deletion syndrome. (*A*) Axial CT image shows an anomalous course of the left carotid canal (*asterisk*) with a lateralized course in close proximity to the cochlea. (*B* and *C*) The incus (*short white arrows*) is abnormally shaped with shortened long and lenticular processes with an abnormally obtuse IS angle. The posterior crus of the stapes is thickened (*long black arrows*) and closely apposed to the shallow sinus tympani and pyramidal eminence. (*D* and *E*) Cleidocranial dysplasia. Axial CT images in 2 different patients showing abnormally thickened stapedial crura. Note the prominent petrosquamosal suture (*short thick black arrow*). (*F*) Cornelia de Lange syndrome. Axial CT showing heart-shaped morphology of the head of the malleus with a bony cleft in the incus body resulting in a V-shaped incudomalleal joint (enclosed in oval). Note the diminutive, malformed stapes (*long black arrow*).

with the inner ear anomalies and lateralized carotid canals are highly characteristic of this disorder.[61] In the differential diagnosis for the SCC and ossicular anomalies seen in 22q11.2 deletion syndrome is Kabuki syndrome.[62]

Miscellaneous Syndromes

Inumerable other syndromes are associated with characteristic anomalies, some of which are described briefly below. For many syndromes associated with CHL the cause of hearing loss is multifactorial related to cleft palate, midface hypoplasia, and alteration in the size and course of the Eustachian tube leading to Eustachian tube dysfunction and otitis media with effusion, in addition to any preexisting external and/or MES and ossicular anomalies.

Cleidocranial dysplasia
Temporal bone findings include EAC stenosis, underdeveloped mastoid air cells, prominent petrosquamosal suture, wide Eustachian tubes, rotated incus and malleus, lateralized tensor tympani

muscle/tendon, and thickened stapedial crura with fusion of stapes to the FNC (see **Figs. 8D–E**).[63] Other craniofacial features include brachycephaly, widened metopic and sagittal sutures with delayed closure, numerous wormian bones, high-arched palate with nasal cavity stenosis, and multiple supernumerary teeth with delayed eruption.

Cornelia de Lange syndrome
Temporal bone features include dysmorphic, large head of the malleus with a bony cleft of the incus body, malformed stapes (see **Fig. 8**G), EAC and IAC narrowing, cochlear malformation with modiolar deficiency, mastoid and/or MEC opacification, and a misshapen vestibule with posteroinferior protrusion.[1,64] Other features include characteristic facial dysmorphism, congenital heart defects, limb anomalies, and growth impairment.[65]

Sclerosing Bone Disorders

Pronounced constriction of the MES sometimes resulting in ossicular ankylosis is seen in several disorders such as fibrous dysplasia, craniometaphyseal dysplasia, and osteopetrosis (Figs. 9A–C).

Radiolucent Disorders

It is unusual to see pronounced ossicular lucency. In our experience, conditions to consider include osteogenesis imperfecta, multifocal lymphatic malformation (Gorham Stout disease), and multifocal venous malformations (eg, blue rubber bleb nevus syndrome) (see Figs. 9 D–F), with a tendency to develop CSF leaks and intracranial hypotension in the latter 2 conditions.[66,67]

Chronic Inflammatory Disorders

In addition to the ossicles, ligaments, and tendons housed within the MES, there are also mucosal folds that transmit blood vessels to the ossicles and these folds help compartmentalize the MES.[68] Aeration between the epitympanum

and mesotympanum occurs via the tympanic isthmi, which are 2 openings in the so-called tympanic diaphragm (malleus head and neck, incus body and short process, and the anterior and lateral mallear and incudal ligaments).[69] Obstruction of the tympanic isthmi is attributed to a variety of processes including thickened or hyperplastic mucosal folds, inflammatory adhesive webs, TM retraction, inflammatory exudate, edematous mucosa, cholesteatoma, and congenital anomalies.[68] Another possible site of obstruction is the aditus at antrum between the epitympanum and mastoid antrum. In conjunction with various other factors (eg, Eustachian tube dysfunction, immunologic disorders, and so forth), middle ear obstruction and inflammation results in chronic disease of the MES including chronic otitis media (often with TM perforation), tympanosclerosis, cholesteatoma, and cholesterol granuloma.

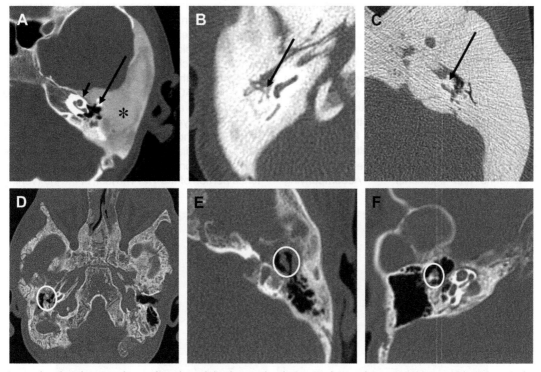

Fig. 9. (A–C). Sclerosing bone disorders. (A) Fibrous dysplasia. CT shows characteristic expansile, ground glass appearance of the left temporal bone due to fibrous dysplasia (asterisk) partially encompassing the ossicles (long black arrow) and narrowing the MES and FNC (short black arrow). Axial CT of (B) craniometaphyseal dysplasia and (C) osteopetrosis demonstrate features of sclerosing bone disorders with severe narrowing of the opacified MESs and ossicular dysmorphism (long black arrows) with partial ankylosis. (D–F). Ossicular lucency on axial CT. (D) Osteogenesis imperfecta with innumerable osseous lucencies as well as Wormian bones. Partial ossicular lucency is shown on the right (enclosed in oval). (E) Gorham stout (vanishing bone) disease with extensive, biopsy proven lymphatic malformation resulting in radiolucent ossicles (enclosed in circle). Note the radiolucency due to lymphatic malformation involving the surrounding petrous and squamous temporal bones with a defect in the anterior attic. (F) Multiple venous malformations involving the right temporal bone with involvement of the right malleus, which is demineralized (enclosed in oval).

Tympanosclerosis

Tympanosclerosis refers to deposition of hyalinized collagen with subsequent dystrophic calcification within the MES.[70] Myringosclerosis refers to associated mineralization of the TM. Tympanosclerosis typically occurs in patients with a history of recurrent acute or chronic otitis media.[71] Myringosclerosis is also seen in the setting of prior tympanostomy tubes and/or tympanoplasty.[72] Although the etiology and pathogenesis of tympanosclerosis is not fully understood, it is an irreversible degenerative inflammatory process related to a possible combination of immunologic reaction, genetic predisposition, long-standing chronic middle ear infection, surgery, trauma, and free oxygen radicles.[71] Tympanosclerosis is associated with significant progressive hearing loss, predominantly CHL, due to interference with sound conduction, transmission, and rarely transduction, attributable to ossicular fixation, TM perforation, and less frequently reduced TM mobility.[70]

CT features of tympanosclerosis include unilateral or multifocal punctate, ovoid, linear or web-like hyperattenuating, calcified or ossified foci in the MES, along ossicles, suspensory ligaments or tendons, and perforation and mineralization of the TM.[70] Thickening of the stapedial crura and footplate, obliteration of the oval window niche, concretions encasing the malleus and incus, ossicular fixation and narrowing of the MES lumen are additional features (Fig. 10).[70] Postinflammatory ossicular fixation can also result from nonmineralized fibrous tissue encasing the ossicles and/or tendons and ligaments.[68,73] Accompanying signs of chronic otitis media include underpneumatized and sometimes opacified mastoid air cells with thickened mastoid trabeculae and surrounding sclerosis (see Fig. 10A).[68] CT provides valuable preoperative information in diagnosing or corroborating the cause of hearing loss, localizing the abnormality, and helping plan operative intervention.

Cholesteatoma

Cholesteatoma is a histologically benign mass formed by keratinizing squamous epithelium in the tympanic cavity and/or mastoid and subepithelial connective tissue with progressive accumulation of keratin debris with or without a surrounding inflammatory reaction. Cholesteatoma is classified as congenital or acquired.[74] Congenital cholesteatoma is defined as a white retrotympanic mass located medial to an intact TM that is presumed to have been present at birth but is usually diagnosed during infancy or in early childhood, without a preceding history of otorrhea, TM perforation, or otologic surgery.[75] However, despite this definition, a history of previous otitis media or effusion does not exclude the diagnosis of congenital cholesteatoma. Cholesteatoma can also occur in the EAC particularly in patients with congenital EAC stenosis, attributed to trapped epithelial cells medial to the stenosis.[76]

The inner layer of the TM is covered by mucosa of the MES, and the outer layer is covered by keratinizing stratified epithelium of the EAC. A middle fibrous supporting layer is present in the pars tensa portion of the TM. The lack of the intervening

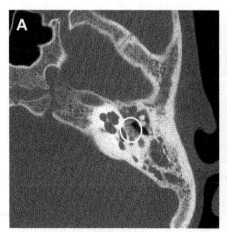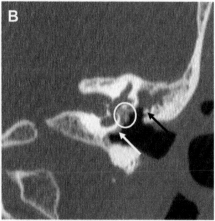

Fig. 10. Tympanosclerosis associated with chronic otitis media. (A) Axial and (B) reformatted coronal CT images. There is decreased mastoid pneumatization with opacified air cells and surrounding sclerosis. Partial opacification of the attic and hazy mineralization/ossification surrounds the stapes (enclosed in circles) and overlies the promontory (*white arrow*, B), consistent with tympanosclerosis. Note the gap between the body of the incus (*black arrow*, B) and stapes consistent with absent/eroded incus long/lenticular process. These findings were confirmed at surgery, which also demonstrated cholesteatoma.

fibrous layer in the posterosuperior pars flaccida portion of the TM is thought to predispose to the formation of a retraction pocket in Prussak space, which can lead to the subsequent development of an acquired pars flaccida cholesteatoma.[68] Acquired cholesteatoma develops less frequently in relation to pars tensa retraction pockets, secondary to TM perforation, or due trauma or iatrogenic causes.[74]

The clinical presentation of cholesteatoma ranges from an incidental finding on routine physical examination to unilateral CHL, otalgia, signs and symptoms related to infection including coalescent mastoiditis and related complications or facial palsy.[74,75] The development of vestibular symptoms, SNHL, meningitis or CSF leak herald the rare complication of otic capsule involvement with resultant labyrinthitis, perilymph fistula, and/or CSF leak.

CT of EAC cholesteatoma is suggested by the presence of a rounded or oval erosive opacity in the EAC. In the setting of a previously stenotic EAC this leads to paradoxic widening the previously stenotic EAC due to osseous remodeling/erosion (see Figs. 3B and D). The appearance is indistinguishable from keratosis obturans which also occurs in stenotic EACs.

CT of congenital MES cholesteatoma demonstrates a rounded or ovoid opacity usually in the mesotympanum (abutting the malleus and cochlear promontory), less commonly in other locations, with ossicular erosion reported in approximately 36% of patients.[77] The goal of imaging is to confirm or determine the diagnosis, detect the extent of disease, and to diagnose ossicular erosion (Fig. 11).

A retraction pocket appears as a small opacity in Prussak space located between the pars flaccida of the TM, the neck of the malleus, scutum and lateral malleal ligament. Progressive enlargement, inferomedial displacement of the malleus, and erosion of the scutum and ossicles are features of pars flaccida cholesteatoma (see Fig 11). Pars tensa acquired cholesteatoma tends to develop medial to the ossicles which are then displaced laterally. Occasionally MES cholesteatoma can erode otic capsule bone leading to perilymph fistula and/or CSF leak (see Fig 11G).

Post-operative evaluation for suspected residual or recurrent cholesteatoma usually consists of CT or MR, or both. Routine MR temporal bone sequences and non echoplanar or multishot echoplanar DWI are invaluable in distinguishing cholesteatoma from granulation tissue, mucosal thickening and/or secretions (hyperintense on T2 with facilitated diffusivity) and from cholesterol granuloma (hyperintense on FS T1 and T2 weighted MR) which may coexist with recurrent or residual cholesteatoma (intermediate to hyperintense on T2 with decreased diffusivity) (see Fig. 11H).

Cholesterol Granuloma

Cholesterol granuloma (CG) is a histologic definition used to describe foreign body giant cell reaction to cholesterol and hemosiderin derived from ruptured erythrocytes.[78] Microscopically CG is composed of cholesterol crystals surrounded and engulfed by multinucleated foreign-body giant cells and embedded in fibrous granulation tissue with histiocytes, round cell infiltrate, macrophages, capillaries, hemorrhage of varying ages and hemosiderin.[79] Isolated CG typically involves the petrous apex and is rarely described in the tympanomastoid region.[80] CG is more commonly encountered in conjunction with cholesteatoma and chronic otitis media or in the context of post-traumatic hemorrhage of the temporal bone related to inciting events such as hemorrhage, impaired drainage and obstructed ventilation.[78,79]

CT depicts the location of the CG but does not discriminate between cholesteatoma and CG. Both CG and cholesteatoma may have well-defined margins, appear of similar attenuation and erode surrounding structures. MR is the exam of choice to help distinguish between CG and cholesteatoma, CG appearing hyperintense relative to surrounding structures on T1, FS T1 and T2 weighted MR and demonstrating facilitated diffusivity (see Fig. 11H).

Masses and Tumors

A variety of benign and malignant tumors occurs in the EAC and MES potentially causing CHL. The type of tumor varies with age and with an increased incidence of specific tumor types in various tumor predisposition syndromes. Tumor types include plexiform neurofibroma, teratoma, choristoma (hairy polyp), infantile hemangioma, Langerhans cell histiocytosis, rhabdomyosarcoma, a wide variety of other primary malignant tumors and metastatic disease. CT and MR provide complimentary information regarding the extent of disease, presence and pattern of osseous destruction (CT) and tumor type (MR) (Fig. 12).

Vascular Lesions

Vascular variants that may be associated with CHL include high and/or dehiscent jugular bulb, anomalous internal carotid artery (ICA), and PSA.[81] Identification of these anomalies is particularly important for patients undergoing surgery on the MES.

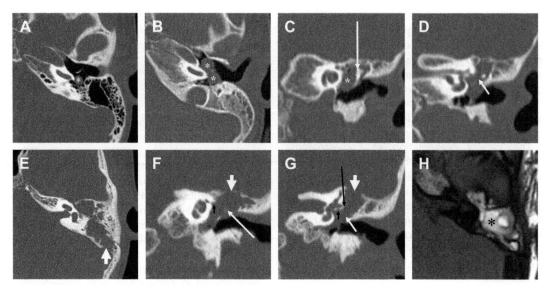

Fig. 11. Cholesteatoma (*A–G*) and cholesterol granuloma (*H*). (*A, B* and *E*) axial and (*C, D, F,* and *G*) reformatted coronal CT images. (*A*) Congenital cholesteatoma. There is a small rounded opacity abutting the cochlear promontory (white *asterisk*), which is typical although not specific for the diagnosis. Congenital cholesteatoma is more frequently seen ventral to the malleus and abutting the promontory. (*B–D*) Larger congenital cholesteatoma in a different patient. (*B*) There is a bilobed, sharply defined opacity surrounding the malleus in the mesotympanum (white *asterisks*). (*C*) The cholesteatoma extends cephalad into the attic, displacing the malleus laterally (long thin *white arrow*). (*D*) There is erosion of the long process of the incus (short thin *white arrow*). Opacified mastoid air cells are likely due to obstruction of the aditus ad antrum. (*E–G*) Acquired cholesteatoma. The MES, mastoid antrum and under pneumatized mastoid air cells are opacified. (*E*) The malleus and incus are not seen in the attic. There is erosion of the posterior mastoid cortex (*short thick white arrow*). (*F, G*) The eroded malleus remnant is displaced inferiorly and medially (*long thin white arrow*) and the scutum is blunted. There is erosion of the tegmen tympani (*short thick white arrows*). There is pronounced erosion of the incus (*short thin white arrow*). There is also erosion of the tympanic segment of the FNC (*short thin black arrows*) and eroded bone over the horizontal SCC (long thin *black arrow*), which resulted in a perilymph fistula. (*H*) Cholesterol granuloma. T1-weighted axial MR image obtained following canal wall up mastoidectomy for cholesteatoma. There is extensive high-signal material in the MES and mastoid (*black asterisk*). Diffusion-weighted images (not shown) showed predominantly facilitated diffusivity surrounding a small focus of decreased diffusivity. At surgery there was extensive cholesterol granuloma encompassing a small focus of recurrent cholesteatoma.

High jugular bulb that is dehiscent into the MES is associated with tinnitus, vertigo, and hearing loss on audiometry (most commonly CHL).[82] On otoscopic examination a blueish mass is visible behind the TM. There is no consensus as to the precise definition of a high-riding jugular bulb with one report describing type 1 high jugular bulb with the dome reaching the inferior part of the round window and type 2 with the dome protruding above the inferior margin of the internal auditory canal.[82] High-riding jugular bulb is readily diagnosed on CT and integrity of the overlying bone should be carefully assessed in order to diagnose dehiscence with respect to the MES, round window niche, vestibular aqueduct, and SCCs (Fig. 13A–C). An increased incidence of high jugular bulb and jugular bulb dehiscence is seen in patients with syndromic craniosynostosis (see Figs. 13A and B). These patients frequently have stenosis or atresia of the jugular veins at

the skull base and markedly enlarged occipito-mastoid emissary veins.[83] High-riding and dehiscent jugular bulb is more frequently seen on the right side and dehiscence into the vestibular aqueduct in pediatric patients is controversial, with some authors reporting that there is not a clearly defined link to hearing loss.[84]

Aberrancy of the ICA is rare. Symptoms and signs include vertigo, pulsatile tinnitus, CHL, and usually a red retrotympanic mass behind the TM on otoscopic examination.[85] This entity is attributed to segmental agenesis of the first embryologic segment of the ICA during fetal life with blood flowing through the inferior tympanic artery. On axial CT, the inferior tympanic artery is smaller than the normal ICA and courses through the inferior tympanic canaliculus, which is adjacent to the jugular bulb. The aberrant vessel then courses across the MES before rejoining the petrous carotid canal (see Fig. 13D).[85,86]

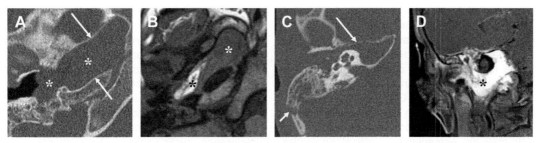

Fig. 12. Masses and tumors. (*A* and *B*) Benign mass. (*A*) Axial CT demonstrates an expansile, tubular mass (*white asterisks*) within the MES, protruding through an osseous defect and remodeling the right petrous apex and sphenoid bone (long *arrows*). (*B*) Axial T1-weighted MR image shows that the mass is partly isointense with brain (white *asterisk*) and partly hyperintense (*black asterisk*), shown to be fat on FS T1-weighted images (not shown). Although histology demonstrated heterotopic neuroglial tissue, the imaging characteristics suggest choristoma or teratoma. (*C* and *D*) Rhabdomyosarcoma. (*C*) Axial CT image shows opacification of the MES and ossicular erosion. There is also erosion of the petrous apex (long *arrow*), suggestive of an aggressive process. Note the opacified mastoid air cells with erosion of the retroauricular mastoid cortex (short *arrow*). The patient initially presented with signs and symptoms of coalescent mastoiditis resulting from obstructed secretions due to the tumor. (*D*) Coronal FS T1 postcontrast MR image shows enhancing tumor (*asterisk*) within the petrous bone and MES with adjacent dural enhancement.

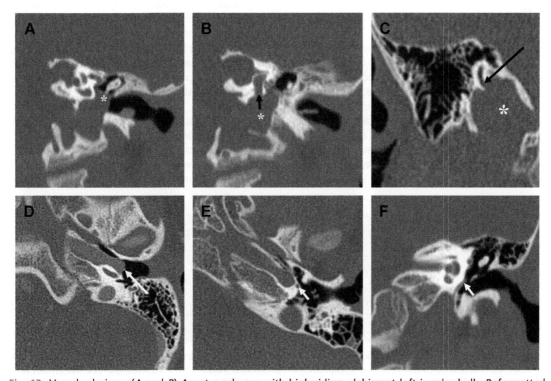

Fig. 13. Vascular lesions. (*A* and *B*) Apert syndrome with high-riding, dehiscent left jugular bulb. Reformatted coronal CT images show the dehiscent jugular bulb (*asterisks*) protruding into the MES and abutting the (*A*) incus and (*B*) occupying the round window niche (*short black arrow*). (*C*) High-riding jugular bulb with SCC dehiscence. Coronal reformatted CT demonstrates a high-riding right jugular bulb (*asterisk*) with posterior SCC dehiscence (long *black arrow*). (*D*) Dehiscent ICA. Axial CT shows the aberrant, dehiscent ICA coursing over the thinned cochlear promontory and abutting the malleus (*long white arrow*). (*E* and *F*) PSA. (*E*) Axial CT shows the tiny PSA emanating from the carotid canal (*short white arrow*). (*F*) Reformatted coronal CT demonstrates the PSA coursing cephalad along the cochlear promontory (*short white arrow*).

The stapedial artery is an embryonic artery that transforms the middle meningeal artery from a branch of the ICA to a branch of the external carotid artery then usually disappears in utero.[87] A PSA is rare and usually asymptomatic but can cause pulsatile tinnitus and impaired movement of the stapes resulting in CHL.[88] PSA sometimes occurs in association with an aberrant ICA and is also seen in PHACE(S) association (posterior fossa malformations, hemangioma, arterial anomalies and aortic coarctation, cardiac anomalies, esophageal and eye anomalies and sternal anomalies and supraumbilical raphe).[89] On CT, the foramen spinosum (which ordinarily transmits the middle meningeal artery) is absent, and the PSA seems as a tiny tubular structure coursing over the cochlear promontory (see Figs. 13 E and F), and sometimes through the obturator foramen of the stapes to enter the FNC through a dehiscence in its wall posterior to the cochleariform process. The PSA then courses anteriorly, exiting the FNC before the geniculate ganglion and travels to the middle cranial fossa to supply the middle meningeal artery.[88] PSA is similarly depicted on brain MRA.

Third Window Disorders

The oval and round windows are 2 mobile windows responsible for normal sound transmission between the middle and inner ears, as described previously. Additional normal "windows" that do not affect sound conduction under normal circumstances include the cochlear and vestibular aqueducts, and numerous foramina transmitting nerves and vessels.[90] By contrast, pathologic third window abnormalities are lesions where there is abnormal communication between the inner and middle ear as well as CSF and vascular structures. The mechanism of action is a reduction in bone conduction hearing thresholds with elevation in air conduction thresholds resulting in an air-bone gap on audiogram. Clinical symptoms depend on cause and include vertigo, dizziness, lightheadedness, oscillopsia, pulsatile or continuous tinnitus, hyperacusis, autophony, motion intolerance, cyclic vomiting, Tullio phenomenon, and CHL or MHL.[2,91] Anatomic locations for third window lesions include dehiscent SCC, large vestibular aqueduct, carotid cochlear dehiscence, X-linked stapes gusher, and other cochlear malformations.[90] In children, third window lesions are rare, and the most frequently encountered causes are enlarged vestibular aqueducts and SCC dehiscence.[91,92] Dehiscent jugular bulb may also impede motion of the round window (see Fig 13B).

Trauma

Temporal bone fracture that results in CHL or MHL is typically orientated in a longitudinal, oblique, or mixed direction with respect to the long axis of the petrous bone. Causes of posttraumatic CHL include trauma to the MES and contents resulting in hemotympanum, fracture, and sometimes ossicular disruption. Pediatric temporal bone fractures are classified as longitudinal (50%), transverse (12.5%), and mixed (37.5%) in orientation with otic capsule violation seen in approximately 5% of longitudinal fractures.[93]

Temporal bone CT demonstrates the fracture trajectory and whether there is evidence of ossicular displacement, fracture, subluxation, or

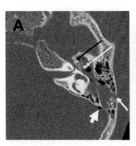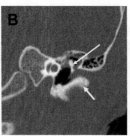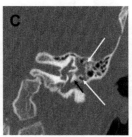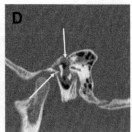

Fig. 14. Temporal bone trauma. (A) Axial CT at the level of the attic shows a mildly diastatic, longitudinal fracture through the mastoid bone (*short thin white arrow*). There is also a fracture fragment (*long thin black arrow*) protruding into the FNC close to the anterior genu. Only the head of the malleus is seen (*long thin white arrow*) at the level of the incudomalleal joint. There is opacification of the MES and mastoid air cells with air fluid levels attributable to hemorrhage. There is a small amount of pneumocephalus in the posterior fossa (short thick *white arrow*). (B) Coronal reformatted CT image shows angulation of the malleus (*long thin white arrow*) and a nondisplaced fracture of the tympanic plate (short thin *white arrow*). (C and D) Reformatted coronal and oblique images shows the avulsed incus (dislocated incudomalleal and IS joints) rotated and displaced inferiorly (short thin *black arrow*). There are additional fractures through the tegmen tympani, scutum, and TMJ (*long thin white arrows*).

dislocation (Fig. 14). The images should also be carefully assessed for fracture of the FNC, carotid canal, jugular foramen, tegmen tympani, and/or tegmen mastoideum. Trauma can also result from penetrating foreign bodies or surgery resulting in subluxation of stapes into the vestibule.

SUMMARY

Childhood CHL is uncommon and imaging plays an essential role in helping determine the cause of HL, providing invaluable information that helps assess prognosis, determine therapeutic options, and highlight potential risks of surgery. Many of the conditions described in this review have characteristic although sometimes subtle imaging findings.

CLINICS CARE POINTS

- Congenital external auditory canal stenosis and atresia are invariably associated with ossicular anomalies and often with hypoplasia or abnormal shape of the middle ear space.

- When oval window atresia or stenosis is present. look for associated aberrancy of the facial nerve canal.

- Temporal bone anomalies associated with micrognathia suggest an underlying, potentially heritable syndrome such as craniofacial microsomia (unilateral or bilateral asymmetric micrognathia) or Treacher Collins syndrome (bilateral symmetric micrognathia).

- External, middle and inner ear anomalies are also suggestive of an underlying syndrome or teratogenic insult, with charachertistic inner ear findings seen in branchio-oto-renal syndrome and CHARGE syndrome.

- White retrotympanic mass is typical of cholesteatoma; look for association ossicular erosion.

- Blue retrotympanic mass suggests jugular bulb dehiscence that may be sporadic or syndromic (e.g. with large emissary veins in syndromic craniosynostosis).

- Red retrotympanic mass suggests aberrant internal carotid artery, a rare anomaly that may be associated with aberrant stapedial artery.

DISCLOSURE

The authors have nothing to disclose.

REFERENCES

1. Foust AM, Poe DS, Robson CD. The Ossicles in Pediatric Conductive Hearing Loss. Neurographics 2020;10(5–6):259–71.

2. Scarpa A, Ralli M, Cassandro C, et al. Inner-Ear Disorders Presenting with Air-Bone Gaps: A Review. J Int Adv Otol 2020;16(1):111–6.

3. Ankamreddy H, Min H, Kim JY, et al. Region-specific endodermal signals direct neural crest cells to form the three middle ear ossicles. Development 2019; 146(2). https://doi.org/10.1242/dev.167965.

4. Whyte J, Cisneros A, Yus C, et al. Development of the dynamic structure (force lines) of the middle ear ossicles in human foetuses. Histol Histopathol 2008;23(9):1049–60.

5. Mukherjee S, Kesser BW, Raghavan P. The "boomerang" malleus-incus complex in congenital aural atresia. AJNR Am J Neuroradiol 2014;35(11): 2181–5.

6. Mortier J, van den Ende J, Declau F, et al. Search for a genetic cause in children with unilateral isolated microtia and congenital aural atresia. Eur Arch Oto-Rhino-Laryngol 2023;280(2):623–31.

7. Lammer EJ, Chen DT, Hoar RM, et al. Retinoic acid embryopathy. N Engl J Med 1985;313(14):837–41.

8. Ewart-Toland A, Yankowitz J, Winder A, et al. Oculoauriculovertebral abnormalities in children of diabetic mothers. Am J Med Genet 2000;90(4): 303–9.

9. Cheung MMY, Tsang TW, Watkins R, et al. Ear Abnormalities Among Children with Fetal Alcohol Spectrum Disorder: A Systematic Review and Meta-Analysis. J Pediatr 2022;242:113–120 e16.

10. Li J, Chen K, Li C, et al. Anatomical measurement of the ossicles in patients with congenital aural atresia and stenosis. Int J Pediatr Otorhinolaryngol 2017; 101:230–4.

11. Shonka DC Jr, Livingston WJ 3rd, Kesser BW. The Jahrsdoerfer grading scale in surgery to repair congenital aural atresia. Arch Otolaryngol Head Neck Surg 2008;134(8):873–7.

12. Jahrsdoerfer RA, Yeakley JW, Aguilar EA, et al. Grading system for the selection of patients with congenital aural atresia. Am J Otol 1992;13(1):6–12.

13. Bachor E, Just T, Wright CG, et al. Fixation of the stapes footplate in children: a clinical and temporal bone histopathologic study. Otol Neurotol 2005; 26(5):866–73.

14. Briggs RJ, Luxford WM. Correction of conductive hearing loss in children. Otolaryngol Clin North Am 1994;27(3):607–20.

15. Stewart JM, Downs MP. Congenital conductive hearing loss: the need for early identification and intervention. Pediatrics 1993;91(2):355–9.

16. Cremers CW, Teunissen E. The impact of a syndromal diagnosis on surgery for congenital minor ear

anomalies. Int J Pediatr Otorhinolaryngol 1991; 22(1):59–74.

17. Totten DJ, Marinelli JP, Carlson ML. Incidence of Congenital Stapes Footplate Fixation Since 1970: A Population-based Study. Otol Neurotol 2020;41(4): 489–93.

18. Teunissen EB, Cremers WR. Classification of congenital middle ear anomalies. Report on 144 ears. Ann Otol Rhinol Laryngol 1993;102(8 Pt 1):606–12.

19. Thomeer HG, Kunst HP, Cremers CW. Congenital stapes ankylosis associated with another ossicular chain anomaly: surgical results in 30 ears. Arch Otolaryngol Head Neck Surg 2011;137(9):935–41.

20. Khoo HW, Choong CC, Yeo SB, et al. High Resolution Computed Tomography (HRCT) Imaging Findings of Oval Window Atresia with Surgical Correlation. Ann Acad Med Singap 2020;49(6): 346–53.

21. Henkemans SE, Smit AL, Stokroos RJ, et al. Congenital Anomalies of the Ossicular Chain: Surgical and Audiological Outcomes. Ann Otol Rhinol Laryngol 2022;131(4):388–96.

22. Cox TC, Camci ED, Vora S, et al. The genetics of auricular development and malformation: new findings in model systems driving future directions for microtia research. Eur J Med Genet 2014;57(8): 394–401.

23. Raposo BK, Ferreira GB, Silva A, et al. Determination of Extra Craniofacial Abnormalities in Patients With Craniofacial Microsomia. J Craniofac Surg 2022;33(1):230–2.

24. Birgfeld C, Heike C. Craniofacial Microsomia. Clin Plast Surg 2019;46(2):207–21.

25. Renkema RW, Caron C, Pauws E, et al. Extracraniofacial anomalies in craniofacial microsomia: retrospective analysis of 991 patients. Int J Oral Maxillofac Surg 2019;48(9):1169–76.

26. Timberlake AT, Griffin C, Heike CL, et al. Haploinsufficiency of SF3B2 causes craniofacial microsomia. Nat Commun 2021;12(1):4680.

27. Rooijers W, Tio PAE, van der Schroeff MP, et al. Hearing impairment and ear anomalies in craniofacial microsomia: a systematic review. Int J Oral Maxillofac Surg 2022;51(10):1296–304.

28. Quiat D, Timberlake AT, Curran JJ, et al. Damaging variants in FOXI3 cause microtia and craniofacial microsomia. Genet Med 2023;25(1):143–50.

29. Horgan JE, Padwa BL, LaBrie RA, et al. OMENS-Plus: analysis of craniofacial and extracraniofacial anomalies in hemifacial microsomia. Cleft Palate Craniofac J 1995;32(5):405–12.

30. Vento AR, LaBrie RA, Mulliken JB. The O.M.E.N.S. classification of hemifacial microsomia. Cleft Palate Craniofac J 1991;28(1):68–76. discussion 77.

31. Keegan CE, Mulliken JB, Wu BL, et al. Townes-Brocks syndrome versus expanded spectrum hemifacial microsomia: review of eight patients and further evidence of a "hot spot" for mutation in the SALL1 gene. Genet Med 2001;3(4):310–3.

32. Marszalek-Kruk BA, Wojcicki P, Dowgierd K, et al. Treacher Collins Syndrome: Genetics, Clinical Features and Management. Genes 2021;12(9). https://doi.org/10.3390/genes12091392.

33. Marszalek-Kruk BA, Wojcicki P. Identification of three novel TCOF1 mutations in patients with Treacher Collins Syndrome. Hum Genome Var 2021;8(1):36.

34. Sanchez E, Laplace-Builhe B, Mau-Them FT, et al. POLR1B and neural crest cell anomalies in Treacher Collins syndrome type 4. Genet Med 2020;22(3): 547–56.

35. Pron G, Galloway C, Armstrong D, et al. Ear malformation and hearing loss in patients with Treacher Collins syndrome. Cleft Palate Craniofac J 1993; 30(1):97–103.

36. Rosa F, Coutinho MB, Ferreira JP, et al. Ear malformations, hearing loss and hearing rehabilitation in children with Treacher Collins syndrome. Acta Otorrinolaringol Esp 2016;67(3):142–7.

37. Bernier FP, Caluseriu O, Ng S, et al. Haploinsufficiency of SF3B4, a component of the pre-mRNA spliceosomal complex, causes Nager syndrome. Am J Hum Genet 2012;90(5):925–33.

38. Ulhaq ZS, Soraya GV, Istifiani LA, et al. SF3B4 Frameshift Variants Represented a More Severe Clinical Manifestation in Nager Syndrome. Cleft Palate Craniofac J 2022;25. https://doi.org/10.1177/10556656221089156. 10556656221089156.

39. Maharana SK, Saint-Jeannet JP. Molecular mechanisms of hearing loss in Nager syndrome. Dev Biol 2021;476:200–8.

40. Fraser FC, Sproule JR, Halal F. Frequency of the branchio-oto-renal (BOR) syndrome in children with profound hearing loss. Am J Med Genet 1980;7(3): 341–9.

41. Chang EH, Menezes M, Meyer NC, et al. Branchio-oto-renal syndrome: the mutation spectrum in EYA1 and its phenotypic consequences. Hum Mutat 2004;23(6):582–9.

42. Klingbeil KD, Greenland CM, Arslan S, et al. Novel EYA1 variants causing Branchio-oto-renal syndrome. Int J Pediatr Otorhinolaryngol 2017;98: 59–63.

43. Ruf RG, Xu PX, Silvius D, et al. SIX1 mutations cause branchio-oto-renal syndrome by disruption of EYA1-SIX1-DNA complexes. Proc Natl Acad Sci U S A 2004;101(21):8090–5.

44. Abdelhak S, Kalatzis V, Heilig R, et al. A human homologue of the Drosophila eyes absent gene underlies branchio-oto-renal (BOR) syndrome and identifies a novel gene family. Nat Genet 1997; 15(2):157–64.

45. Propst EJ, Blaser S, Gordon KA, et al. Temporal bone findings on computed tomography imaging

in branchio-oto-renal syndrome. Laryngoscope 2005;115(10):1855–62.

46. Juliano AF, D'Arco F, Pao J, et al. The Cochlea in Branchio-Oto-Renal Syndrome: An Objective Method for the Diagnosis of Offset Cochlear Turns. AJNR Am J Neuroradiol 2022;43(11):1646–52.

47. Pao J, D'Arco F, Clement E, et al. Re-Examining the Cochlea in Branchio-Oto-Renal Syndrome: Genotype-Phenotype Correlation. AJNR Am J Neuroradiol 2022;43(2):309–14.

48. Robson CD. Congenital hearing impairment. Pediatr Radiol 2006;36(4):309–24.

49. Moccia A, Srivastava A, Skidmore JM, et al. Genetic analysis of CHARGE syndrome identifies overlapping molecular biology. Genet Med 2018;20(9):1022–9.

50. Vissers LE, van Ravenswaaij CM, Admiraal R, et al. Mutations in a new member of the chromodomain gene family cause CHARGE syndrome. Nat Genet 2004;36(9):955–7.

51. van Ravenswaaij-Arts C, Martin DM. New insights and advances in CHARGE syndrome: Diagnosis, etiologies, treatments, and research discoveries. Am J Med Genet C Semin Med Genet 2017;175(4):397–406.

52. Lewis MA, Juliano A, Robson C, et al. The spectrum of cochlear malformations in CHARGE syndrome and insights into the role of the CHD7 gene during embryogenesis of the inner ear. Neuroradiology 2023;65(4):819–34.

53. Morimoto AK, Wiggins RH 3rd, Hudgins PA, et al. Absent semicircular canals in CHARGE syndrome: radiologic spectrum of findings. AJNR Am J Neuroradiol 2006;27(8):1663–71.

54. Vesseur AC, Verbist BM, Westerlaan HE, et al. CT findings of the temporal bone in CHARGE syndrome: aspects of importance in cochlear implant surgery. Eur Arch Oto-Rhino-Laryngol 2016;273(12):4225–40.

55. Hoch MJ, Patel SH, Jethanamest D, et al. Head and Neck MRI Findings in CHARGE Syndrome. AJNR Am J Neuroradiol 2017;38(12):2357–63.

56. Botto LD, May K, Fernhoff PM, et al. A population-based study of the 22q11.2 deletion: phenotype, incidence, and contribution to major birth defects in the population. Pediatrics 2003;112(1 Pt 1):101–7.

57. Du Q, de la Morena MT, van Oers NSC. The Genetics and Epigenetics of 22q11.2 Deletion Syndrome. Front Genet 2019;10:1365.

58. Jiramongkolchai P, Kumar MS, Chinnadurai S, et al. Prevalence of hearing loss in children with 22q11.2 deletion syndrome. Int J Pediatr Otorhinolaryngol 2016;87:130–3.

59. Kruszka P, Addissie YA, McGinn DE, et al. 22q11.2 deletion syndrome in diverse populations. Am J Med Genet 2017;173(4):879–88.

60. Loos E, Verhaert N, Willaert A, et al. Malformations of the middle and inner ear on CT imaging in 22q11 deletion syndrome. Am J Med Genet 2016;170(11):2975–83.

61. Verheij E, Elden L, Crowley TB, et al. Anatomic Malformations of the Middle and Inner Ear in 22q11.2 Deletion Syndrome: Case Series and Literature Review. AJNR Am J Neuroradiol 2018;39(5):928–34.

62. Stadelmaier RT, Kenna MA, Barrett D, et al. Neuroimaging in Kabuki syndrome and another KMT2D-related disorder. Am J Med Genet 2021;185(12):3770–83.

63. Gonzalez GE, Caruso PA, Small JE, et al. Craniofacial and temporal bone CT findings in cleidocranial dysplasia. Pediatr Radiol 2008;38(8):892–7.

64. Kim J, Kim EY, Lee JS, et al. Temporal bone CT findings in Cornelia de Lange syndrome. AJNR Am J Neuroradiol 2008;29(3):569–73.

65. Avagliano L, Parenti I, Grazioli P, et al. Chromatinopathies: A focus on Cornelia de Lange syndrome. Clin Genet 2020;97(1):3–11.

66. Alomari MH, Shahin MM, Fishman SJ, et al. Cerebrospinal fluid leak in epidural venous malformations and blue rubber bleb nevus syndrome. J Neurosurg Spine 2022;1–7. https://doi.org/10.3171/2022.1.SPINE2138.

67. Aouad P, Young NM, Saratsis AM, et al. Gorham Stout disease of the temporal bone with cerebrospinal fluid leak. Childs Nerv Syst 2022;38(2):455–60.

68. Mafee MF, Aimi K, Kahen HL, et al. Chronic otomastoiditis: a conceptual understanding of CT findings. Radiology 1986;160(1):193–200.

69. Proctor B. Attic-aditus block and the tympanic diaphragm. Ann Otol Rhinol Laryngol 1971;80(3):371–5.

70. Larem A, Abu Rajab Altamimi Z, Aljariri AA, et al. Reliability of high-resolution CT scan in diagnosis of ossicular tympanosclerosis. Laryngoscope Investig Otolaryngol 2021;6(3):540–8.

71. Forseni M, Bagger-Sjoback D, Hultcrantz M. A study of inflammatory mediators in the human tympanosclerotic middle ear. Arch Otolaryngol Head Neck Surg 2001;127(5):559–64.

72. Tos M, Stangerup SE. Hearing loss in tympanosclerosis caused by grommets. Arch Otolaryngol Head Neck Surg 1989;115(8):931–5.

73. Swartz JD, Wolfson RJ, Marlowe FI, et al. Postinflammatory ossicular fixation: CT analysis with surgical correlation. Radiology 1985;154(3):697–700.

74. Yung M, Tono T, Olszewska E, et al. EAONO/JOS Joint Consensus Statements on the Definitions, Classification and Staging of Middle Ear Cholesteatoma. J Int Adv Otol 2017;13(1):1–8.

75. Denoyelle F, Simon F, Chang KW, et al. International Pediatric Otolaryngology Group (IPOG) Consensus Recommendations: Congenital Cholesteatoma. Otol Neurotol 2020;41(3):345–51.

76. Chan CY, Karmali SA, Arulanandam B, et al. Cholesteatoma in Congenital Aural Atresia and External Auditory Canal Stenosis: A Systematic Review.

Otolaryngol Head Neck Surg 2022. https://doi.org/10.1177/01945998221094230. 1945998221094230.

77. Reuven Y, Raveh E, Ulanovski D, et al. Congenital cholesteatoma: Clinical features and surgical outcomes. Int J Pediatr Otorhinolaryngol 2022;156:111098.

78. Pace A, Iannella G, Riminucci M, et al. Tympano-Mastoid Cholesterol Granuloma: Case Report and Review of the Literature. Clin Med Insights Case Rep 2020;13. https://doi.org/10.1177/1179547620958728. 1179547620958728.

79. Rinaldo A, Ferlito A, Cureoglu S, et al. Cholesterol granuloma of the temporal bone: a pathologic designation or a clinical diagnosis? Acta Otolaryngol 2005;125(1):86–90.

80. Angeletti D, Pace A, Iannella G, et al. Tympanic Cholesterol Granuloma and Exclusive Endoscopic Approach. Am J Case Rep 2020;21:e925369.

81. Raveh E, Hu W, Papsin BC, et al. Congenital conductive hearing loss. J Laryngol Otol 2002;116(2):92–6.

82. Sayit AT, Gunbey HP, Fethallah B, et al. Radiological and audiometric evaluation of high jugular bulb and dehiscent high jugular bulb. J Laryngol Otol 2016;130(11):1059–63.

83. Robson CD, Mulliken JB, Robertson RL, et al. Prominent basal emissary foramina in syndromic craniosynostosis: correlation with phenotypic and molecular diagnoses. AJNR Am J Neuroradiol 2000;21(9):1707–17.

84. Kupfer RA, Hoesli RC, Green GE, et al. The relationship between jugular bulb-vestibular aqueduct dehiscence and hearing loss in pediatric patients. Otolaryngol Head Neck Surg 2012;146(3):473–7.

85. Yanmaz R, Okuyucu S, Burakgazi G, et al. Aberrant Internal Carotid Artery in the Tympanic Cavity. J Craniofac Surg 2016;27(8):2001–3.

86. Song YS, Yuan YY, Wang GJ, et al. Aberrant internal carotid artery causing objective pulsatile tinnitus and conductive hearing loss. Acta Otolaryngol 2012;132(10):1126–30.

87. Hitier M, Zhang M, Labrousse M, et al. Persistent stapedial arteries in human: from phylogeny to surgical consequences. Surg Radiol Anat 2013;35(10):883–91.

88. Goderie TPM, Alkhateeb WHF, Smit CF, et al. Surgical Management of a Persistent Stapedial Artery: A Review. Otol Neurotol 2017;38(6):788–91.

89. Quatre R, Manipoud P, Schmerber S. Persistent stapedial artery in PHACE syndrome. Eur Ann Otorhinolaryngol Head Neck Dis 2019;136(3):215–7.

90. Merchant SN, Rosowski JJ. Conductive hearing loss caused by third-window lesions of the inner ear. Otol Neurotol 2008;29(3):282–9.

91. Dasgupta S, Ratnayake S, Crunkhorn R, et al. Audiovestibular Quantification in Rare Third Window Disorders in Children. Front Neurol 2020;11:954.

92. Sarioglu FC, Pekcevik Y, Guleryuz H, et al. The Relationship Between the Third Window Abnormalities and Inner Ear Malformations in Children with Hearing Loss. J Int Adv Otol 2021;17(5):387–92.

93. Wexler S, Poletto E, Chennupati SK. Pediatric Temporal Bone Fractures: A 10-Year Experience. Pediatr Emerg Care 2017;33(11):745–7.

Syndromic Hearing Loss in Children

Martin Lewis, MD[a], Caroline D. Robson, MBChB[b], Felice D'Arco, MD[a],*

KEYWORDS

- Syndromic hearing loss • Sensorineural hearing loss (SNHL) • Deafness • CHARGE
- Pendred syndrome • Branchiootorenal syndrome

INTRODUCTION

The estimated prevalence of permanent bilateral hearing loss (HL) in children is 1.33 per 1000 live births, increasing to 3.5 per 1000 adolescents, presumably reflecting additional patients owing to progressive, acquired, or late-onset genetic causes.[1] HL can be environmental, genetic or mixed, with pure genetic causes making up approximately 50% of deafness in infants.[2,3] For most genetic causes, HL is an isolated finding without the involvement of other organ systems (non-syndromic HL).

Syndromic HL refers to hearing impairment that is associated with abnormalities affecting other organs/systems. Up to 20% of hereditary HL is syndromic and there are currently over 400 known syndromes associated with HL and affecting various other systems of the body.[4] This article will review the radiological findings and clinical presentation of the most common causes of syndromic sensorineural HL (SNHL) focusing on the radiological appearances that may suggest a specific syndrome (pattern recognition approach) and associated findings outside of the temporal bone.

EMBRYOLOGY

Development of the ear requires contributions from all 3 germ layers with the involvement of 2 largely distinct developmental processes involving the otic placodes, which form the inner ear, and 1st/2nd branchial arch development, which form the outer/middle ear structures. Embryological development of the ear is complex, but critical in understanding the difference in radiological phenotypes characteristic of different syndromes. A complete embryological description of the ear development is outside the scope of this article, and we defer to the pivotal work done by Peter Som and colleagues.[5]

As a general rule (with some exceptions) useful for the radiological assessment of complex ear anomalies, malformations of the pinna, external auditory canal (EAC) are usually associated with abnormalities of the middle ear space and contents. While anomalies of the inner ear and nerves may be found in isolation. Of course, in the context of syndromic causes of HL external/middle and internal ear compartments can be involved to varying extents.

PATTERN RECOGNITION IN SYNDROMIC HEARING LOSS

The following section describes the radiological, genetic, pathophysiological, and clinical features of the more common causes of syndromic HL, as well as rare but important causes, the understanding of which is enhanced by recent genetic discoveries.

CHARGE Syndrome

Gene
Autosomal dominant (AD); CDH7 gene present in ≈ 2/3 of cases (>1000 mutations identified).[6,7]

Pathophysiology
CHD7 is a chromatin remodeling protein involved in the epigenetic regulation of gene expression,[8]

[a] Department of Radiology, Great Ormond Street Hospital for Children NHS Foundation Trust, Great Ormond St. London, London, WC1N3JH, UK; [b] Department of Radiology, Boston Children's Hospital, Harvard Medical School, Boston, MA, USA
* Corresponding author.
E-mail address: felice.d'arco@gosh.nhs.uk

Neuroimag Clin N Am 33 (2023) 563–580
https://doi.org/10.1016/j.nic.2023.05.007

mutation of which results in the disturbance of chromatin remodeling in many developmental pathways, particularly involving neural crest-derived structures.[9,10] CHD7-related sensorineural hearing loss (SNHL) is characterised by abnormal anatomical morphology of the inner ear and cochlear or vestibulocochlear nerves and abnormal regulation of hair cells.[11,12]

Diagnosis

Established with suggestive clinical and imaging findings (Blake and Verloes diagnostic criteria) (Table 1) ± molecular confirmation of a *CDH7* heterozygous pathological variant or deletion in a proband.[7,13]

Clinical characteristics

HL is seen in 60% to 90% of patients and may be conductive, SNHL, or mixed, with anomalies involving every segment of the auditory system from the external ear to the brainstem.[14] Additional clinical findings range in severity from fatal to subclinical and reflect end-organ involvement from the constellation of findings seen in the acronym plus updated minor criteria. The CHARGE mnemonic was introduced in the pre-molecular era, with the phenotypic spectrum expanded, following the identification of the CHD7 gene, to include rhomboencephalic dysfunction (mental retardation, seizures), disorders of the hypothalamic-hypophyseal axis (pituitary hormone deficiency), mediastinal organs (leading to organ failure with cardiovascular collapse and/or difficulties with feeding/aspiration secondary to tracheoesophageal anomalies), urogenital (renal failure, genital hypoplasia), cleft lip/palate and cranial nerve palsy.[15,16]

Temporal bone

Findings are bilateral, with variable degrees of asymmetry. The most common finding is the total or near-total absence of the semicircular canals (SCC) associated with hypoplasia of the vestibule and variable cochlear hypoplasia (seen in >90%) (Fig. 1).[17–19] Cochlear hypoplasia manifests with variable severity and dysmorphism (mild phenotype being the most prevalent) frequently with associated cochlear nerve aplasia/hypoplasia and cochlear aperture stenosis/atresia.[17] Visualization of the cochlear nerve is critical for cochlear implant planning and magnetic resonance imaging (MRI) should always be performed.[20] Funnel-shaped enlargement of the vestibular aqueduct is sometimes present.

The characteristic appearance of the "CHARGE" ear, is a small, low set, anteverted, misshapen pinna seen in 95% to 100% of cases and variably associated with EAC stenosis.[4]

The middle ear cavities are often underdeveloped with malformation/hypoplasia of the ossicles, particularly the stapedial superstructure, usually associated with oval window atresia.[17] The ossicles may be ankylosed to the anterior epitympanic wall. The stapedius muscle may be absent.[4] There may be the absence of the pyramidal eminence and atresia/hypoplasia of the round window.

There is a variable aberrancy of the facial nerve canal.[18,21] Dilated occipitomastoid emissary veins frequently course through or posterior to the temporal bones.

Other findings[4]

Ocular: coloboma.[22]

Brain: olfactory bulb hypoplasia or aplasia, vermis/pons/cerebellar hypoplasia or malformation (Fig. 2), pituitary gland abnormalities (small anterior gland, absent stalk, ectopic posterior gland), Chiari 1 malformation.[10,20] More recently reported findings include persistent trigeminal arteries.[23]

Head/neck: choanal atresia, cleft lip and palate, facial and, skull base malformation (J shaped sella, basioccipital hypoplasia, short and dorsally angulated clivus, coronal clival cleft, platybasia with basilar invagination), aplastic/hypoplastic parotid glands, persistent petro-squamous sinus.[20]

Chest: congenital heart disease,[24] tracheoesophageal atresia.[25]

Urinary system; duplex or solitary kidney.[26]

Teaching points

- Complete or near-complete absence of the semicircular canals in the presence of hypoplastic cochlea/cochlear nerve is almost pathognomonic of CHARGE.
- In the presence of choanal atresia or other systemic manifestation of CHARGE look at the semicircular canals.
- In case of inner ear findings suggestive of CHARGE, look at the posterior fossa and olfactory bulbs.

Branchiootorenal Spectrum Disorder

Gene

Heterozygous pathogenic variants in the *EYA1* gene and *SIX* homolog family (AD). Approximately 40% with branchiootorenal (BOR) phenotypes have mutations of the *EYA1* gene and 4% in the *SIX* homolog family.[29–32]

Pathophysiology

Both *EYA1* and *SIX1* are expressed in the ventral part of otic capsule (cochlear development pole).[33] EYA1 has a role in the developing ear, branchial arches, eye, and kidney (development

Table 1
Diagnostic criteria for CHARGE syndrome.[27,28]

Blake Criteria:		Verloes Criteria:	
Definite: 4 major or 3 major and 3 minor criteria		Typical: 3 major, or 2 major and 2 minor criteria	
Probable/possible: 1 or 2 major and several minor criteria		Partial/incomplete: 2 major and 1 minor criteria	
Occasional criteria[a]		Atypical: 2 major, or 1 major and 3 minor criteria	
Major Criteria (4C's):	**Includes:**	**Major Criteria (3C's):**	**Includes:**
Coloboma	Iris, choroid, disc, microphthalmia	Coloboma	Iris, choroid, ± microphthalmia
Choanal atresia	Unilateral/bilateral; membranous/osseous; stenosis/atresia	Choanal atresia	
Cranial nerve (CN)	I anosmia; VII facial palsy; VIII SNHL and vestibular problems; IX and/or X swallow dysfunction	Canals	Hypoplastic semi-circular canals
Characteristic ear anomalies	External ear – "CHARGE ear"; middle ear (ossicular malformations and chronic serous otitis); mixed deafness; cochlear defects		
Minor Criteria:	**Includes:**	**Minor Criteria:**	**Includes:**
Genital hypoplasia	Micropenis; cryptorchidism; hypoplastic labia; delayed puberty	Rhombencephalic dysfunction	Brainstem dysfunctions cranial nerve VII to XII palsies; SNHL
Developmental delay	Delayed motor milestones; hypotonia	Hypothalamo-hypophyseal dysfunction	GH and gonadotrophin deficiencies
Cardiovascular malformations	Varied but commonly conotruncal defects, atrio-vestibular (AV) cushion defects, and arch anomalies	Abnormal middle or external ear	
Growth deficiency	Short stature	Malformation of mediastinal organs	Heart; esophagus
Orofacial cleft	Cleft lip and/or palate	Mental retardation	
Tracheoesophageal fistula	All types		
Characteristic face	Characteristic face		

[a] Includes additional renal, hand, abdominal, spinal, general, thymic anomalies not directly applicable for diagnosis but used as supportive findings.

of metanephric cells surrounding ureteric buds).[34] SIX1 encodes a homeobox protein involved in the inner ear, limb development, nephrogenesis and development of the ureteric collecting system. EYA1 also functions as a transcription co-activator for SIX1 which provides a plausible explanation for the more pronounced phenotype seen with EYA1 (and by extension BOR).[35]

Diagnosis: BOR spectrum disorder comprises branchiootorenal (BOR) and brachiootic syndrome (BOS), that differ by the presence or absence of a renal abnormality. Evaluating phenotype is essential as causative gene mutations are recognized in only 36% to 72% of clinically diagnosed individuals with BOR spectrum disorder.[36] Clinical diagnosis depends on major and minor criteria (Table 2).[37,38] Genetic testing includes a multigene panel (EYA1, SIX1, SIX5) when the phenotype is suggestive or comprehensive genomic testing when the phenotype is atypical.

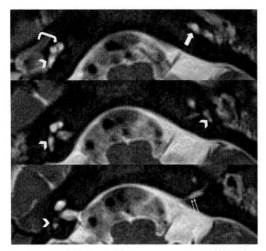

Fig. 1. Characteristic inner ear MRI findings in CHARGE syndrome. Axial, high resolution heavily T2-weighted DRIVE sequence (same patient) of the temporal bone shows: small vestibule (*arrowheads*) the semicircular canals (SCCs) are absent bilaterally. The internal auditory canal (IAC) on the left is very small (double *arrow*) and the VIII cranial nerve is not present bilaterally. There is asymmetric cochlear hypoplasia with only half of basal turn seen on the left (thick *arrow*) and a more developed cochlea on the right, with complete basal turn and hypoplastic upper portion of the cochlea (curved *arrow*).

Clinical characteristics

The estimated prevalence is 1 in 40,000 and accounts for about 2% of profoundly deaf children.[32,39]

Branchiootorenal (BOR) syndrome is characterized by malformations of the external, middle and inner ear with associated hearing disability, branchial apparatus anomalies (eg, tags, pits, sinuses, fistulae, cysts, and squamous remnants) and renal malformations. Brachiootic (BO) syndrome is similar but with the lower frequency of branchial apparatus anomalies and absent renal pathology.[40]

HL is present in >90% and can be SNHL (≈50%), conductive (≈33%) or mixed.[41] HL is progressive in ≈ 30% and if so, correlates with the presence of a dilated vestibular aqueduct (VA) on computed tomogrpahy (CT).[42]

Renal anomalies can progress to end-stage renal failure in later life.[43]

These clinical characteristics mandate annual/semiannual surveillance of audiologicalical and renal function.[44]

Temporal bone

The classically described cochlear malformation, of the "offset" or "unwound" cochlea, is seen most specifically in the EYA1 mutation and appears as an anteromedial offset of the hypoplastic middle/apical turns away from the tapered basal cochlear turn[45,46] (Fig. 3A). Associated anomalies include funnel-shaped VA enlargement, medially displaced labyrinthine segment of the facial nerve canal, widened internal auditory canal (IAC), patulous/dilated Eustachian tube, ossicular anomalies, misshapen middle ear space and mild EAC stenosis.[42,47]

A different cochlear phenotype, demonstrating irregular "thorny," apical turn, but otherwise normal cochlea, is seen specifically in the SIX1 mutation and demonstrates less or near total absence of associated temporal findings[46] (Fig. 3B). Although other recently described genetic causes of hearing loss may present with abnormalities involving the upper turns of the cochlea,[48] the combination of the "thorny" cochlea and associated BOR findings in other organ-systems is very suggestive of an underlying SIX1 mutation.

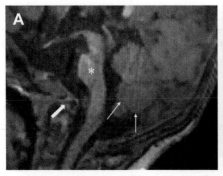
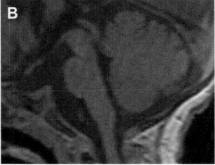

Fig. 2. Posterior fossa findings in CHARGE syndrome. Sagittal T1 weighted-sequence on the midline in CHARGE patient (*A*) and normal control (*B*). There is hypoplastic pons (*asterisk*) in the CHARGE patient, the vermis is uplifted with inferior vermian hypoplasia (*thin arrows*). Note the hypoplastic, cleft basi-occiput (*thick arrow*) and deep set pituitary fossa. There is a partially imaged C2-3 fusion anomaly.

Table 2
Diagnostic criteria for BOR syndrome.[38]

Diagnostic criteria: 3 major, 2 major plus 2 minor, or 1 major with an Affected First Degree Relative who meets criteria for BOR	
Major Criteria	**Minor Criteria**
Branchial anomalies	External ear anomalies
Deafness	Middle ear anomalies
Preauricular pits	Inner ear anomalies
Renal anomalies	Preauricular tags
	Other: facial asymmetry, palate anomalies

Other findings

2nd branchial apparatus anomalies[32,38,49]
Preauricular tags, pits, cervical sinus tracts, fistulae, cysts, or squamous remnants.

Renal anomalies

A spectrum of renal anomalies, from fatal (renal agenesis with death in utero) to moderate (hypoplasia), is seen in ≈ 2/3 of cases of BOR. Associated with ureteropelvic junction obstruction, calyceal cyst/diverticulum, caliectasis/pelviectasis/hydronephrosis/vesico-ureteric junction reflux.

Head/neck (rare)

Lacrimal duct aplasia, short/cleft palate, retrognathia, euthyroid goiter, facial nerve palsy.

Teaching points

- *"Unwound" (anterior off-set) cochlea is a typical phenotype of EYA1-BOR.*

- *SIX1-BOR has an almost normal cochlea with irregular superior margin described as "thorny" cochlea.*
- *In case of suspected BOR it is important to evaluate for renal problems, branchial apparatus anomalies, and associated malformations in the middle and external ear compartments.*

Pendred Syndrome

Genes
SLC26A4 (autosomal recessive, AR) on chromosome 7 is mutated in 50% of cases and encodes the protein pendrin.[50] Patients can harbor 2 pathogenic variants of *SLC26A4* : one pathogenic variant of *SLC26A4* with a CEVA haplotype (M1 plus CEVA) or infrequently (<1%), digenic inheritance with one pathogenic variant *SLC26A4* and one pathogenic variant in *FOXI1,* or rarely *EPHA2.*[51] These associated genes may interact with the *SLC26A4* gene or directly with pendrin, modifying its function.

Pathophysiology
SLC26A4 is expressed in the inner ear, thyroid, kidney, and airway epithelium.[52] Pendrin acts as a chloride/bicarbonate exchanger in the inner ear and is involved in endolymph homoeostasis, critical for the function of hair cells,[53] with the loss of the endocochlear potential as the cause of HL in these patients. In the thyroid, it mediates the efflux of iodide from thyroid follicular cells into the lumen.[54] Mutation results in the loss of function of these processes.

Diagnosis
The diagnosis is suggested by SNHL, characteristic temporal bone findings (see later discussion),

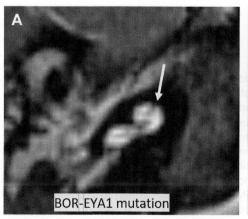 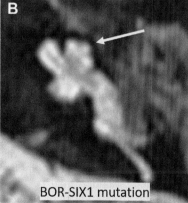

Fig. 3. Characteristic inner ear MR findings in BOR patients; axial, high resolution heavily T2-weighted DRIVE sequence focused on the cochlea. (*A*) "unwound" EYA1-BOR cochlea with anterior offset of the second half of the basal turn and upper part of the cochlea (*arrow*). (*B*) "thorny" cochlea in SIX1-BOR with irregular and prominent superior profile of the upper turn (*arrow*).

and biochemical evidence of thyroid endocrine abnormality. Goiter is an associated clinical finding especially in areas where iodine is deficient in the diet. This is supported but not defined by (as the detection rate is limited at ≈ 50%), the molecular diagnosis of biallelic pathogenic *SLC26A4* variants, or double heterozygosity for one variant in *SLC26A4* and *FOXI1*.[52]

Clinical characteristics

Pendred syndrome is considered the most common cause of syndromic congenital SNHL (7.5%–15%).[14]

Deafness, as an almost constant feature, may be present at birth or progress during childhood aggravated by head trauma, barotrauma or acoustic trauma.[55] Biallelic *SLC26A4* variants demonstrate an earlier age of HL onset, more severe HL and have a higher incidence of thyroid abnormality. Vertigo can precede or accompany hearing loss[56] with a range of vestibular dysfunction seen in ≈ 67% of patients.

Goiter is seen in ≈ 75% of patients,[57] develops in late childhood or early adult life, and are mostly euthyroid, unless they have an associated deficient dietary in iodine, resulting in small numbers of hypothyroid cases.[58] The goiter continues to increase in size with each decade.[58]

Despite confirmed *SLC26A4* expression in the kidney, clinical abnormalities are infrequently observed.

Of note, mutation in the FOXI1 gene is associated with the Pendred ear phenotype with distal tubular acidosis instead of thyroid dysfunction.[59] In these cases, association between acidosis, deafness, and typical inner ear appearances (see later) is very helpful in suggesting a FOXI1 gene mutation.[60]

Surveillance includes lifelong monitoring of hearing and thyroid function.

Temporal bone

Enlarged vestibular aqueduct (EVA) on thin section temporal bone CT is the most characteristic finding and can be associated with incomplete partition type 2 (deficient interscalar septum between the upper cochlear turns and flattened lateral profile of the cochlear upper turns resembling a "baseball cap"[61]), and sometimes vestibular enlargement is present (this combination was formerly called "Mondini triad").[14,60,62] No clear difference in imaging findings has been demonstrated between the different genotypes (**Fig. 4**).

When evaluating the size of VA, it is important to refer to normal VA measurements available in the literature; the measurements can be taken on the axial or in Poshl's plane.[63,64]

Other findings

Head/neck: euthyroid goiter (30%–70%) apparent after age 10.[65] The goiter continues to increase in size with each decade.[58]

Genito-urinary: In cases with FOXI1 gene mutation, there is renal tubular acidosis.[59]

Waardenburg syndrome - WS (Type 1–4 and PCWH)

Genes

There are multiple causative variants within the *PAX3*, *SOX10*, *EDNRB*, and *MITF* genes,[66] with some genotype-phenotype correlation reported. Inheritance is AD (types 1 and 3), AR (type 4) or mixed (type 2) among the different genes, specific phenotypes have been reported for *SOX10*.[67]

Pathophysiology

Pigment disorder secondary to the abnormal distribution of neural crest-derived elements during embryogenesis (neurocristopathy),[68] with loss of pigmentary cells in eyes, skin, cochlea, and hair. Specifically, the melanocyte depletion of the otic vesicle affects the stria vascularis of the cochlea,[69] resulting in atrophy of the spiral ganglion and absence of the organ of Corti and deafness.[70]

Diagnosis

Diagnosis of type 1 is primarily clinical with major and minor criteria (**Table 3**).

Once suspected, this diagnosis is supported by mutational subgrouping,[72] with 4 subtypes recognized depending on the presence of associated findings and the gene involved. In the case of type 1 identification of a pathogenic variant in PAX3 is diagnostic if clinical features are inconclusive. The addition or absence of specific phenotypic features will determine types 2, 3, and 4 (see later in discussion), which are more genetically heterogeneous. It may also be diagnosed as a part of a complex syndrome (PCWH – peripheral demyelinating neuropathy, central dysmyelinating leukodystrophy, Waardenburg syndrome, Hirschsprung disease related to SOX10 mutation and called type 2E).

Clinical characteristics

WS is characterized by variable presentations of SNHL and pigmentation anomalies after birth. SNHL is seen in > 90% and is mostly bilateral. Of note, SNHL often exists without radiological abnormality of the temporal bone in all other than the SOX10-related subtypes.

Characteristic clinical signs including facial abnormalities (square jaw, patent metopic suture), hypopigmentation of hair and skin, iris

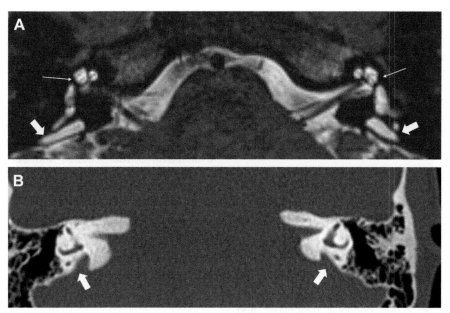

Fig. 4. Characteristics MRI and CT temporal findings in Pendred syndrome. (A) axial high resolution heavily T2-weigthed DRIVE sequence showing enlarged endolymphatic sac (*thick arrows*) and flattening of the external profile of the cochlea (*thin arrow*) in keeping with incomplete partition type 2. (B) Axial temporal bone CT shows the dilatation of the vestibular aqueduct (thick *arrows*). Note that the vestibular aqueduct on CT corresponds to endolymphatic sac on MRI.

heterochromia, and dystopia canthorum.[72] Anomalies of the limbs and digits sometimes occur.[67] The pigmentary disturbances and limb anomalies are characteristically absent in the SOX10 subtypes which usually present with SNHL and constipation due to Hirschsprung disease.[73]

Cerebellar ataxia may rarely present with associated brain findings (see later in discussion).

Temporal bone
Abnormalities are variable (17%–100% in case series). Malformed SCCs is the most common finding ± vestibular malformation ± enlargement of the vestibular duct (seen in ≈ 50%).[74] Cochlear malformations are variable but when present,

include moderate-severe hypoplasia or a hypoplastic modiolus.

The presence of a type SOX10 mutation is associated with a more characteristic appearance with agenesis/hypoplasia of one SCC (most commonly the posterior SCC), and variable malformation of the other SCCs occasionally with complete agenesis of all 3. Cochlear malformations are characterized by variable cochlear hypoplasia but all turns are present (the cochlea looks slightly smaller on caudocranial dimension and has been described as a "hammered" cochlea) and there maybe hypoplasia/absence of CN VII and VIII. Narrowing of the internal auditory meati (IAMs) may be present, middle ear abnormalities are uncommon.[74,75]

Table 3
Diagnostic criteria for Waardenburg syndrome[71]

Diagnostic criteria: Type 1: 2 major or 1 major plus 2 minor	
Major Criteria	Minor Criteria
Heterochromia	Broad nasal root
SNHL	White macules/patches
White forelock	Synophrys
Lateral displacement of the inner canthi of the eye	Premature greying of scalp hairs
1st degree relative with WS	Hypoplasia of nasal alae

Other findings

Brain : white matter signal abnormality, enlarged perivascular spaces (PVS), delay in myelin maturation, agenesis/hypoplasia of the olfactory bulbs, and rarely cerebellar malformation.[74]

Head/neck : parotid/lacrimal gland absence or hypoplasia.[74]

*Musculoskeletal (MSK):*limb/digit abnormalities – type 3 only.[67]

Gastro-intestinal tract (GI): Hirschsprung disease.

The combination of olfactory bulb hypoplasia, Hirschsprung disease, and typical inner anomalies is almost pathognomonic of SOX10 mutation[60,76] (Fig. 5).[73] In these patients, hypoplastic lacrimal and parotid glands are also often present.

Teaching point

- *Combination of Hirschprung disease, deafness with anomalies of the semicircular canals + subtle cochlear hypoplasia and absence/hypoplasia of the olfactory bulbs strongly suggests Waardenburg disease due to SOX10 mutation.*

Alfa Dystroglycanopathies

Genes

Mutations in at least 18 genes involved in the glycosylation of alpha-dystroglycan have been described without a precise genotype-phenotype correlation.[77]

Pathophysiology

All mutations result in a functional defect in the glycosylation of alpha-dystroglycan, a cellular membrane adhesive molecule expressed in the central nervous system (CNS), retina and cochlea, which is critical for neuronal migration, organization of synapses and development of the basement membrane.[78] This results in variable-sized gaps in the pial basement membrane and overmigration of neuronal cells resulting in cortical malformations.[79]

Diagnosis

They are considered a clinicoradiological spectrum with multiple phenotypes demonstrating overlapping clinical features and severity, supported by genetic analysis. Previous attempts to distinguish between different mutations based on brain imaging findings alone have been largely unsuccessful.[77] Among the most severe phenotypes Walker-Warburg syndrome (WWS), muscle-eye-brain disease (MEB), and Fukuyama congenital muscular disorder (FCMD)[80] all are characterized by cobblestone brain malformations.

Clinical characteristics

Often present with muscular dystrophy, ± brain malformations, and ± ocular abnormalities leading to variable epilepsy, motor/language deficits, and visual disturbances. HL is less frequently reported most likely because of the serious neurological symptoms. Variable severity is demonstrated from mild adult-onset limb girdle muscular dystrophy to early onset severe dystrophy with eye and brain involvement.[77]

Temporal bone

Severe forms (eg, WWS) are almost universally associated with cochlear hypoplasia with only the basal turn present and very small and anteriorly located upper part (an "extremely unwound" form of cochlear hypoplasia-Fig. 6A, B), with milder forms (eg, MEB/FCMB) demonstrating less frequent and

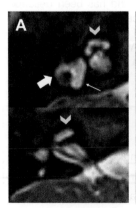
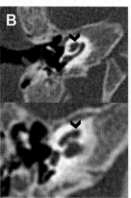
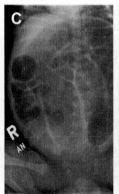
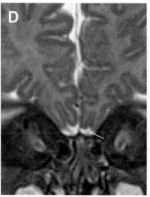

Fig. 5. Typical constellation of findings in SOX10-mutation. (*A*) axial high resolution heavily T2-weigthed DRIVE sequence and (*B*) axial temporal bone CT, showing slightly hypoplastic cochlea with all turns present but smaller than expected ("hammered cochlea," *arrowheads*), absent posterior semicircular canal (*thin arrow, A*) and dysplastic lateral semicircular canal (*thick arrow in A*). (*C*) X-ray of the stomach showing marked bowel dilatation (in keeping with Hirschsprung disease). (*D*) coronal T2 WI showing hypoplastic olfactory bulbs (*arrow*).

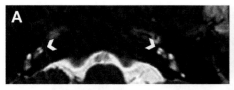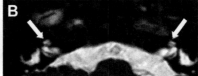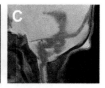

Fig. 6. Inner ear and posterior fossa MR findings in a patient with Walker-Warburg syndrome, axial high resolution heavily T2-weigthed DRIVE sequence (*A* and *B*), shows marked cochlear hypoplasia with normal first half of the basal turn (*arrowheads, A*) and extremely hypoplastic and anteriorly located upper portion of the cochlea (*arrows, B*). (*C*) Sagittal T2 weighted images at the level of the craniovertebral junction show typical Z-shaped brainstem.

less severe cochlear malformations.[80] Interestingly the SCCs are normal, suggesting that these genes are only involved in cochlear development.

Other findings
Brain[81,82] – malformations of cortical development including cobblestone lissencephaly/polymicrogyria-like cortex seen (seen with severe forms), pontocerebellar hypoplasia/dysplasia and Z-shaped brainstem in sagittal (**Fig. 6**C).

Teaching points

- *Cochlear malformations in patients with Alfa Dystroglicanopathies are overshadowed by the significant brain anomalies and neurological symptoms,*
- *The apparently isolated cochlear anomaly which is found mainly in patients with WWS may shed light on the role of the responsible genes in the linked development between the ear and the brain.*

Oculo-Auriculo-Vertebral Spectrum - OAVS (Goldenhar Syndrome)

Genes
Mostly sporadic[83] and associated with multifactorial etiology with some chromosomal abnormalities described.[84,85]

Pathophysiology
A multifactorial etiology with mainly environmental causes has been proposed. The most widely accepted theory is that the disorder results from a pathological embryonic vascular supply and/or drug abuse in gestation. The condition involves malformations of head and neck structures originating from the 1st/2nd branchial apparatus.[86] It may occasionally have alterations originating from other structures for example, neural tube, neural crest, or notochord.[87]

Diagnosis
Diagnosis is clinical: there are variable grades of severity and different phenotypic subtypes, the most severe form is called Goldenhar syndrome

and has variable involvement of the spine, ± eye abnormalities.[88] The "expanded Goldenhar complex" is used when unusual extrafacial abnormalities are seen such as involving the central nervous and respiratory systems.[89]

Clinical characteristics
The clinical phenotype is highly variable and consists of HL, developmental/motor delay plus a range of end-organ effects depending on the phenotype (see later in discussion).

Temporal bone
External ear involvement is constant, ranging from isolated tags/pits/appendages and EAC stenosis to complete anotia with EAC atresia.[90]

Middle ear
Underdevelopment of the tympanic cavity, ossicular anomalies, absence of tensor tympani muscle, anomalous course of facial nerve canal, and round/oval window stenosis/atresia.[91]

Inner ear
Hypoplastic cochlea, common cavity, vestibular enlargement, absence/fusion of SCC, EAV and duplicated, short, enlarged, narrowed or absent IAM, labyrinthine aplasia.[92,93]

Cranial nerves: often involved to a different degree with the fusion of the V and VII nerves and small or absent cochlear nerve (**Fig. 7**).[94]

Other findings
Ocular: epibulbar/limbal dermoid, lipodermoid, coloboma (also of lid), microphthalmia/anophthalmia, ptosis, strabismus, lacrimal duct stenosis classified into 4 categories.[83]

Brain[85]*:* vast range of structural abnormalities including diffuse cerebral hypoplasia, dilated ventricles, midline anomalies (corpus callosum agenesis/lipoma, absence of septum pellucidum, hypothalamic hamartoma), non-specific white matter abnormalities, microcephaly, aqueduct stenosis, Chiari 1/2, encephaloceles, IAMs abnormalities, tegmental cap dysplasia, cerebellar dysplasia. Various functional deficits such as

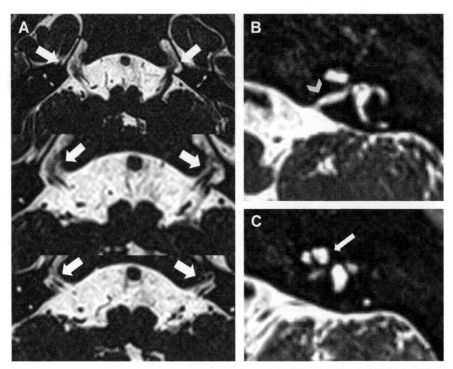

Fig. 7. MR findings in OAVS. Axial high resolution heavily T2-weigthed DRIVE sequence shows enlarged Meckel's cave fused with VII nerve canal (*arrows* in *A* – note that the fibers of the VII nerve on both sides seem to come from the trigeminal nerve). On the left, the IAC extremely hypoplastic (*arrowhead, B*), the cochlear nerve is absent, and the cochlea is dysplastic (*arrow, C*).

autism spectrum, developmental delay, speech/hearing/visual abnormalities.

Neuro-vascular[95]: internal carotid artery agenesis/hypoplasia.

Head/neck[95 96]: hemifacial microsomia (common), skull base/foraminal abnormalities (along with CN hypoplasia/aplasia or partial/complete fusion).

Genito-urinary system[97]: Renal agenesis, hydronephrosis, ectopic and fused kidneys, polycystic kidney, double and hydroureter.

Cardiovascular system[98]: TOF, ASD, VSD, persistent truncus arteriosus, TOGV, dextrocardia, conotruncal defects, situs inversus, vascular rings with respiratory compromise.

Gastro-intestinal system (GI)[87]: rectal atresia, and esophageal atresia.

MSK system: radial ray anomalies, vertebral defects (hemivertebra, hypoplasia, or butterfly vertebra), club foot.[96]

Teaching point

- *The spectrum of malformations (fusion, hypoplasia and absence) involving the VII, VIII, and V cranial nerves with abnormal Meckel's caves and IAMs, in association with ocular and vertebral abnormalities, suggest OAVS.*

X-linked Deafness with Progressive Gusher (POU3F4)

Gene
X-linked; *PO3F4* mutations (DFNX2) in ≈ 50%; occasionally *COL4A6* [60].

Pathophysiology
Congenital, progressive, profound, mixed hearing loss – the SNHL component is due to symmetrical cochlear malformation (incomplete partition, IP-3) and conductive component due to fixed stapes/third window phenomenon.[99] There is a speculative theory that IP-3 is caused by a defect in the vascular supply for the middle ear, impairing the formation of the 2 outer layers of the otic capsule.[100]

Diagnosis
Typical Imaging Features (Bilateral IP-3 Virtually Pathognomonic).

Clinical characteristics
Accounts for 2% of inner ear malformations. Typically presents with profound, mixed HL in males.[101]

Temporal bone
Bilateral, symmetrical cochlear malformation (IP-3, giving a "corkscrew" appearance) (Fig. 8A). The

IAM is enlarged and bulbous leading to the abnormal connection between subarachnoid space and perilymph with increased perilymphatic pressure. There can be vestibular and SCC abnormalities and aberrant course of facial nerve.[102]

Other findings

Brain:dysmorphic hypothalamus, ranging from lumpy-bumpy appearance to a frank hamartoma[102,103] (Fig. 8B). This is probably related to the role of the POU gene family in the development of the brain.

Interestingly, the association between cochlear malformations, hypothalamic hamartomas, and polydactyly has been described in Pallister-Hall syndrome, suggesting a link between the development of the ear and hypothalamus.[104]

SYNDROMIC CAUSES WITH PROMINENT INVOLVEMENT OF THE LATERAL SEMICIRCULAR CANALS
Down Syndrome

Gene

Sporadic in most cases; caused by trisomy 21 (nondisjunction or translocation in >95%, mosaicism and partial trisomy 21 less common).[105]

Pathophysiology

Disrupts multiple cellular pathways. The additional copy of trisomy 21 leads to elevated expression of many genes on the chromosome with variable gain of function.[106]

Diagnosis

Characteristic clinical features and karyotyping.

Clinical characteristics

Conductive hearing loss is commonly seen in 53% to 88% of patients due to chronic otitis media and Eustachian tube dysfunction. Mixed HL or SNHL is seen in 4% to 55%.[107]

Wide range of other features include intellectual disability/early onset AD, congenital heart disease (A-V cushion defects most common), hematological problems (risk of leukemia and immune dysfunction), GI, MSK, and ophthalmic complaints.[108]

Temporal bone

External ear: external canal stenosis.[109]

Middle and inner ear: lateral SCC malformation ranging from a small bone island to persistent SCC anlage, superior SCC dehiscence, ossicular anomalies, decreased cartilage density, and enlarged vestibular aqueduct (Fig. 9).[110] Narrow IAM, stenosis of the cochlear nerve canal (CNC) and cochlear nerve hypoplasia or aplasia have also been reported.

Other findings

Brain[111]: prominent extra axial spaces, vermian and pontine hypoplasia, simplified gyration of frontal lobes.

Cardiovascular[112]:atrial and/or vestibular septal defects.

GI[113]: Hirschsprung disease, duodenal stenosis, imperforate anus.

MSK[111]: atlantoaxial and joint instability.

Ocular[114]:cataracts, glaucoma.

Apert Syndrome (a.k.a Acrocephalosyndactyly Type 1)

Gene

At lea 10 mutations in the FGFR2 gene have been found to cause Apert syndrome, with >98% caused by 2 mutations (Ser252Trp and Pro253Arg).[115]

Pathophysiology

Mutations lead to the gain of function of the fibroblast growth factor receptor 2 protein with cells maturing too quickly and abnormal development.[116]

Diagnosis

Classical clinical characteristics (multisuture craniosynostosis, midface hypoplasia and retrusion, and syndactyly) and/or heterozygous pathogenic

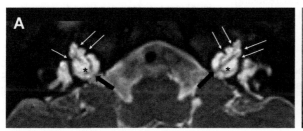
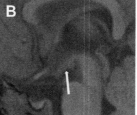

Fig. 8. MR findings in POU3F4 mutations. (*A*) Axial high resolution heavily T2-weigthed DRIVE sequence shows the typical IP-3 "corkscrew" cochlea, with deficient internal structure (asterixis) and preserved external cochlear profile (i.e. interscalar septi, thin *arrows*), enlarged cochlear nerve canal and IAC (*thick black arrows*). (*B*) sagittal T1 weighted images of the brain show thee dysmorphic hypothalamus noted on sagittal T1 weighted (*arrow*).

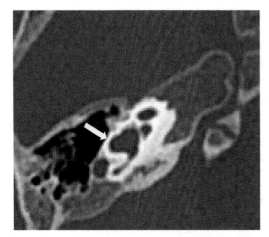

Fig. 9. Temporal bone CT of a patient with Down syndrome showing a dysplastic lateral SCC (*arrow*). The complete absence of the bony island with the fusion between the lateral SCC and thee vestibule is called "persistent anlage" of the canal. Similar findings are found in Apert syndrome.

variant in FGFR2 and phenotypic features consistent with Apert.[117]

Clinical characteristics
Demonstrates phenotypic overlap with other FGFR-2-associated craniosynostoses, the classical defining feature is the presence of syndactyly.

Craniosynostosis is almost universal with characteristic underdeveloped and retruded midface, shallow orbits, downslanting palpebral fissures, and dental abnormalities. There is variable high arched/cleft palate leading to feeding abnormalities.[118]

HL is seen ≈ 80% and is typically conductive secondary to middle ear disease, ossicular abnormalities, ECA stenosis/atresia.[119]

The characteristic Apert hand/foot includes the fusion of the middle 3 digits, ± thumb/5th digit with more severe involvement of the upper limb.[117]

There is a high prevalence of cervical spinal fusions (≈67%), most commonly at C5-C6, resulting in scoliosis with variable atlanto-axial subluxation and C1 spina bifida occulta.[117,118]

Temporal bone
Most frequently anomalies described are small lateral SCC bone islands or persistent SCC anlage.[120]

Other findings

Head/neck: Mid nasal cavity stenosis, midface retrusion, high arched/cleft palate, tracheal cartilaginous sleeves, concave ethmoid roof.[117]

Ocular: Exorbitism, downslanting palpebral fissures, strabismus, refractive error, anisometropia, exposure keratopathy, corneal scarring, optic atrophy.

MSK.- syndactyly hand/foot, synostosis of the radius/humerus, polydactyly of hand/foot, broad distal phalanx of the thumb/hallux.

Spine: cervical fusions, scoliosis, atlanto-axial subluxation, C1 spina bifida occulta.

Brain[118]: Jugular foraminal stenosis (>90%), non-progressive ventriculomegaly (≈67%) with 10% hydrocephalic, abnormalities of the corpus callosum, absent septum pellicidum, Chiari 1, posterior fossa arachnoid cyst, and limbic malformations. There is a range of normal to severe intellectual impairment.

Cardiovascular: Ventricular septal defect, overriding aorta.

GI: intestinal malrotation, distal esophageal stenosis, pyloric stenosis, ectopic anus.

Genitourinary system: Hydronephrosis, cryptorchidism.

22q11

Gene
22q11 microdeletion with deleted genes (*SMARCB1, HIRA, COMT, TBX1*).[121]

Pathophysiology
Most common congenital microdeletion in humans (1:6000–1:2000 live births). TBX1 inactivation disrupts inner ear development and is responsible for the otologic and cardiovascular findings.[121]

Diagnosis
Characteristic clinical and genetic findings.

Clinical characteristics
There is phenotypic variability resulting in syndromes known as DiGeorge, velocardiofacial (VCF), and Shprintzen syndrome with HL (mostly conductive ≈ 2/3, mixed or SNHL ≈ 1/3), with clinical features as determined by end-organ involvement (as described later in discussion) plus neurological/psychiatric disorders.

Temporal bone
External ear: aural atresia, stenosis or normal (some overlap in appearance with OAVS).[121,122]

Middle ear: dense stapedial superstructure (≈36%), abnormal ossicular orientation, fusion of the malleus with incus, monopod stapes.[123,124]

Inner ear: small lateral SCC bone island (≈1/3), or lateral SCC anlage anomaly, vestibular malformation. Variable cochlear malformations ± dilated vestibular aqueduct.

Other findings

Cardiovascular: congenital heart disease.

Head/neck:velopharyngeal insufficiency, cleft palate, thymic hypoplasia.

Immune system: immunodeficiency, hypoparathyroidism with hypocalcaemia.[4]

Teaching point

- *Lateral SCC malformation or persistent anlage is a non-specific abnormality noted in several syndromic (such as Down and Apert syndromes) or isolated causes of hearing impairment.*

SYNDROMIC CAUSES WITH A HIGH RATE OF COMPLETE LABYRINTHINE APLASIA

LAMM Syndrome (Labyrinthine Aplasia, Microtia, and Microdontia)

Genes

Autosomal recessive; *FGF3* gene (multiple loss of function mutations)

Pathophysiology

Variable and incomplete penetrant inner ear malformations involving dorsal otic patterning. The most severe form representing arrest before the formation of the otocyst (3rd week). FGF3 is also required for tooth stellate reticulum cells (dental core).

Diagnosis

Clinical findings.

Clinical characteristics

Profound SNHL from birth. Motor delay but cognitively intact.

Temporal

Labyrinthine aplasia – complete absence of inner ear structures (complete membranous aplasia) usually with otic capsule and petrous apex hypoplasia and microtia. Some variability in the inner ear phenotypes has been described,[125] but labyrinthine aplasia with microdontia and microtia is extremely suggestive of LAMM syndrome (Fig. 10).

Extratemporal

Microdontia with small widely spaced teeth.

HOXA 1 Mutation-Associated Syndromes (Bosley-Salih-Alorainy Syndrome & Athabascan Brainstem Dysgenesis Syndrome)

Gene

Homozygous *HOXA1* truncating mutations; (175–176 insG guainin base pair insertions, 84C > G nonsense) causing Bosley-Salih-Alorainy syndrome

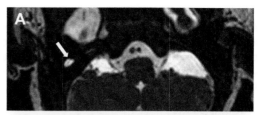

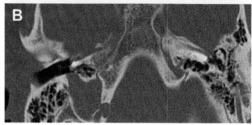

Fig. 10. Axial high resolution heavily T2-weigthed DRIVE sequence (*A*) and temporal bone CT (*B*) in 2 patients with LAMM syndrome. Image A shows complete left labyrinthine aplasia and a right rudimentary otocyst (*arrow*). Image B shows the complete absence of the labyrinth bilaterally with hypoplastic otic capsules.

(BSAS) or Athabascan Brainstem Dysgenesis Syndrome (ABDS).[126,127]

Pathophysiology

HOXA1 is critical for the development of hindbrain rhombomeres. Inner ear/deafness in HOXA1 likely sequela of abnormal inductive signals from hindbrain neuroectoderm. Suggestion that HOXA1 has an effect on aortic sac and paired dorsal aorta/arches similar to DiGeorge syndrome from loss of TBX1.[126,127]

Diagnosis

Suggested by clinical features plus genetic profiling.

Clinical characteristics

HOXA1 spectrum with SNHL and horizontal gaze restriction considered cardinal features in both BSAS and ABDS.

Cognitive abnormality/motor delay, central hypoventilation, and congenital heart disease in ABDS. Variable facial, bulbar, and respiratory abnormalities imply brainstem development abnormalities.

Cerebrovascular anomalies, autism and somatic disorder in BSAS.

Temporal bone

Variability in the spectrum of inner ear anomalies but the majority of the cases described show complete labyrinthine aplasia.[126,127]

al

575

..dings

...ies of the cerebrovascular system, ..ding internal carotid aplasia have been ...scribed. In the right clinical context, these vascular findings together with complete labyrinthine aplasia may suggest genetic diagnosis.

Teaching points

- In the presence of complete labyrinthine aplasia (Michel anomaly), think of LAMM syndrome or HOXA1 mutations and look for associated systemic findings.
- Variability in the ear anomalies with milder forms of inner ear malformation do not exclude the diagnosis.

SUMMARY

In recent years several characteristic temporal bone anomalies, and in particular inner ear radiological phenotypes, have been associated with specific syndromes or genetic anomalies. Knowledge of these patterns, and constellation of associated abnormalities in other organs/systems, is a powerful tool for the diagnostic radiologist. As a final remark, it is important to note that, while bilateral and symmetrical inner ear anomalies strongly suggest an underlying genetic cause, asymmetrical findings can be found in both genetic and environmental (early gestational) causes of hearing loss.

FUNDING

Research reported in this publication was supported by the National Institute of Health Biomedical Research Center at GreatOrmond Street Hospital, London UK (unfunded).

DISCLOSURE

The authors have nothing to disclose.

REFERENCES

1. Morton CC, Nance WE. Newborn hearing screening–a silent revolution. N Engl J Med 2006; 354(20):2151–64.
2. Korver AMH, Smith RJH, Van Camp G, et al. Congenital hearing loss. Nat Rev Dis Primers 2017;3:16094.
3. Wilson C, Roberts A, Stephens D. Aetiological investigation of sensorineural hearing loss in children. Arch Dis Child 2005;90(3):307–9.
4. D'Arco F, Youssef A, Ioannidou E, et al. Temporal bone and intracranial abnormalities in syndromic causes of hearing loss: an updated guide. Eur J Radiol 2020;123:108803.
5. Som PM, Curtin HD, Liu K, et al. Current embryology of the temporal bone, part I: the inner ear. Neurograph 2016;6(4):250–65.
6. Qin Z, Su J, Li M, et al. Clinical and genetic analysis of CHD7 expands the genotype and phenotype of CHARGE syndrome. Front Genet 2020;11:592.
7. Bergman JEH, Janssen N, Hoefsloot LH, et al. CHD7 mutations and CHARGE syndrome: the clinical implications of an expanding phenotype. J Med Genet 2011;48(5):334–42.
8. Reddy NC, Majidi SP, Kong L, et al. CHARGE syndrome protein CHD7 regulates epigenomic activation of enhancers in granule cell precursors and gyrification of the cerebellum. Nat Commun 2021;12(1):5702.
9. Bérubé-Simard F-A, Pilon N. Molecular dissection of CHARGE syndrome highlights the vulnerability of neural crest cells to problems with alternative splicing and other transcription-related processes. Transcription 2019;10(1):21–8.
10. Pauli S, Bajpai R, Borchers A. CHARGEd with neural crest defects. Am J Med Genet C Semin Med Genet 2017;175(4):478–86.
11. Blake KD, Prasad C. CHARGE syndrome. Orphanet J Rare Dis 2006;1:34.
12. Green GE, Huq FS, Emery SB, et al. CHD7 mutations and CHARGE syndrome in semicircular canal dysplasia. Otol Neurotol 2014;35(8):1466–70.
13. Sanlaville D, Verloes A. CHARGE syndrome: an update. Eur J Hum Genet 2007;15(4):389–99.
14. Huang BY, Zdanski C, Castillo M. Pediatric sensorineural hearing loss, part 2: syndromic and acquired causes. AJNR Am J Neuroradiol 2012; 33(3):399–406.
15. Aramaki M, Udaka T, Kosaki R, et al. Phenotypic spectrum of CHARGE syndrome with CHD7 mutations. J Pediatr 2006;148(3):410–4.
16. Aramaki M, Udaka T, Torii C, et al. Screening for CHARGE syndrome mutations in the CHD7 gene using denaturing high-performance liquid chromatography. Genet Test 2006;10(4):244–51.
17. Lewis MA, Juliano A, Robson C, et al. The spectrum of cochlear malformations in CHARGE syndrome and insights into the role of the CHD7 gene during embryogenesis of the inner ear. Neuroradiology 2023. https://doi.org/10.1007/s00234-023-03118-9.
18. Vesseur AC, Verbist BM, Westerlaan HE, et al. CT findings of the temporal bone in CHARGE syndrome: aspects of importance in cochlear implant surgery. Eur Arch Oto-Rhino-Laryngol 2016; 273(12):4225–40.
19. Ha J, Ong F, Wood B, et al. Radiologic and Audiologic Findings in the Temporal Bone of Patients with CHARGE Syndrome. Ochsner J 2016;16(2):125–9.
20. Hoch MJ, Patel SH, Jethanamest D, et al. Head and neck MRI findings in CHARGE syndrome. AJNR Am J Neuroradiol 2017;38(12):2357–63.

21. Morimoto AK, Wiggins RH, Hudgins PA, et al. Absent semicircular canals in CHARGE syndrome: radiologic spectrum of findings. AJNR Am J Neuroradiol 2006;27(8):1663–71.

22. George A, Cogliati T, Brooks BP. Genetics of syndromic ocular coloboma: CHARGE and COACH syndromes. Exp Eye Res 2020;193:107940.

23. Siddiqui A, Touska P, Josifova D, et al. Persistent trigeminal artery: A novel imaging finding in CHARGE syndrome. AJNR Am J Neuroradiol 2021;42(10):1898–903.

24. Corsten-Janssen N, Scambler PJ. Clinical and molecular effects of CHD7 in the heart. Am J Med Genet C Semin Med Genet 2017;175(4):487–95.

25. Ranza E, Le Gouez M, Guimier A, et al. Retrospective evaluation of clinical and molecular data of 148 cases of esophageal atresia. Am J Med Genet 2023;191(1):77–83.

26. Ragan DC, Casale AJ, Rink RC, et al. Genitourinary anomalies in the CHARGE association. J Urol 1999; 161(2):622–5.

27. Blake KD, Davenport SL, Hall BD, et al. CHARGE association: an update and review for the primary pediatrician. Clin Pediatr (Phila) 1998;37(3):159–73.

28. Verloes A. Updated diagnostic criteria for CHARGE syndrome: a proposal. Am J Med Genet 2005; 133A(3):306–8.

29. Song MH, Kwon T-J, Kim HR, et al. Mutational analysis of EYA1, SIX1 and SIX5 genes and strategies for management of hearing loss in patients with BOR/BO syndrome. PLoS One 2013;8(6):e67236.

30. Krug P, Morinière V, Marlin S, et al. Mutation screening of the EYA1, SIX1, and SIX5 genes in a large cohort of patients harboring branchio-oto-renal syndrome calls into question the pathogenic role of SIX5 mutations. Hum Mutat 2011;32(2): 183–90.

31. Kochhar A, Orten DJ, Sorensen JL, et al. SIX1 mutation screening in 247 branchio-oto-renal syndrome families: a recurrent missense mutation associated with BOR. Hum Mutat 2008;29(4):565.

32. Morisada N, Nozu K, Iijima K. Branchio-oto-renal syndrome: comprehensive review based on nationwide surveillance in Japan. Pediatr Int 2014;56(3): 309–14.

33. Shah AM, Krohn P, Baxi AB, et al. Six1 proteins with human branchio-oto-renal mutations differentially affect cranial gene expression and otic development. Dis Model Mech 2020;13(3). https://doi.org/10.1242/dmm.043489.

34. Kalatzis V, Sahly I, El-Amraoui A, et al. Eya1 expression in the developing ear and kidney: towards the understanding of the pathogenesis of Branchio-Oto-Renal (BOR) syndrome. Dev Dyn 1998;213(4):486–99.

35. Ruf RG, Xu P-X, Silvius D, et al. SIX1 mutations cause branchio-oto-renal syndrome by disruption of EYA1-SIX1-DNA complexes. Proc Natl Acad Sci USA 2004;101(21):8090–5.

36. Feng HF, Xu GE, Chen B, et al. [Branchio-oto-renal syndrome or branchio-oto syndrome: the clinical and genetic analysis in five Chinese families]. Zhonghua er bi yan hou tou jing wai ke za zhi 2022;57(12):1433–41.

37. Lindau TA, Cardoso ACV, Rossi NF, et al. Anatomical Changes and Audiological Profile in Branchio-oto-renal Syndrome: A Literature Review. Int Arch Otorhinolaryngol 2014;18(1):68–76.

38. Chang EH, Menezes M, Meyer NC, et al. Branchio-oto-renal syndrome: the mutation spectrum in EYA1 and its phenotypic consequences. Hum Mutat 2004;23(6):582–9.

39. Fraser FC, Sproule JR, Halal F. Frequency of the branchio-oto-renal (BOR) syndrome in children with profound hearing loss. Am J Med Genet 1980;7(3):341–9.

40. Biggs K, Crundwell G, Metcalfe C, et al. Anatomical and audiological considerations in branchiootorenal syndrome: A systematic review. Laryngoscope Investig Otolaryngol 2022;7(2):540–63.

41. Kemperman MH, Stinckens C, Kumar S, et al. Progressive fluctuant hearing loss, enlarged vestibular aqueduct, and cochlear hypoplasia in branchio-oto-renal syndrome. Otol Neurotol 2001;22(5): 637–43.

42. Kemperman MH, Koch SMP, Joosten FBM, et al. Inner ear anomalies are frequent but nonobligatory features of the branchio-oto-renal syndrome. Arch Otolaryngol Head Neck Surg 2002;128(9):1033–8.

43. David JJ, Shanbag P. Branchio-oto-renal syndrome presenting with syndrome of hyporeninemic hypoaldosteronism. Saudi J Kidney Dis Transpl 2017; 28(5):1165–8.

44. Smith RJ. Branchiootorenal Spectrum Disorder. In: Adam MP, Ardinger HH, Pagon RA, et al, editors. GeneReviews®. Seattle: University of Washington; 1993.

45. Hsu A, Desai N, Paldino MJ. The Unwound Cochlea: A Specific Imaging Marker of Branchio-Oto-Renal Syndrome. AJNR Am J Neuroradiol 2018;39(12):2345–9.

46. Pao J, D'Arco F, Clement E, et al. Re-Examining the Cochlea in Branchio-Oto-Renal Syndrome: Genotype-Phenotype Correlation. AJNR Am J Neuroradiol 2022;43(2):309–14.

47. Ceruti S, Stinckens C, Cremers CWRJ, et al. Temporal bone anomalies in the branchio-oto-renal syndrome: detailed computed tomographic and magnetic resonance imaging findings. Otol Neurotol 2002;23(2):200–7.

48. D'Arco F, Biswas A, Clement E, et al. Subtle malformation of the cochlear apex and genetic abnormalities: beyond the "thorny" cochlea. AJNR Am J Neuroradiol 2023;44(1):79–81.

49. Unzaki A, Morisada N, Nozu K, et al. Clinically diverse phenotypes and genotypes of patients with branchio-oto-renal syndrome. J Hum Genet 2018;63(5):647–56.

50. Danilchenko VY, Zytsar MV, Maslova EA, et al. Selection of diagnostically significant regions of the SLC26A4 gene involved in hearing loss. Int J Mol Sci 2022;23(21). https://doi.org/10.3390/ijms232113453.

51. Li M, Nishio S-Y, Naruse C, et al. Digenic inheritance of mutations in EPHA2 and SLC26A4 in Pendred syndrome. Nat Commun 2020;11(1):1343.

52. Ito T, Choi BY, King KA, et al. SLC26A4 genotypes and phenotypes associated with enlargement of the vestibular aqueduct. Cell Physiol Biochem 2011;28(3):545–52.

53. Bassot C, Minervini G, Leonardi E, et al. Mapping pathogenic mutations suggests an innovative structural model for the pendrin (SLC26A4) transmembrane domain. Biochimie 2017;132:109–20.

54. Tamma G, Dossena S. Functional interplay between CFTR and pendrin: physiological and pathophysiological relevance. Front Biosci (Landmark Ed). 2022;27(2):75.

55. Wémeau J-L, Kopp P. Pendred syndrome. Best Pract Res Clin Endocrinol Metab 2017;31(2):213–24.

56. Sugiura M, Sato E, Nakashima T, et al. Long-term follow-up in patients with Pendred syndrome: vestibular, auditory and other phenotypes. Eur Arch Oto-Rhino-Laryngol 2005;262(9):737–43.

57. Reardon W, Coffey R, Phelps PD, et al. Pendred syndrome–100 years of underascertainment? QJM 1997;90(7):443–7.

58. Madeo AC, Manichaikul A, Pryor SP, et al. Do mutations of the Pendred syndrome gene, SLC26A4, confer resistance to asthma and hypertension? J Med Genet 2009;46(6):405–6.

59. Enerbäck S, Nilsson D, Edwards N, et al. Acidosis and Deafness in Patients with Recessive Mutations in FOXI1. J Am Soc Nephrol 2018;29(3):1041–8.

60. D'Arco F, Sanverdi E, O'Brien WT, et al. The link between inner ear malformations and the rest of the body: what we know so far about genetic, imaging and histology. Neuroradiology 2020;62(5):539–44.

61. Robson CD. Congenital hearing impairment. Pediatr Radiol 2006;36(4):309–24.

62. Ganaha A, Kaname T, Yanagi K, et al. Pathogenic substitution of IVS15 + 5G > A in SLC26A4 in patients of Okinawa Islands with enlarged vestibular aqueduct syndrome or Pendred syndrome. BMC Med Genet 2013;14:56.

63. Juliano AF, Ting EY, Mingkwansook V, et al. Vestibular aqueduct measurements in the 45° oblique (pöschl) plane. AJNR Am J Neuroradiol 2016;37(7):1331–7.

64. D'Arco F, Talenti G, Lakshmanan R, et al. Do measurements of inner ear structures help in the diagnosis of inner ear malformations? A review of literature. Otol Neurotol 2017;38(10):e384–92.

65. Tesolin P, Fiorino S, Lenarduzzi S, et al. Pendred syndrome, or not pendred syndrome? that is the question. Genes 2021;12(10). https://doi.org/10.3390/genes12101569.

66. Lee C-Y, Lo M-Y, Chen Y-M, et al. Identification of nine novel variants across PAX3, SOX10, EDNRB, and MITF genes in Waardenburg syndrome with next-generation sequencing. Mol Genet Genomic Med 2022;10(12):e2082.

67. Pingault V, Ente D, Dastot-Le Moal F, et al. Review and update of mutations causing Waardenburg syndrome. Hum Mutat 2010;31(4):391–406.

68. Inoue K, Khajavi M, Ohyama T, et al. Molecular mechanism for distinct neurological phenotypes conveyed by allelic truncating mutations. Nat Genet 2004;36(4):361–9.

69. Steel KP, Barkway C. Another role for melanocytes: their importance for normal stria vascularis development in the mammalian inner ear. Development 1989;107(3):453–63.

70. Bommakanti K, Iyer JS, Stankovic KM. Cochlear histopathology in human genetic hearing loss: State of the science and future prospects. Hear Res 2019;382:107785.

71. Gowda VK, Srinivas S, Srinivasan VM. Waardenburg syndrome type I. Indian J Pediatr 2020;87(3):244.

72. Sil A, Panigrahi A. Visual dermatology: waardenburg syndrome type II. J Cutan Med Surg 2020;24(3):305.

73. Sham MH, Lui VC, Fu M, et al. SOX10 is abnormally expressed in aganglionic bowel of Hirschsprung's disease infants. Gut 2001;49(2):220–6.

74. Elmaleh-Bergès M, Baumann C, Noël-Pétroff N, et al. Spectrum of temporal bone abnormalities in patients with Waardenburg syndrome and SOX10 mutations. AJNR Am J Neuroradiol 2013;34(6):1257–63.

75. Bogdanova-Mihaylova P, Alexander MD, Murphy RPJ, et al. Waardenburg syndrome: a rare cause of inherited neuropathy due to SOX10 mutation. J Peripher Nerv Syst 2017;22(3):219–23.

76. Pingault V, Bodereau V, Baral V, et al. Loss-of-function mutations in SOX10 cause Kallmann syndrome with deafness. Am J Hum Genet 2013;92(5):707–24.

77. Martin PT. The dystroglycanopathies: the new disorders of O-linked glycosylation. Semin Pediatr Neurol 2005;12(3):152–8.

78. Gao QQ, McNally EM. The dystrophin complex: structure, function, and implications for therapy. Compr Physiol 2015;5(3):1223–39.

79. Nickolls AR, Bönnemann CG. The roles of dystroglycan in the nervous system: insights from animal

models of muscular dystrophy. Dis Model Mech 2018;11(12). https://doi.org/10.1242/dmm.035931.

80. Talenti G, Robson C, Severino MS, et al. Characteristic Cochlear Hypoplasia in Patients with Walker-Warburg Syndrome: A Radiologic Study of the Inner Ear in α-Dystroglycan-Related Muscular Disorders. AJNR Am J Neuroradiol 2021;42(1):167–72.

81. Alharbi S, Alhashem A, Alkuraya F, et al. Neuroimaging manifestations and genetic heterogeneity of Walker-Warburg syndrome in Saudi patients. Brain Dev 2021;43(3):380–8.

82. Shenoy AM, Markowitz JA, Bonnemann CG, et al. Muscle-Eye-Brain disease. J Clin Neuromuscul Dis 2010;11(3):124–6.

83. Barisic I, Odak L, Loane M, et al. Prevalence, prenatal diagnosis and clinical features of oculo-auriculo-vertebral spectrum: a registry-based study in Europe. Eur J Hum Genet 2014;22(8):1026–33.

84. Davide B, Renzo M, Sara G, et al. Oculo-auriculo-vertebral spectrum: going beyond the first and second pharyngeal arch involvement. Neuroradiology 2017;59(3):305–16.

85. Tasse C, Böhringer S, Fischer S, et al. Oculo-auriculo-vertebral spectrum (OAVS): clinical evaluation and severity scoring of 53 patients and proposal for a new classification. Eur J Med Genet 2005; 48(4):397–411.

86. Johnson JM, Moonis G, Green GE, et al. Syndromes of the first and second branchial arches, part 1: embryology and characteristic defects. AJNR Am J Neuroradiol 2011;32(1):14–9.

87. Cohen N, Cohen E, Gaiero A, et al. Maxillofacial features and systemic malformations in expanded spectrum Hemifacial Microsomia. Am J Med Genet 2017;173(5):1208–18.

88. Bogusiak K, Puch A, Arkuszewski P. Goldenhar syndrome: current perspectives. World J Pediatr 2017;13(5):405–15.

89. Zelante L, Gasparini P, Castriota Scanderbeg A, et al. Goldenhar complex: a further case with uncommon associated anomalies. Am J Med Genet 1997;69(4):418–21.

90. Ashokan CS, Sreenivasan A, Saraswathy GK. Goldenhar syndrome - review with case series. J Clin Diagn Res 2014;8(4):ZD17–9.

91. Rosa RFM, Silva AP da, Goetze TB, et al. Ear abnormalities in patients with oculo-auriculo-vertebral spectrum (Goldenhar syndrome). Braz J Otorhinolaryngol 2011;77(4):455–60.

92. Hennersdorf F, Friese N, Löwenheim H, et al. Temporal bone changes in patients with Goldenhar syndrome with special emphasis on inner ear abnormalities. Otol Neurotol 2014;35(5):826–30.

93. Bisdas S, Lenarz M, Lenarz T, et al. Inner ear abnormalities in patients with Goldenhar syndrome. Otol Neurotol 2005;26(3):398–404.

94. Manara R, Brotto D, Ghiselli S, et al. Cranial Nerve Abnormalities in Oculo-Auriculo-Vertebral Spectrum. AJNR Am J Neuroradiol 2015;36(7):1375–80.

95. Renkema RW, Spivack OKC, ERN CRANIO Working Group on Craniofacial Microsomia. European guideline on craniofacial microsomia: A version for patients and families. J Craniofac Surg 2022; 33(1):11–4.

96. Renkema RW, Caron CJJM, Pauws E, et al. Extracraniofacial anomalies in craniofacial microsomia: retrospective analysis of 991 patients. Int J Oral Maxillofac Surg 2019;48(9):1169–76.

97. Ritchey ML, Norbeck J, Huang C, et al. Urologic manifestations of Goldenhar syndrome. Urology 1994;43(1):88–91.

98. Nakajima H, Goto G, Tanaka N, et al. Goldenhar syndrome associated with various cardiovascular malformations. Jpn Circ J 1998;62(8):617–20.

99. Smeds H, Wales J, Karltorp E, et al. X-linked Malformation Deafness: Neurodevelopmental Symptoms Are Common in Children With IP3 Malformation and Mutation in POU3F4. Ear Hear 2022;43(1):53–69.

100. Sennaroglu L. Histopathology of inner ear malformations: Do we have enough evidence to explain pathophysiology? Cochlear Implants Int 2016; 17(1):3–20.

101. Mei X, Zhou Y, Amjad M, et al. Next-Generation Sequencing Identifies Pathogenic Variants in HGF, POU3F4, TECTA, and MYO7A in Consanguineous Pakistani Deaf Families. Neural Plast 2021; 2021:5528434.

102. Siddiqui A, D'Amico A, Colafati GS, et al. Hypothalamic malformations in patients with X-linked deafness and incomplete partition type 3. Neuroradiology 2019;61(8):949–52.

103. Prat Matifoll JA, Wilson M, Goetti R, et al. A Case Series of X-Linked Deafness-2 with Sensorineural Hearing Loss, Stapes Fixation, and Perilymphatic Gusher: MR Imaging and Clinical Features of Hypothalamic Malformations. AJNR Am J Neuroradiol 2020;41(6):1087–93.

104. Avula S, Alam N, Roberts E. Cochlear abnormality in a case of Pallister-Hall syndrome. Pediatr Radiol 2012;42(12):1502–5.

105. Hernandez D, Fisher EM. Down syndrome genetics: unravelling a multifactorial disorder. Hum Mol Genet 1996;5:1411–6.

106. Krivega M, Storchova Z. Consequences of trisomy syndromes - 21 and beyond. Trends Genet 2023; 39(3):172–4.

107. Kreicher KL, Weir FW, Nguyen SA, et al. Characteristics and Progression of Hearing Loss in Children with Down Syndrome. J Pediatr 2018;193:27–33.e2.

108. Tsou P-Y, Cielo CM, Xanthopoulos MS, et al. The impact of obstructive sleep apnea on bronchiolitis severity in children with Down syndrome. Sleep Med 2021;83:188–95.

109. Intrapiromkul J, Aygun N, Tunkel DE, et al. Inner ear anomalies seen on CT images in people with Down syndrome. Pediatr Radiol 2012;42(12):1449–55.

110. Blaser S, Propst EJ, Martin D, et al. Inner ear dysplasia is common in children with Down syndrome (trisomy 21). Laryngoscope 2006;116(12): 2113–9.

111. Rodrigues M, Nunes J, Figueiredo S, et al. Neuroimaging assessment in Down syndrome: a pictorial review. Insights Imaging 2019;10(1):52.

112. Dimopoulos K, Constantine A, Clift P, et al. Cardiovascular complications of down syndrome: scoping review and expert consensus. Circulation 2023;147(5):425–41.

113. Holmes G. Gastrointestinal disorders in Down syndrome. Gastroenterol Hepatol Bed Bench 2014; 7(1):6–8.

114. Haseeb A, Huynh E, ElSheikh RH, et al. Down syndrome: a review of ocular manifestations. Ther Adv Ophthalmol 2022;14. 25158414221101720.

115. Azoury SC, Reddy S, Shukla V, et al. Fibroblast growth factor receptor 2 (FGFR2) mutation related syndromic craniosynostosis. Int J Biol Sci 2017; 13(12):1479–88.

116. Ibrahimi OA, Chiu ES, McCarthy JG, et al. Understanding the molecular basis of Apert syndrome. Plast Reconstr Surg 2005;115(1):264–70.

117. Khan QA, Farkouh C, Uzair M, et al. Clinical manifestations of Apert syndrome. Clin Case Rep 2023; 11(2):e6941.

118. Wenger TL, Hing AV, Evans KN. Apert Syndrome. In: Adam MP, Ardinger HH, Pagon RA, et al, editors. GeneReviews®. Seattle: University of Washington; 1993.

119. Agochukwu NB, Solomon BD, Muenke M. Hearing loss in syndromic craniosynostoses: otologic manifestations and clinical findings. Int J Pediatr Otorhinolaryngol 2014;78(12):2037–47.

120. Zhou G, Schwartz LT, Gopen Q. Inner ear anomalies and conductive hearing loss in children with Apert syndrome: an overlooked otologic aspect. Otol Neurotol 2009;30(2):184–9.

121. Fomin ABF, Pastorino AC, Kim CA, et al. DiGeorge Syndrome: a not so rare disease. Clinics 2010; 65(9):865–9.

122. Verheij E, Elden L, Crowley TB, et al. Anatomic malformations of the middle and inner ear in 22q11.2 deletion syndrome: case series and literature review. AJNR Am J Neuroradiol 2018;39(5):928–34.

123. Bohm LA, Zhou TC, Mingo TJ, et al. Neuroradiographic findings in 22q11.2 deletion syndrome. Am J Med Genet 2017;173(8):2158–65.

124. Loos E, Verhaert N, Willaert A, et al. Malformations of the middle and inner ear on CT imaging in 22q11 deletion syndrome. Am J Med Genet 2016;170(11): 2975–83.

125. Al Yassin A, D'Arco F, Morín M, et al. Three new mutations and mild, asymmetrical phenotype in the highly distinctive LAMM syndrome: A report of eight further cases. Genes 2019;10(7). https://doi.org/10.3390/genes10070529.

126. Bosley TM, Alorainy IA, Salih MA, et al. The clinical spectrum of homozygous HOXA1 mutations. Am J Med Genet 2008;146A(10):1235–40.

127. Higley MJ, Walkiewicz TW, Miller JH, et al. Bilateral complete labyrinthine aplasia with bilateral internal carotid artery aplasia, developmental delay, and gaze abnormalities: a presumptive case of a rare HOXA1 mutation syndrome. AJNR Am J Neuroradiol 2011;32(2):E23–5.

Imaging of Pediatric Cervical Lymphadenopathy

Jennifer A. Vaughn, MD[a,b,c,d],*

KEYWORDS

- Pediatric • Cervical lymph nodes • Lymphadenopathy • Neck infection • Neck malignancy
- Reactive nodes • Imaging

INTRODUCTION

Pediatric cervical adenopathy is common occurring in up to 90% of children between the ages of 4 and 8 year old.[1] The most common cause is reactivity to a variety of viral agents, and the second most common cause is due to bacterial infection. The overall rate of malignancy in pediatric cervical adenopathy is low, less than 5%.[2] With the expanding capabilities of various imaging modalities and the discovery of new disease entities, deciding when to image and what modality to select remains a challenge for clinicians in the workup of children with suspected cervical adenopathy. This review aims to compare the strengths and limitations of the various imaging modalities available, provide guidance on when to image patients, and highlight the imaging appearance of a variety of pathologies affecting the cervical nodes in children.

PROTOCOLS
Modality Strengths and Limitations

Ultrasound, contrast-enhanced computed tomography (CT), and contrast-enhanced MR imaging are all given high ratings according to the American College of Radiology (ACR) appropriateness criteria for evaluating children with single or multiple neck masses with or without fever.[3] PET-CT, or PET-MR imaging where available, are reserved for children with known malignancy including for both the initial staging and following treatment response. Each modality has strengths and limitations, and often modalities are complimentary in

the workup of cervical adenopathy. More recently in adult populations, deep learning techniques have been applied to distinguish among nodes.[4] This technology may be applicable to the evaluation of pediatric cervical adenopathy as well in the future.

Ultrasound is an excellent screening modality given it is available, uses no radiation and is done without sedation. It is extremely useful in helping to determine whether a palpable abnormality is a normal node or not. Ultrasound (US) can delineate whether the mass or node in question is solid or cystic, can assess the vascularity, and allows one to do real-time biopsy in the cooperative patient. US is somewhat limited, however, in its ability to evaluate the overall anatomic extent of the process, evaluate the deep neck spaces, and to image nodes adjacent to the airway or osseous structures. A typical US for assessment of cervical nodes will be performed using a high-frequency linear transducer to include targeted gray scale and color Doppler imaging of any palpable or concerning masses with additional bilateral nodal mapping of all cervical stations possible depending on the clinical indication.

CT with contrast is excellent for evaluating the acutely ill child suspected of having infectious adenitis which may have progressed to an abscess and require surgical management. CT can evaluate the overall extent of the adenopathy including the deep neck spaces and whether nodes are calcified, which can help refine the differential. We do of course want to be cautious about radiation exposure in children, though scans

No financial disclosures.
[a] Department of Radiology, Phoenix Children's Hospital, Phoenix, AZ, USA; [b] Radiology, University of Arizona College of Medicine, Phoenix, AZ, USA; [c] Radiology, Creighton University School of Medicine, Phoenix, AZ, USA; [d] Barrows Neurological Institute, Phoenix, AZ, USA
* Corresponding author. Department of Radiology, 1919 East Thomas Road, Phoenix, AZ 85016.
E-mail address: jvaughn2@phoenixchildrens.com

at most large pediatric hospitals are being performed at well managed radiation doses typically without the need for sedation as the scanner technology and protocols now enable very fast scanning.[5] A typical CT protocol with intravenous contrast would include coverage from the infraorbital rim to the aortic arch following the administration of a nonionic agent either using a monophasic or biphasic injection technique. Reconstructions ideally consist of soft tissue images in axial, sagittal, and coronal planes and thin axial bone algorithm images. Many institutions will place markers on the skin at the site of palpable concern to aid the radiologist and clinician in correlating particular regions.

MR imaging with and without contrast including the use of diffusion-weighted imaging (DWI) can help identify small subcentimeter nodes due to the high signal relative to the background on the DWI sequence. Like the DWI appearance of other malignancies, metastatic cervical lymph nodes also tend to have relatively lower apparent diffusion coefficient values when compared with benign lymph nodes and can be useful in developing a differential.[6] MR imaging confers the same advantages in evaluation of overall anatomic extent and deep neck spaces as CT and it is also useful for follow-up when repeated examinations may be required due to the absence of radiation. One major limitation of MR imaging is that the examinations are often rather lengthy so may not be appropriate for acute ill children with suspected airway compromise, and in young children, sedation is typically necessary. Typical soft tissue neck MR imaging with and without contrast will consist of multiplanar T2-weighted imaging with at least one series obtained with fat saturation (eg, short tau inversion recovery [STIR], MDIXON), axial DWI, axial pre-contrast T1 without fat saturation, and post-contrast multiplanar T1-weighted imaging with fat saturation.

IMAGING FINDINGS/PATHOLOGY

When evaluating a patient presenting with cervical adenopathy, there are some key clinical and imaging features useful to formulating a differential diagnosis. The age of the patient and an attempt to ascertain the acuity of onset, the quality of the nodes on physical examination, whether the adenopathy is localized to the cervical nodes or more generalized and whether there are systemic symptoms, can all help not only to decide if imaging is warranted, but also which disease entities are most likely. Nodes which are subacute or chronic in onset, fixed and immobile, enlarging and in a patient experiencing weight loss, fatigue, persistent

fever, and night sweats are more likely to be malignant in nature.[7 1] All these pieces of clinical information may not be available to the radiologist at the time of interpretation; therefore, a practical approach to imaging interpretation also relies on certain imaging features including nodal size, shape, station, laterality, and whether the nodes are cystic, calcified, or hyper-enhancing. Additional clues in the non-nodal organs imaged on cross-sectional imaging should be sought and can help narrow the differential when the nodes themselves are nonspecific in appearance.

LARGE NODES

Large nodes are typically the greatest concern to clinicians with the ultimate question being whether the nodes reflect malignancy or not. Size is not a reliable predictor of malignancy in children and attempting to apply a size cutoff from adult literature will result in a high false positive rate. In addition, small nodes may be malignant and large nodes can result from a number of infectious and inflammatory processes.[8] For this reason, in cases of large nodes, evaluating the nodal shape, internal character, and station can be useful.

Reactive Adenopathy

Pediatric reactive adenopathy can have several morphologic patterns, of which follicular hyperplasia is the most common. A great number of non-neoplastic reactive etiologies can generate these different patterns, but in general, they are secondary to infectious entities or autoimmune/autoinflammatory disorders including things that may present in the pediatric population such as toxoplasmosis, human immunodeficiency virus (HIV)-associated lymphadenopathy, infectious mononucleosis, Kimura disease, Sjogren syndrome, and Kawasaki disease among many others.[9] These nodes can be very large; however, in many of these disease entities, they will maintain normal ovoid morphology and appear identical in their density, echogenicity, and signal to the normal appearing nodes on the various imaging modalities. Reactive nodes typically involve the upper more often than the lower nodal stations, draining sites of common pediatric infections. Bilateral diffuse cervical involvement can occur with reactive adenopathy as well and has been reported in the setting of immune-mediated reaction to anti-seizure drugs such as lamotrigine[10] among other causes. Reactive nodes can be confusing in that a single node may also enlarge out of proportion to the others (Fig. 1). For practical purposes, for these otherwise well patients with suspected reactive cervical adenopathy, one can follow the nodes

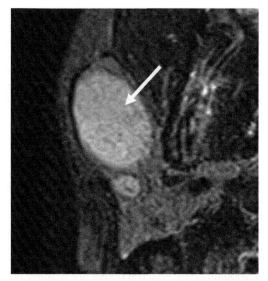

Fig. 1. Axial T2 fat-saturated MR image demonstrating an enlarged ovoid right intraparotid node (*arrow*). The node is isointense in signal to an adjacent small intraparotid node. Progressive enlargement of the node over a 6-week period led to biopsy which demonstrated follicular hyperplasia in a benign reactive node.

for 4 to 6 weeks to evaluate for resolution and consider biopsy if the node or nodes persist or progressively grow.

Malignancy

Patients with either primary or metastatic malignancy may present with chronic cervical adenopathy. In children under the age of 6 years, the most common malignancies are neuroblastoma, leukemia, rhabdomyosarcoma, and non-Hodgkin lymphoma. After age 6, Hodgkin lymphoma becomes most common.[11] Imaging plays an important role in the diagnosis, staging, and follow-up in cervical malignancy.

Hodgkin Lymphoma

Pediatric Hodgkin lymphoma is most commonly a disease of adolescents and rarely seen in young children. Imaging is crucial to correct staging, which facilitates appropriate management, with higher stages requiring more aggressive treatment regimens. The staging system for Hodgkin lymphoma is the Ann Arbor system with Cotswold modifications, and the imaging criteria most widely used in the United States are those used by the Children's Oncology Group (COG).[12] In the neck, it is important to evaluate for cervical airway compromise which has crucial clinical ramifications if present. Contrast-enhanced CT or MR imaging can be used to evaluate the size of the nodes which by COG criteria are abnormal if they measure greater than 2 cm in longest dimension. The cervical nodal group is the most common location of nodes in Hodgkin lymphoma.[12] The nodes may involve any nodal station, be unilateral or bilateral, and are typically rounded in morphology and homogeneous in density before therapy. Nodes between 1 and 2 cm may also be considered abnormal if they are fluorodeoxyglucose (FDG)-PET avid. Bulk nodal disease is defined by nodal mass measuring $\geq$ 6 cm in maximal length in any plane and is a poor prognostic factor. On CT, the nodes are typically homogeneous, round, and large. They may be unilateral or bilateral and tend to involve the lower cervical chain and mediastinum (Fig. 2). Bone involvement in Hodgkin lymphoma is defined as either structural lesions or marrow infiltration and confers Stage IV disease. Focal lesions may be either lytic and/or sclerotic on CT and present as marrow edema on MR imaging. In the absence of a discrete structural lesion, FDG-PET avidity has also been shown to have some correlation with marrow infiltration though imperfectly and COG trials still perform bone marrow biopsy.[12],[13] When evaluating cross-sectional neck imaging, lesions may be seen in the spine, more often the thoracic than the cervical, as well as in the imaged ribs and sternum, so the osseous structures should be scrutinized using bone windows.

Non-Hodgkin Lymphoma

Non-Hodgkin Lymphoma is less frequent in children than in adults but still more common overall than Hodgkin lymphoma in children with the principal subtypes affecting children being Burkitt, T cell, diffuse large B cell, and anaplastic large cell. Staging is with the St Jude Classification by Murphy or the more recently revised in 2015 International Pediatric Non-Hodgkin Lymphoma Staging System which accounts for advances in imaging techniques and new findings of organ involvement. In the neck, the imaging criteria described for Hodgkin lymphoma can be applied to non-Hodgkin lymphoma as well. Non-Hodgkin lymphoma may present as a single-dominant large node or as multiple more mildly enlarged nodes (Fig. 3A). Non-Hodgkin lymphoma is also more likely to have bone involvement as well as extranodal involvement in other sites including the spinal cord and gentral nervous system (CNS) compared with Hodgkin lymphoma. Ultimately, there is overlap in the presentation of Hodgkin lymphoma and non-Hodgkin lymphoma, with the two entities being indistinguishable on imaging alone and requiring tissue sampling for definitive diagnosis. The tissues of Waldeyer's ring reflect an

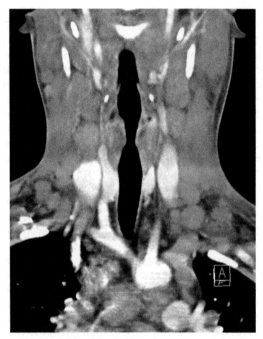

Fig. 2. CT with intravenous contrast coronal plane image of the neck demonstrating numerous round large bilateral mid and lower cervical chain, supraclavicular and mediastinal nodes in a teenage patient with Hodgkin lymphoma.

additional potential extra-nodal site of involvement in both Hodgkin and non-Hodgkin lymphoma though remains a difficult area to assess in pediatric patients who frequently have inflammatory changes in these tissues in the absence of oncologic disease which can also cause FDG-PET avidity and enlargement. The assessment of the architecture of the tissue can help which may be extremely distorted and asymmetric when involved with disease, with abnormal signal on both T2-weighted and DWI/apparent diffusion coefficient (ADC) sequences when MR imaging is performed (Fig. 3B). Response evaluation is now largely based on decreased FDG uptake rather than size criteria for both Hodgkin and non-Hodgkin lymphoma cervical nodes.

Histiocytic and Lymphoproliferative

Outside of malignancy, there are several additional disease entities in children which can present with big nodes including histiocytic and lymphoproliferative diseases. Rosai-Dorfman or non-Langerhans cell histiocytosis typically presents with systemic symptoms and bilateral painless often massive adenopathy (Fig. 4A). The nodes are typically homogeneous, though cystic nodes are possible. Patients are frequently thought to have lymphoma with biopsy ultimately required to make the diagnosis. Extra-nodal disease can be seen in 30% to 50% of patients at sites including the sinonasal cavity, dura, orbits, and other sites (Fig. 4B).[14] PET avidity is seen in both the nodes and extra-nodal sites of disease (Fig. 4C).

Lymphadenopathy may be present in up to 20% of patients with the multifocal uni-system and multisystem forms of Langerhans cell histiocytosis with the cervical nodal group being the most involved. There are no specific nodal imaging features with the nodes being variable in size and either homogeneous or cystic in nature. Clues to the diagnosis may be present on cross-sectional imaging in the form of lytic osseous skull lesions.

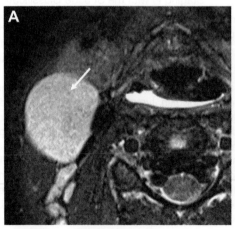
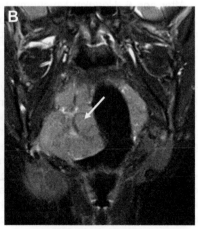

Fig. 3. (A) Axial T2 fat-saturated MR image demonstrating a dominant enlarged round right level 2 node (arrow, A) in a patient with non-Hodgkin lymphoma. (B) Coronal T2 fat-saturated MR image in the same patient demonstrating markedly enlarged and irregular right palatine tonsil (arrow, B) reflecting extra-nodal involvement in the tissue of Waldeyer's ring.

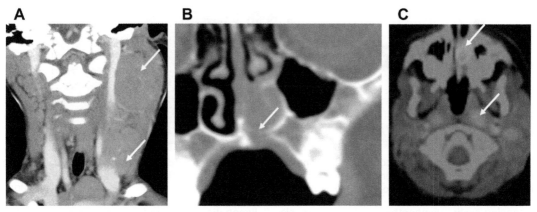

Fig. 4. (A) CT with intravenous contrast coronal plane image of the neck demonstrating numerous round large left upper, mid, and lower cervical chain nodes (*arrows, A*) in a patient with Rosai-Dorfman disease. (*B*) Coronal bone window image in the same patient demonstrating a left nasal cavity mass with erosion of the nasal cavity floor (*arrow, B*). (*C*) Axial PET-CT image in the same patient demonstrating PET avidity in both the cervical nodes and the left sino-nasal cavity extra-nodal disease (*arrows, C*).

Kikuchi disease, also known as Kikuchi histio-cytic necrotizing lymphadenitis, is an additional idiopathic disease which can present in children and young adults with systemic symptoms and cervical lymphadenopathy which is more commonly unilateral and homogeneous but may be bilateral and rarely cystic. Perinodal infiltration is a common imaging finding and the nodes can range in size from small to very large.[15] Homogeneous hypoechogenicity has been reported as a sonographic feature with the highest diagnostic accuracy in differentiating Kikuchi disease from other common infectious lymphadenitis.[16]

Castleman's disease is a rare lymphoprolifera-tive disorder which most commonly manifests in the unicentric hyaline vascular subtype as a hyper-vascular nodal mass (Fig. 5).[17] The cervical nodes are much less commonly involved than the abdominal or thoracic locations. Although imaging can be suggestive, for all these diseases described above, biopsy is ultimately necessary to make a definitive diagnosis.

CYSTIC AND CALCIFIED NODES

Cystic cervical nodes have a broad differential including infection with typical and atypical bacteria, parasitic and fungal species, and malignancies potentially presenting in this fashion. The acuity of onset, character of the nodes, and presence of systemic symptoms in these patients can help refine the differential.

Infectious Adenitis

Bacterial adenitis
Acute bacterial adenitis, with or without suppuration, remains the second most common cause of cervical adenopathy in children. The most common pathogens involved are *Staphylococcus aureus* and *Streptococcus* species. Children typically present acutely with fever and a swollen, erythematous neck with limited range of motion. Ultrasound and contrast-enhanced CT are both appropriate for the initial workup of these children. If there is clinical suspicion of progression to an abscess or for those infections involving the deep neck spaces, CT is preferred. On CT, the nodes may show varying degrees of necrosis manifested by internal hypodensity as well as changes related to concomitant tonsillitis, parotitis, sinusitis, or pharyngitis with soft tissue inflammatory stranding and reactive retropharyngeal effusions.

The remaining infectious entities that can present with cystic nodes tend to do so in a subacute fashion. Cat scratch disease caused by infection with *Bartonella henselae* most commonly presents as regional subacute tender adenopathy with the location of the involved nodes dependent on the site of inoculation, though the neck and axilla are the most common (Fig. 6).[18] Atypical manifestations of cat scratch disease are rarer and may present with or without lymphadenopathy with potential involvement of many different organs including the orbits, liver, brain, skin, and bones.[19]

Atypical Bacterial Adenitis

Mycobacterial infection including both nontuberculous mycobacterial disease (NTM) and tuberculosis (TB) both can also present with subacute cystic adenopathy in children that goes on to calcify chronically. NTM classically occurs in afebrile younger children as painless rim

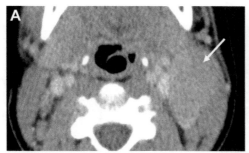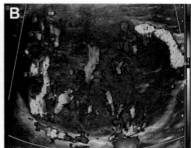

Fig. 5. (*A*) CT with intravenous contrast axial plane image of the upper neck demonstrating an irregular in shape, hyper-enhancing, left level 2 cervical nodal mass (*arrow, A*) in a patient with Castleman's disease. (*B*) The node demonstrates hypervascularity on Doppler ultrasound.

enhancing/cystic adenopathy unilaterally in levels 1 and 2 with variable surrounding inflammatory stranding, typically minimal (Fig. 7). The nodes may contact the skin surface and yield a purplish discoloration of the overlying skin. Occasionally, internal stippled calcifications may be present.[20] In contrast, TB adenitis most frequently presents in ill children who have concomitant pulmonary disease (Fig. 8A) with the cervical nodes being a common site in pediatric extra-pulmonary TB. Cystic conglomerate necrotic nodal masses most often are in levels 2 and 5 and the supraclavicular region. The nodes may fistulize to the skin surface and frequently have perinodal infiltration and surrounding stranding (Fig. 8B). Chronically or following treatment, the nodes may calcify, though less commonly than in the mediastinum and hila.[21]

Fungal Adenitis

Coccidioidomycosis, also known as valley fever, is an entity which can be seen in the south-west United States, Central and South America. It results from the inhalation of the spores of the *Coccidioides* fungal species. Cervical or supraclavicular nodal disease can be from direct

lymphatic drainage of a primary pulmonary infection or a manifestation of disseminated disease which is very rare and more often encountered in immunocompromised patients.[22] The most common sites of extrapulmonary involvement are in the central nervous system, bones, and soft tissues. The reported cases of nodal disease most frequently are cystic and may involve any cervical nodal station including the supraclavicular nodes (Fig. 9).[23] Fistula formation from cervical adenitis has also been reported.[22]

Malignancy

In contrast to adults, where the presence of cystic cervical adenopathy is strongly suggestive of metastatic malignancy, cystic nodes in pediatric patients are only rarely indicative of metastases.

Thyroid carcinoma

Like adults, when papillary thyroid carcinoma metastasizes in children and young adults, it can yield cystic cervical nodes, and up to 60% to 80% of patients with thyroid carcinoma present with regional lymph node involvement.[24] Though classically involving the infrahyoid visceral space

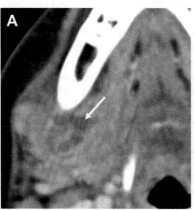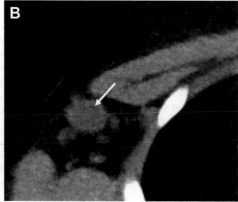

Fig. 6. (*A*) CT with intravenous contrast axial plane images of the upper neck and (*B*) lateral chest in a patient with cat scratch disease demonstrating cystic adenopathy involving the right submandibular (*arrow, A*) and axillary nodes (*arrow, B*).

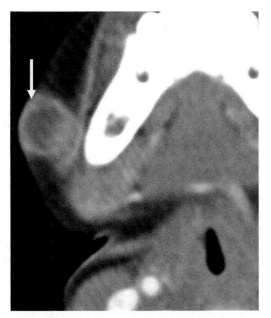

Fig. 7. CT with intravenous contrast axial plane images of the upper neck demonstrating a small cystic node with minimal surrounding stranding in the right submandibular region which contacts the skin surface (*arrow*) in a patient with nontuberculous mycobacterial disease.

nodes, metastatic papillary carcinoma can present with cystic nodes in any cervical nodal station including in level 2 (Fig. 10).[25] The nodes are variable in size ranging from less than 1 cm to over 3 cm and are also variable in morphology on cross-sectional imaging, with nodal intrinsic T1 shortening on MR imaging,[26] microcalcification, and hyper-enhancement all possible (see Fig. 10). It is important to remember that the thyroid may appear normal on cross-sectional imaging in these patients, so a normal appearing thyroid should not dissuade you from this diagnosis.[26] Less common variants of thyroid malignancy including the very rare medullary thyroid carcinoma, which is frequently genetic when

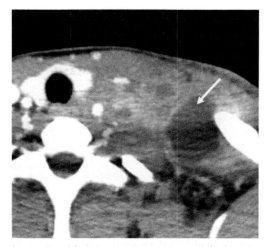

Fig. 9. CT with intravenous contrast axial plane images of the lower neck demonstrating numerous cystic left supraclavicular nodes (*arrow*) with perinodal stranding in a patient with coccidioidomycosis and primary pulmonary infection.

seen in the pediatric population, can also present with necrotic cervical adenopathy.[27]

Other carcinomas

Very rarely in children, head and neck carcinomas can present with cystic cervical adenopathy including nasopharyngeal carcinoma (NPC) and NUT carcinoma. NPC accounts for less than 1% of all childhood cancers with higher rates in southern Asia and the Mediterranean.[28] Pediatric NPC also has a closer association with the Epstein–Barr virus than adults. In children, the most common clinical presentation of NPC is cervical lymphadenopathy.[29] On imaging, the nodes may be homogenous, irregular, large, and/or demonstrate internal necrosis (Fig. 11). Determining sites of nodal involvement is important to treatment planning as radiation therapy is given not only to the primary tumor but also to the involved nodal sites.[29]

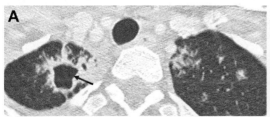
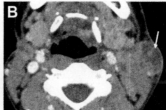

Fig. 8. (*A*) CT with intravenous contrast axial plane images of the chest and (*B*) upper neck, in a patient with tuberculosis demonstrating lung disease in the form of bilateral upper lobe reticulonodular densities and a right apical cavity (*arrow*, *A*) and concomitant cystic adenopathy involving the bilateral upper cervical nodes with perinodal stranding around a large left nodal mass which fistulizes to the skin surface (*arrow*, *B*).

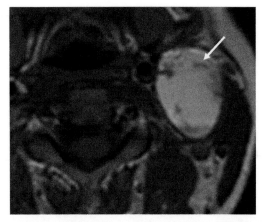

Fig. 10. MR imaging pre-contrast axial T1-weighted image without fat saturation demonstrating a cystic left level 2a nodal mass with internal septations and intrinsic T1 shortening (*arrow*) in a patient with metastatic papillary thyroid carcinoma.

NUT carcinoma, previously known as NUT midline carcinoma, is a rare and aggressive malignancy which is defined by the presence of a specific gene rearrangement and can occur in adults, adolescents, and children. The primary tumor can present in various sites of the head and neck and the mediastinum as well as other sites of the body with a predilection toward a midline location though not exclusively.[30] Regional lymph node involvement and distal metastases are possible with overall very poor patient prognosis and no established and effective treatment regimen.[31] Typically, the mass appears as locally aggressive and invasive. In the head and neck, the tumor can involve the sino-nasal cavity, aero-digestive tract, or salivary glands. Regional nodal involvement can present as necrotic conglomerate nodes or homogeneous nodal enlargement (**Fig. 12**).

CLINICAL APPLICATIONS

When deciding when it is appropriate to image children presenting with adenopathy, we can broadly divide patients into three categories: acute, occurring for less than 2 weeks; subacute, occurring for 2 to 6 weeks; and chronic, occurring for more than 6 weeks. In the acute category, patients can then be divided into those that are well and those that are unwell. Most children fall into this first category of well children presenting with acute adenopathy, which is likely reactive in nature and no imaging is required. A smaller subset of children with acute adenopathy are unwell, and in these patients, imaging can be performed to answer a specific clinical question, for example, has bacterial adenitis progressed to an abscess or in patients with suspected Kawasaki disease to fulfill one of the five diagnostic criteria. Imaging, therefore, is largely reserved for patients presenting with subacute and chronic adenopathy with the goal of aiding management in a specific clinical scenario such as guiding alternate antibiotic or chemotherapeutic treatment; confirming a node is the cause of a persistent palpable abnormality; assessing for involvement of the deep neck spaces; evaluating for concerning nodal imaging features or progressive enlargement; planning surgery, nodal excision or biopsy; and to follow known malignancies.

DIFFERENTIAL DIAGNOSIS

Cervical lymphadenopathy is just one potential cause of a neck mass in a child with the differential including congenital, neoplastic, and vascular entities. When distinguishing among these possibilities, it is useful to consider the location in the neck (midline or lateral), the focality of the process

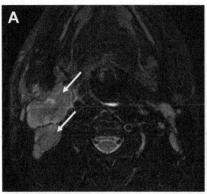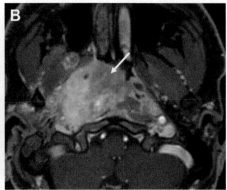

Fig. 11. (*A*) Axial T2 fat-saturated MR image demonstrating large irregular right upper cervical chain nodes (*arrows, A*). (*B*) Axial post-contrast fat-saturated T1-weighted image in the same patient demonstrating a large, enhancing, invasive ipsilateral nasopharyngeal mass (*arrow, B*) in a patient with nasopharyngeal carcinoma.

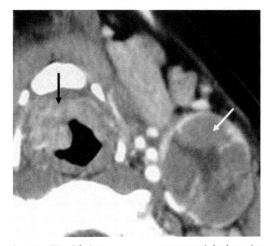

Fig. 12. CT with intravenous contrast axial plane images of the neck at the level of the hyoid demonstrating an irregular enhancing mass of the epiglottis (*black arrow*) and a necrotic left mid-cervical chain nodal mass (*white arrow*) in a patient with metastatic NUT carcinoma.

(unifocal, multifocal, or trans-spatial), the character of the mass (cystic vs solid), and physical examination findings and vascularity. Although it is beyond the scope of this review to delineate the workup of all neck masses in children, in general, nodes tend to be lateral in location and multifocal in nature. If one encounters a unifocal midline cystic neck mass, a congenital lesion such as a thyroglossal duct cyst, dermoid cyst, or foregut duplication cyst should be strongly considered. In the lateral neck, the differential for a unifocal cystic mass includes not only isolated adenopathy with the entities described above but also congenital lesions such as branchial apparatus anomalies and thymic cysts, vascular masses such as lymphatic malformations and venolymphatic malformations, and neoplasms such as pilomatrixoma and teratoma. A solid, unifocal neck mass should prompt one to consider neoplasms such as rhabdomyosarcoma, teratoma, neuroblastoma, neurogenic tumors, or solitary fibrous tumor among others as well as vascular tumors like a hemangioma with assessment of other internal characteristics and vascularity important in refining the differential.

SUMMARY

The variety of disease entities in children which can present with adenopathy is vast and includes a different spectrum of pathology than is seen in adults. The radiologist interpreting pediatric cervical imaging must be familiar with the typical imaging appearance of lymph nodes on the variety of different imaging modalities deemed appropriate for workup by the ACR as well as the assortment of neck masses in pediatric patients which may present similarly. Furthermore, the radiologist can play a key role in helping to guide clinicians in not only the selection of the most appropriate imaging modality but also in making recommendations on when it is appropriate to image this population in general.

CLINICS CARE POINTS

- Pediatric cervical lymphadenopathy is common and most often secondary to infectious entities with an overall very low rate of malignancy.
- Most otherwise well children with acute cervical adenopathy do not require imaging with imaging reserved for unwell children or those with persistent adenopathy to answer a specific clinical question.
- Ultrasound and contrast-enhanced CT are both appropriate for the initial workup of a patient with suspected adenopathy. MR imaging with and without contrast can be useful for problem-solving and follow-up of patients with known adenopathy. PET-CT and PET-MR imaging are reserved for patients with known malignancy and certain other disease entities.
- Nodal size is not a reliable predictor of malignancy in children; therefore, evaluating other nodal features such as shape, station, laterality, and internal character is useful when formulating a differential.

DISCLOSURES

No financial disclosures.

REFERENCES

1. Weinstock MS, Patel NA, Smith LP. Pediatric Cervical Lymphadenopathy. Pediatr Rev 2018;39(9): 433–43.
2. Deosthali A, Donches K, DelVecchio M, et al. Etiologies of Pediatric Cervical Lymphadenopathy: A Systematic Review of 2687 Subjects. Glob Pediatr Health 2019;6. https://doi.org/10.1177/2333794X19865440.
3. Aulino JM, Kirsch CFE, Burns J et al. ACR Appropriateness Criteria® Neck Mass/Adenopathy. Available at https://acsearch.acr.org/docs/69504/Narrative/. American College of Radiology. Accessed 9/27/22.
4. Onoue K, Fujima N, Andreu-Arasa VC, et al. Cystic cervical lymph nodes of papillary thyroid carcinoma, tuberculosis and human papillomavirus positive

oropharyngeal squamous cell carcinoma: utility of deep learning in their differentiation on CT. Am J Otolaryngol 2021;42(5):103026.

5. Kanal KM, Butler PF, Chatfield MB, et al. U.S. Diagnostic Reference Levels and Achievable Doses for 10 Pediatric CT Examinations. Radiology 2021;26:211241.

6. Suh CH, Choi YJ, Baek JH, et al. The Diagnostic Value of Diffusion-Weighted Imaging in Differentiating Metastatic Lymph Nodes of Head and Neck Squamous Cell Carcinoma: A Systematic Review and Meta-Analysis. AJNR 2018;39(10):1889–95.

7. Celenk F, Gulsen S, Baysal E, et al. Predictive factors for malignancy in patients with persistent cervical lymphadenopathy. Eur Arch Oto-Rhino-Laryngol 2016;273(1):251–6.

8. Hoang JK, Vanka J, Ludwig BJ, et al. Evaluation of cervical lymph nodes in head and neck cancer with CT and MRI: tips, traps, and a systematic approach. AJR 2013;200(1):W17–25.

9. Weiss L, O'Malley D. Benign lymphadenopathies. Mod Pathol 2013;26(Suppl 1):S88–96.

10. Mulroy E, Walker E. Lamotrigine-related pseudolymphoma presenting as cervical lymphadenopathy. Epilepsy Behav Case Rep 2017;7:40–1.

11. Leung AK, Robson WL. Childhood cervical lymphadenopathy. J Pediatr Health Care 2004 Jan 1;18(1):3–7.

12. McCarten KM, Nadel HR, Shulkin BL, et al. Imaging for diagnosis, staging and response assessment of Hodgkin lymphoma and non-Hodgkin lymphoma. Pediatr Radiol 2019;49(11):1545–64.

13. Adams HJ, Kwee TC. Is FDG-PET/CT a sensitive and specific method for the detection of extranodal involvement in diffuse large B-cell lymphoma? Am J Hematol 2016;91(2):E1–2.

14. Mantilla JG, Goldberg-Stein S, Wang Y. Extranodal Rosai-Dorfman Disease: Clinicopathologic Series of 10 Patients With Radiologic Correlation and Review of the Literature. Am J Clin Pathol 2016;145(2):211–21.

15. Kwon SY, Kim TK, Kim YS, et al. CT Findings in Kikuchi Disease: Analysis of 96 Cases. AJNR 2004;25(6):1099–102.

16. Park S, Kim JY, Ryu YJ, et al. Kikuchi Cervical Lymphadenitis in Children: Ultrasound Differentiation From Common Infectious Lymphadenitis. J Ultrasound Med 2021;40(10):2069–78.

17. Bonekamp D, Horton KM, Hruban RH, et al. Castleman disease: the great mimic. Radiographics 2011;31(6):1793–807.

18. Ridder GJ, Boedeker CC, Technau-Ihling K, et al. Role of Cat-Scratch Disease in Lymphadenopathy in the Head and Neck. Clin Infect Dis 2002;35(Issue 6):643–9.

19. Hopkins KL, Simoneaux SF, Patrick LE, et al. Imaging manifestations of cat-scratch disease. AJR 2013;166(2):435–8.

20. Robson CD, Hazra R, Barnes PD, et al. Nontuberculous mycobacterial infection of the head and neck in immunocompetent children: CT and MR findings. AJNR Am J Neuroradiol 1999;20(10):1829–35.

21. Ludwig BJ, Wang J, Nadgir RN, et al. Imaging of cervical lymphadenopathy in children and young adults. AJR Am J Roentgenol 2012;199(5):1105–13.

22. Loudin M, Clayburgh DR, Hakki M. Coccidioides immitis Cervical Lymphadenitis Complicated by Esophageal Fistula. Case Rep Infect Dis 2016;2016:8715405.

23. Biller JA, Scheuller MC, Eisele DW. Coccidioidomycosis causing massive cervical lymphadenopathy. Laryngoscope 2004;114(11):1892–4.

24. La Quaglia MP, Black T, Holcomb GW 3rd, et al. Differentiated thyroid cancer: clinical characteristics, treatment, and outcome in patients under 21 years of age who present with distant metastases. A report from the Surgical Discipline Committee of the Children's Cancer Group. J Pediatr Surg 2000;35:955–9 [discussion: 60].

25. Attard A, Paladino N, Lo Monte A, et al. Skip metastases to lateral cervical lymph nodes in differentiated thyroid cancer: a systematic review. BMC Surg 2019;18:112.

26. Hoang JK, Branstetter BF 4th, Gafton AR, et al. Imaging of thyroid carcinoma with CT and MRI: approaches to common scenarios. Cancer Imag 2013;13(1):128–39.

27. Moley JF. Medullary thyroid carcinoma: management of lymph node metastases. J Natl Compr Cancer Netw : JNCCN. 2010;8:549–56.

28. Claude L, Jouglar E, Duverge L, et al. Update in pediatric nasopharyngeal undifferentiated carcinoma. Br J Radiol 2019;92(1102):20190107.

29. Cheuk DK, Billups CA, Martin MG, et al. Prognostic factors and long-term outcomes of childhood nasopharyngeal carcinoma. Cancer 2011;117:197–206.

30. Moreno V, Saluja K, Pina-Oviedo S. NUT Carcinoma: Clinicopathologic Features, Molecular Genetics and Epigenetics. Front Oncol 2022;16(12):860830.

31. Prasad M, Baheti A, Ramadwar M, et al. Pediatric NUT Carcinoma Is a Rare and Challenging Tumor: Single Center Experience of Five Children. Oncol 2019;24(11):e1232–5.

Congenital Cystic Neck Masses

Timothy N. Booth, MD

KEYWORDS

• Congenital • Cyst • Pediatric • Imaging • Branchial • Thyroglossal • Dermoid • Lymphatic

KEY POINTS

- Determination of cystic versus solid using imaging is important in evaluating children with neck masses.
- Location is of paramount importance in formulating a differential diagnosis and guiding surgical intervention.
- Ultrasound (US) is the accepted initial modality for the evaluation of a suspected superficial neck mass in children.
- Computed tomography or MR imaging is often needed to determine the extent and deep involvement.

INTRODUCTION

Neck masses are common reason for imaging of the neck in the pediatric population, and these are often cystic. Historical information is key to improve the ability to diagnose including onset of symptoms, duration, cutaneous findings, as well as any syndromic associations. Initial evaluation is performed using ultrasound (US). Defining a lesion as cystic is an important task for the radiologist on any modality used for evaluation (Table 1). Computed tomography (CT) and MR imaging are useful to confirm cystic nature and determine extent.

Age is also important in constructing limited differential diagnosis with certain entities presenting in the fetus and first weeks of life. These entities may also present later in childhood.

Fetal and Neonatal Presentation

- Foregut duplication cyst
- Third to fourth branchial pouch cyst (Thymopharyngeal duct remnant)
- Lymphatic malformation
- Cystic teratoma
- Meningocele

Location is an invaluable tool in evaluating children with a congenital cystic neck mass with thyroglossal, branchial cleft, and pouch-related cysts following distinct embryologic pathways (Table 2).

GENERAL IMAGING CONSIDERATIONS
Ultrasound

High-frequency linear transducers are preferred (9–15 MHz) for lesion evaluation, and curvilinear or extended field transducer is suggested to determine the overall location. Doppler flow analysis is necessary to assess for the internal flow and confirm a cystic nature. This modality is most useful for superficial masses: although, diagnostic accuracy may be limited.[1,2]

Computed Tomography

CT has the advantages of availability and usually does not require sedation or anesthesia with the major disadvantage of exposure to ionizing radiation. The study is performed with intravenous contrast administration and precontrast imaging should be avoided due to additional radiation dose. In the future, dual-energy

University of Texas Southwestern, Children's Health of Texas, 1935 Medical District Drive, Dallas, TX 75235, USA
E-mail address: Timothy.booth@utsouthwestern.edu

Neuroimag Clin N Am 33 (2023) 591–605
https://doi.org/10.1016/j.nic.2023.05.009
1052-5149/23/© 2023 Elsevier Inc. All rights reserved.

Table 1
Cystic characteristics on imaging modalities

Ultrasound	Computed Tomography	MR Imaging
Homogenous echogenicity	Homogenous density	Homogenous signal intensity
No Doppler flow	No contrast enhancement	No contrast enhancement
Fluid–fluid level	Fluid–fluid level	Fluid–fluid level
Absent solid components	Well-defined	Well-defined

CT may be of use in providing a virtual noncontrast image to better determine the presence of enhancement but there is limited published data of pediatric applications in the neck.[3] Reconstructed sagittal and coronal plane to improve anatomic localization and extent of the cystic mass.[4]

Magnetic Resonance Imaging

MR imaging is the preferred imaging modality after initial US due to the improved contrast resolution, tissue characterization, and multiplanar capabilities. The main drawback with MR imaging is the accessibility and the need for sedation/anesthesia in the younger child. Axial and coronal T1-weighted images (T1WIs), T2-weighted images (T2WIs) with fat suppression (Short Tau inversion recovery [STIR] or Dixon preferred). Postgadolinium T1WIs with fat saturation (chemical or Dixon) is often useful to define a lesion as cystic without enhancing solid component.[4,5] Diffusion-weighed images are helpful as cystic lesions will show facilitated diffusion in most circumstances; however, restricted diffusion may be present in a dermoid or associated with infection or hemorrhage.[6]

Pathology

Anterior midline location

Thyroglossal duct cyst   Thyroglossal duct cysts are a commonly encountered congenital neck cyst and represent most midline neck masses in children. Movement with tongue protrusion can be a helpful finding on physical examination due to the connection to the posterior tongue. They are cystic on imaging but may be superinfected and have a secondary cutaneous fistula. Location is usually infrahyoid and associated with the hyoid bone. A suprahyoid is less common. Ultimately, the cysts can occur anywhere along the course to the thyroglossal duct, which extends inferiorly from the foramen cecum, surrounds the anterior body of the hyoid bone, and extends to the thyroid gland (Fig. 1).[7]

In the infrahyoid region, the cyst is usually within or deep to the adjacent strap musculature. Typically, thyroglossal duct cysts (TGDCs) are midline and para midline in location and deform the laryngeal cartilage (Fig. 2).[7] These lesions may be associated with ectopic thyroid tissue and rarely associated with the development of thyroid papillary carcinoma, which is more common in adults. The presence of calcification in the solid

Table 2
Differential diagnosis of congenital cystic neck masses based on location

Anterior Midline	Anterior Lateral	Posterior	Periauricular	Tongue
TGDC	Second BCC	LM	First BCC	Foregut duplication cyst
Dermoid	Third or fourth branchial pouch remnant	Dermoid (midline)	Dermoid	Dermoid
Foregut duplication cyst	LM	Third BCC	LM	LM
	Cystic lymph node, infection or tumor (acquired)		Cystic lymph node or neoplasm (acquired)	Ranula

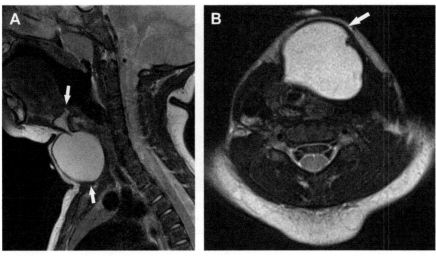

Fig. 1. A 5-year-old child with a midline neck mass and TGDC. Sagittal midline T2WI (*A*) demonstrates a cyst extending from foramen cecum to the thyroid gland (*arrows*). T2WI at the level of the thyroid gland (*B*) shows the infrahyoid cyst posterior to the strap musculature (*arrow*).

component of the cyst may help to diagnose the presence of malignancy (Fig. 3).[8] Secondary infection occurs commonly and may alter the imaging appearance with increased enhancement and surrounding inflammation.

The cyst will usually have homogenous internal echogenicity on US with absent internal Doppler flow (Fig. 4). The relationship with the hyoid bone should be stressed and may be better demonstrated on CT and MR imaging with the cyst extending along the inferior and posterior aspect of the bone. A defect or notch within the anterior hyoid may also be seen (Fig. 5).[9] It is important to document the presence of orthotopic thyroid

gland on imaging to avoid hypothyroidism as an unexpected complication after surgery. A TGCD at the level of the foramen cecum seems like a vallecular cyst, which is located slightly more posterior and displaces the epiglottis (Fig. 6). The diagnosis of TGDC is important because the entire track and anterior body of the hyoid bone needs to be removed at surgery (Sistrunck procedure) to decrease the rate of recurrence.[10]

Thyroglossal duct cyst
- Midline, para midline along expected location of thyroglossal duct
- Associated with hyoid

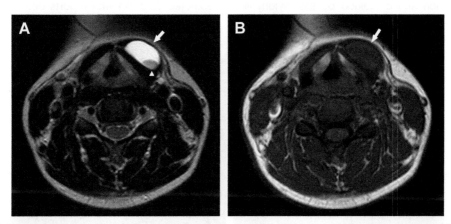

Fig. 2. An 8-year-old child with infrahyoid anterior neck mass and TGDC. Axial T2WI above the thyroid gland (*A*) demonstrates a cyst within the adjacent strap musculature (*arrow*) and a focus of decreased T2 signal posteriorly (*arrowhead*) consistent with debris, which was nonenhancing (not shown). There is slight mass effect on the adjacent thyroid cartilage. Axial T1WI at a similar level (*B*) shows mild increased T1 signal in comparison with muscle compatible with protein or hemorrhage (*arrow*).

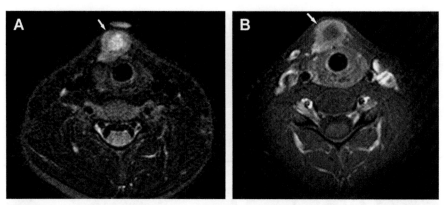

Fig. 3. A 13-year-old child with slowly growing infrahyoid midline mass in the lower neck and papillary thyroid carcinoma originating in a thyroglossal remnant. Axial STIR images slightly above the thyroid gland (A) shows a mass with fluid centrally (arrow). Thick enhancing margins are present on postgadolinium T1WI with fat saturation (B) (arrow).

- Infrahyoid within of posterior to strap musculature

Dermoid cyst

A dermoid cyst presents as a palpable mass and is a benign neoplasm composed of 2 components, mesoderm and ectoderm. The cysts tend to grow slowly over time and can present at any age but most commonly under the age of 5 years. They form along embryonic fusion lines with a propensity for hyoid and suprasternal location in the anterior neck; however, they can be located anywhere from the anterior fontanelle to the suprasternal area. Nasal and occipital dermoid cysts may have an intracranial communication and a thorough evaluation of the intracranial contents is recommended.[11] When the dermoid cyst is within the floor of the mouth, the cyst is commonly submental in location and contained by the mylohyoid sling, which affects surgical approach.

US shows these lesions as well-defined homogenous soft tissue echogenicity with Doppler evaluation demonstrating no internal flow (Fig. 7). Fat density (negative Hounsfield units) may be a helpful imaging finding on CT but is not always encountered. Due to the presence of fat globules in the lesion, a sack of marbles appearance may be present and is best seen on MR imaging and is specific for the diagnosis (Fig. 8). Helpful imaging findings on MR imaging include T1 shortening due to variable fat component with decreased signal when using fat saturation techniques.[12] The sagittal plane is helpful in evaluating position and the presence or intracranial extension with nasal and occipital locations (Fig. 9). When located adjacent to a bone or cartilage, there may be associated regional mass effect and subtle erosion. Diffusion-weighted images may show restricted diffusion with reports demonstrating a threshold apparent diffusion coefficient value of

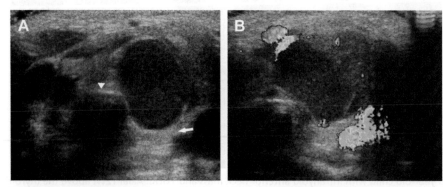

Fig. 4. An 8-year-old child with paramidline neck mass and TGDC. Transverse US image above the level of the thyroid (A) demonstrates a well-defined mass with through sound transmission (arrow) anterior and left of the trachea (arrowhead). The cyst has mild homogeneous internal echogenicity. Doppler image (B) shows no internal flow with only peripheral Doppler flow.

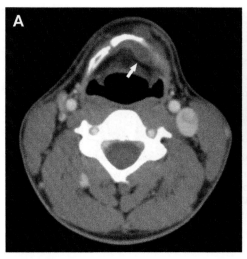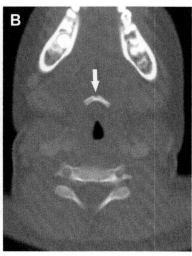

Fig. 5. Two different children with neck masses and TGDCs at the level of the hyoid. Axial postcontrast CT (*A*) demonstrates a cystic lesion anterior and posterior to the left aspect of the hyoid bone (*arrow*). In the second patient, bone windows on an axial postcontrast CT (*B*) shows a subtle defect along the midbody of the hyoid bone (*arrow*) with a small cyst demonstrated inferior (not shown).

in the range of 1.62×10^{-3} mm^2/s, below being a dermoid cyst and above TGDC (Fig. 10).[13]

Dermoid
- Anterior fontanelle to suprasternal region
- May appear solid on US, no internal flow
- Diffusion-weighted sequences show low apparent diffusion coefficient

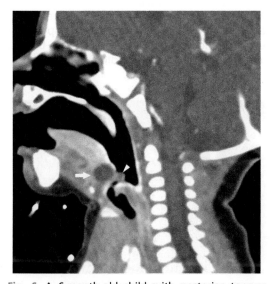

Fig. 6. A 6-month-old child with posterior tongue mass and vallecular cyst. Midline sagittal contrast-enhanced CT demonstrates a posterior tongue cyst (*arrow*) with mass effect on the adjacent epiglottis (*arrowhead*). Marsupialization was performed at surgery.

Foregut duplication cysts
The foregut is composed of the pharynx, lower respiratory tract, and upper gastrointestinal tract. Heterotopic rests of the foregut can persist giving rise to cysts. Pathologically, they must have a smooth muscle layer, contain epithelium, and be attached to a foregut derivative, usually fibrous. In the neck, they are in variable locations but most commonly within the anterior tongue and neck. When located in the anterior tongue, the clinical symptoms relate to poor feeding an inability to latch and are commonly encountered in the neonate. Typical cystic appearance is seen on imaging with no enhancement (Figs. 11 and 12).[14,15] Differential diagnosis includes a dermoid cyst, ranula (rarely congenital), and lymphatic malformation (LM).

Anterior lateral neck location
Second branchial cleft cyst Remnants of the second branchial cleft and may be classified as a sinus (internal or external opening), fistula (internal and external opening), or a cyst (no opening). The course of a complete fistula is important with the external cutaneous fistula within the anterior lateral neck at the junction between the upper two-thirds and lower one-third, then extends superiorly along the anterior medial margin of the sternocleidomastoid muscle posterior to the submandibular gland. The fistula then travels medially between the internal and external carotid arteries opening into the tonsillar fossa. The most common location for a second branchial cleft cyst (BCC) is between the submandibular gland and

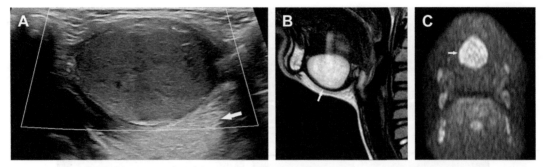

Fig. 7. A 7-year-old child presented with a submental mass and dermoid. A well-defined lesion is identified on transverse US with Doppler (*A*), which shows uniform echogenicity, good through sound transmission (*arrow*), and no internal Doppler flow. Midline sagittal T2WI (*B*) demonstrates the cyst to be confined by the mylohyoid sling (*arrow*) and axial diffusion-weighed image (*C*) shows the cyst to be increase in signal on trace image with an ADC of 0.9 × 10^{-3} mm^2/s (*arrow*).

sternocleidomastoid muscle but they may be located more inferiorly, protrude between the internal and external carotid or be entirely para-pharyngeal.[16,17] Syndromic associations include Branchio-oto-renal syndrome, especially if multiple (Fig. 13).[18]

Imaging features can vary due to protein content and presence of infection. Homogeneous, good through sound transmission, and no Doppler flow on US and imaging features consistent with a cyst on CT and MR imaging. The location is an important factor when considering the diagnosis of a second BCC (Fig. 14).

Differential diagnosis is important to consider, especially if the location for a BCC is not typical. A neck abscess or conglomerate suppurative lymph-adenopathy can seem similar to an infected second BCC and is more common. Additionally, cystic nodal metastases from Human Papilloma Virus

(HPV)-related oropharyngeal carcinoma may present as a unilocular cyst without surrounding inflammation; however, this is uncommonly encountered in children.[19]

Second BCC

- Most common along anterior medial margin of sternocleidomastoid
- Evaluate for medial extension between internal and external carotid
- Multiple may be associated with branchio-oto-renal syndrome

Thymopharyngeal duct remnant (third and fourth branchial pouch remnant)

These are typically cysts or sinuses that occur along the expected course of the thymopharyngeal duct and may be mistaken for BCCs both at imaging with the nomenclature inconsistent.[20]

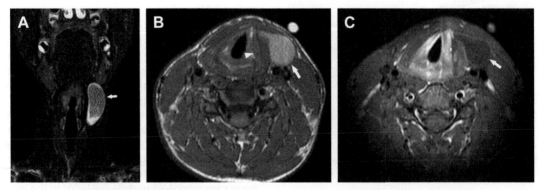

Fig. 8. A 9-year-old child with left paramidline neck mass and dermoid. Axial T2WI (*A*) demonstrates a well-defined mass T2 hyperintense lesion with numerous foci of relatively decreased signal, a sack of marble appearance. The sublingual gland (*arrowhead*) and submandibular gland (*arrow*) are present along the anterior and lateral margin, respectively. Axial T1WI (*B*) shows heterogenous increased T1 signal (*arrow*) and mass effect on the thyroid cartilage (*arrowhead*). There is signal suppression on the postgadolinium fat-saturated T1WI (*C*) and no enhancement (*arrow*). A marker is present at the level of the palpable abnormality.

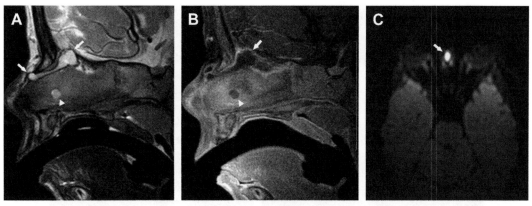

Fig. 9. An 18-month-old child with nasal mass and dermoid. Midline sagittal T2WI (*A*) demonstrates a cystic mass extending from the inferior nasal bridge to the foramen cecum (*arrows*) with a similar satellite lesion in the nasal septum (*arrowhead*). In both lesions, minimal peripheral enhancement (*arrow, arrowhead*) is present on sagittal postgadolinium fat-saturated T1WI (*B*). Restricted diffusion is present (*arrow*) on the axial trace diffusion-weighted image (*C*).

The sinus begins at the level of the piriform sinus (apex or base) and extends along the airway to the mediastinum. These are mostly left-sided, intimately associated with the thyroid gland. Interestingly, this entity presents differently depending on age. Neonates present with large cysts and children present with recurrent neck abscesses due to the presence of a sinus. The diagnosis should be suggested in a child with recurrent neck abscesses and involvement of the thyroid. Imaging demonstrates suppurative thyroiditis and paraglottic inflammation extending superiorly to the level of the piriform sinus. Air may be seen within the sinus but is uncommon (Fig. 15).[20]

Neonates present as large unilocular cysts and airway compromise. These may contain thymic tissue and, if present, designated pathologically as thymic cysts. They are unilocular and are located along the expected course of the thymopharyngeal duct. Mediastinal involvement and a typical medial extension (beak) can be present along the superior margin and project into the retropharyngeal space are helpful in establishing the diagnosis.[21] Superinfection and hemorrhage can occur with fluid–fluid levels present (Fig. 16). Diffusion-weighted images can show restricted diffusion due to the presence of purulent material likely due to airway communication. Direct laryngoscopy for visualization of the opening within the piriform sinus is recommended in both neonates and children with cauterization or complete surgical resection as surgical options. Drainage

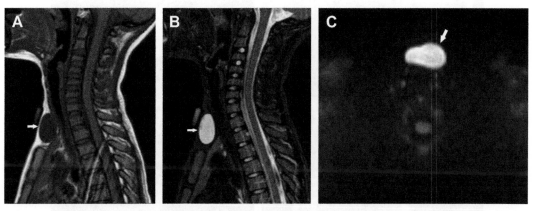

Fig. 10. A 6-year-old child with suprasternal mass and dermoid. Midline sagittal T1WI (*A*) and STIR image (*B*) demonstrates a homogeneous T1 hypointense and T2 hyperintense lesion (*arrows*). No enhancement is present (not shown) and axial trace diffusion-weighted image (*C*) shows increased signal (*arrow*) with an ADC of 1.1×10^{-3} mm^2/s.

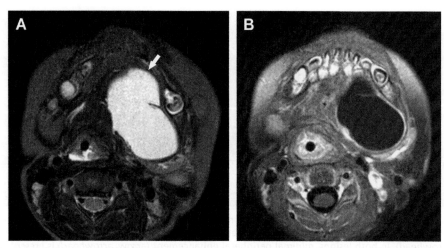

Fig. 11. Neonate with mass involving the floor of the mouth and diagnosis of submental foregut duplication cyst. Axial STIR image of the tongue (A) demonstrates an essentially unilocular homogeneously T2 hyperintense lesion within the floor of the mouth extending into the submandibular space (*arrow*). Minimal peripheral enhancement is present on postgadolinium axial fat-saturated T1WI (B).

may be performed as a temporizing treatment before resection.

Differential diagnosis would include a LM, which is typically are multilocular. A cervical teratoma may also present in this age group as a cystic multilocular mass. Enhancing solid components are key to the diagnosis along with the absence of fluid–fluid levels are useful findings to differentiate from a thymopharyngeal remnant cyst or LM. Fat signal (T1 shortening) may be absent depending on the differentiation of the teratoma (Fig. 17).[22]

Thymopharyngeal duct remnant

- Different presentation depending on age
- Neonates present with large unilocular cyst

- Mediastinal extension and retropharyngeal beak

Posterior Location

Lymphatic malformation

These are slow flow vascular malformations and are typically associated with a posterior lateral location and extend into the retropharyngeal space but can be located throughout the head and neck. Syndromic associations include Noonan, Turner, Down, CLOVES, and Klippel-Trenaunay syndromes. The exact cause of a LM is unknown but may be partially related to *PIK3CA*-activating mutations. Children may present at any age with a neck mass, sometimes rapidly enlarging due to

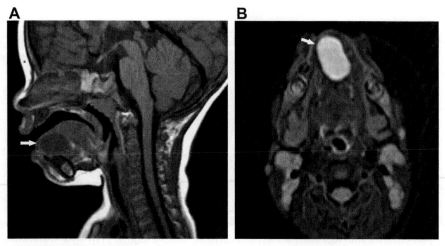

Fig. 12. Neonate with difficulty latching and foregut duplication cyst. Midline sagittal T1WI (A) and axial STIR image (B) although the tongue demonstrates a homogenously T1 hypointense and T2 hyperintense cyst anteriorly within the oral cavity (*arrows*).

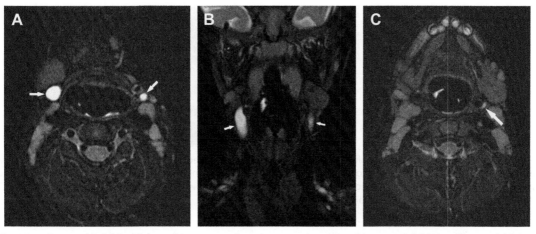

Fig. 13. A 3-year-old child with branchio-oto-renal syndrome and anterior skin tags. Axial (*A*) and coronal (*B*) STIR image at the level of the submandibular glands demonstrates bilateral BCCs, right larger than left (*arrows*), in a typical location anterior medial to the sternocleidomastoid muscle and posterior to the submandibular glands. Axial STIR image (*C*) slightly more superior demonstrates a tail of the cyst extending between the internal and external carotid arteries (*arrow*).

the presence of infection or internal hemorrhage. LMs are commonly trans-spacial and may cause airway compromise due to regional mass effect. Macrocytic and microcystic types have distinctly different imaging features.[23]

Macrocytic LMs are characteristically cystic on all modalities, multilocular, with internal septae. These septations are echogenic on US and helpful to the diagnosis.[1] The septations show enhancement on contrast-enhanced CT and MR imaging without the presence of nodularity. Fluid–fluid levels may also be present usually indicating earlier hemorrhage or infection (**Figs. 18** and **19**). Microcystic LMs can be more solid in appearance but usually have a macrocytic component to aid in the diagnosis (**Fig. 20**).[24] LMs are typically treated with sclerotherapy with surgical resection a second-line treatment, and microcystic LMs may

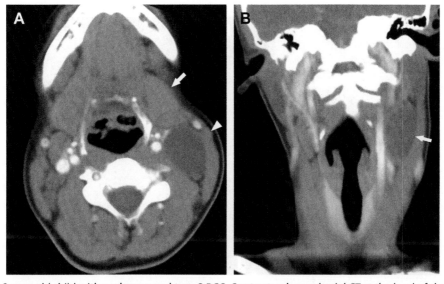

Fig. 14. A 9-year-old child with neck mass and type 2 BCC. Contrast-enhanced axial CT at the level of the hyoid (*A*) shows a cyst between the submandibular gland (*arrow*) and sternocleidomastoid muscle (*arrowhead*), most common location. Coronal CT reconstruction (*B*) shows the superior to inferior extend of the cyst along the medial margin of the sternocleidomastoid muscle (*arrow*).

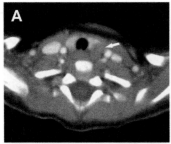
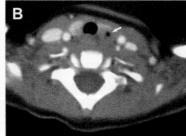
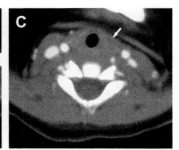

Fig. 15. A 6-year-old child with left-sided neck swelling and documented thymopharyngeal duct remnant with a piriform sinus opening documented on direct laryngoscopy. Contrast-enhanced axial CT image at the level of the thyroid (*A*) shows inflammation along the left lobe of the thyroid (*arrow*). Axial CT images more superiorly (*B, C*) shows paraglottic inflammation an air within the sinus track (*arrows*).

be less responsive to sclerotherapy. Posttreatment grading using MR imaging may be of benefit to access response.[25]

Lymphatic malformation
- Commonly posterior lateral neck but can be in all locations
- Echogenic, enhancing septae
- Fluid–fluid levels

Dermoid cyst
A dermoid can occur posterior in the midline of para-midline location. It important to evaluate for intracranial and intraspinal extension with MR imaging (sagittal plane).[11] Congenital occipital and cervical meningoceles can also occur in this location as well (**Fig. 21**).

Third branchial cleft cyst
These are extremely rare lesions with cystic characteristics on imaging. In contradistinction to second BCCs, these are located posterior to the carotid sheath and along the posterior medial margin of the sternocleidomastoid muscle.[6,26]

Periauricular Location

First branchial cleft cyst
The first branchial cleft forms the external auditory canal. These cysts present with a periauricular mass and may be associated with a skin tag and are most commonly anterior and inferior to the external auditory canal but may be postauricular. These may be seen with atresia of the external canal and well-associated syndromes

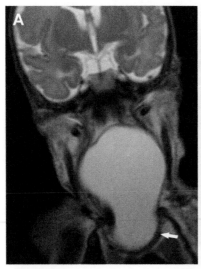
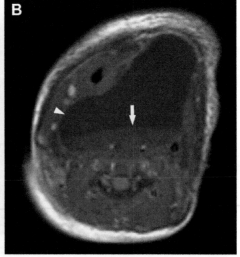

Fig. 16. Newborn with a large neck mass and diagnosed thymic cyst (thymopharyngeal duct remnant). Coronal T2WI (*A*) demonstrates a large unilocular cyst within the neck extending into the mediastinum (*arrow*). Axial T1WI (*B*) at the level of the glottis shows a displaced airway and prominent fluid–fluid level compatible with hemorrhage (*arrow*). There is medial retropharyngeal extension or beak (*arrowhead*).

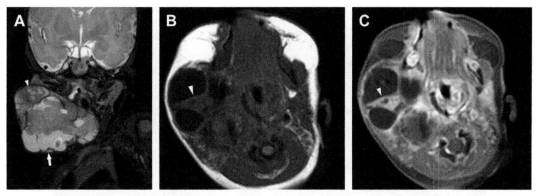

Fig. 17. Newborn with respiratory distress and a large immature teratoma. Coronal T2WI (*A*) demonstrated a cystic mass in the right neck with macrocystic (*arrow*) and microcystic components (*arrowhead*). No fluid–fluid levels were present. Axial T1WI (*B*) and postcontrast fat-saturated T1WI (*C*) shows solid enhancement superiorly (*arrowheads*) and no evidence of fat within the lesion.

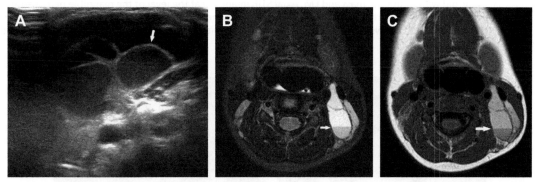

Fig. 18. An 8-year-old with left posterior lateral neck mass and LM. Transverse US image (*A*) demonstrates a multi-locular cystic mass with echogenic septations (*arrow*) characteristic of LM. Axial STIR image (*B*) and axial T1WI (*C*) shows a fluid–fluid level (*arrows*) and T1 shortening anteriorly due to hemorrhage and layering effect.

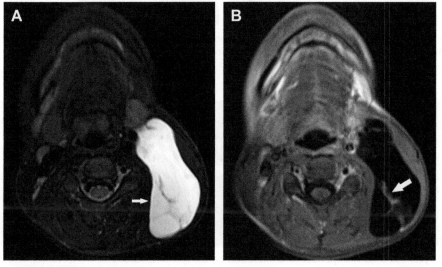

Fig. 19. A 2-year-old child with a left posterior lateral neck mass and LM. Axial STIR image (*A*) demonstrates a homogeneous cystic mass with internal septations (*arrow*), which enhance on the axial postgadolinium fat-saturated T1WI (*B*) (*arrow*).

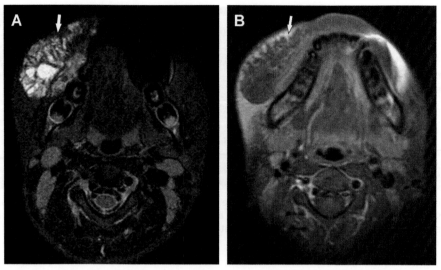

Fig. 20. A 3-year-old with right neck mass and LM. Axial STIR image (*A*) at the level of the mandible demonstrates a microcystic component anteriorly (*arrow*). A macrocystic component is present posteriorly. Axial postgadolinium fat-saturated T1WI (*B*) shows enhancing septae within the microcystic component (*arrow*) giving a more solid appearance.

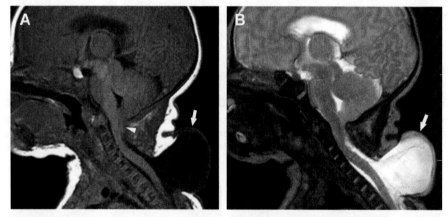

Fig. 21. Neonate with posterior cystic mass and meningocele. Sag T1WI (*A*) and T2WI (*B*) show a large fluid collection communicating with the dorsal cervical CSF space (*arrows*). There is an associated Chiari I deformity (*arrowhead*).

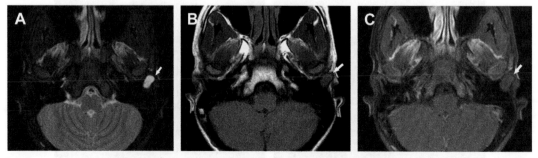

Fig. 22. A 3-year-old child with periauricular mass and type 1 first BCC. Axial STIR (*A*), T1WI (*B*), and postgadolinium fat-saturated T1WI (*C*) images demonstrate a homogeneous T1 and T2 hyperintense and nonenhancing cystic mass along the anterior superior cartilaginous external canal. A peripheral hypointense rim is present (*arrows*).

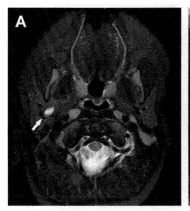
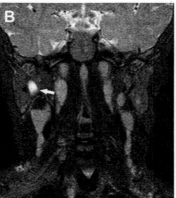
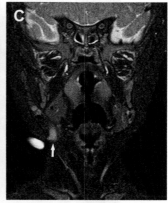

Fig. 23. A 5-year-old child with right cheek mass and type 2 first BCC. Axial STIR image (*A*) demonstrates a cyst anterior and inferior to the external canal within the deep lobe of the parotid gland (*arrow*). The cyst has surrounding low T2 signal. Coronal STIR images, posterior to anterior, (*B, C*) show the cyst to extend inferiorly into the right cheek at the mandibular angle (*arrows*). MR imaging marker denotes the palpable abnormality.

such as Goldenhar. Cholesteatomas may also be found and may be differentiated using diffusion-weighted imaging.[27,28] Multiple classification systems have been developed with the Work classification designating Type I as a duplicated external canal (**Fig. 22**) and type II extending anterior and inferior toward the angle of the mandible. Type I has only ectodermal elements and type II both ectoderm and mesoderm. With type II, presentation may be a cheek mass, and it is important to evaluate for an extension toward the external auditory canal (**Fig. 23**).[29] There does not seem to be a significant association with work type and postoperative facial nerve paralysis with newer classifications showing promise.[30,31]

MR imaging is optimal in these patients as the extent of the cyst can more easily be ascertained as well as the relationship with important regional structures including the parotid gland and expected location of the facial nerve, lateral to the retromandibular vein.[32] The cyst can have a thick wall, which is low signal on T2WIs, possibly relating to cartilaginous component.[6] First BCCs are surgically treated with facial nerve injury, a significant associated complication.[30] The differential in this region also includes parotid lymphoepithelial cyst and cystic pilomatricoma. Additionally, necrotic lymph nodes, and cystic neoplasms within and around the parotid may have a similar appearance (**Fig. 24**).[33]

First branchial cleft cyst
- Anterior and inferior to external auditory canal (maybe postauricular)
- Type 1 parallels external auditory canal
- Type 2 extends toward angle of mandible, may present with cheek mass

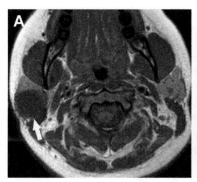
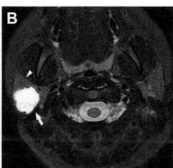
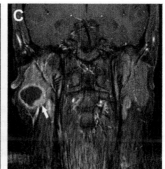

Fig. 24. A 15-year-old child with right parotid mass and cystic mucoepidermoid carcinoma. Axial T1WI (*A*), STIR (*B*) images demonstrates a cystic mass (*arrows*) within the superficial lobe of the right parotid gland (*arrowhead*). Coronal postgadolinium fat-saturated image T1WI (*C*) shows thick peripheral enhancement with concerning nodular enhancement inferiorly (*arrow*).

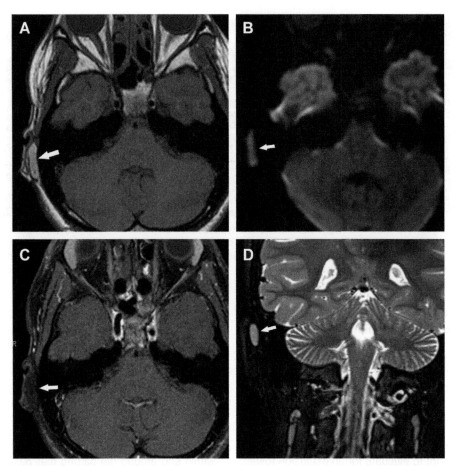

Fig. 25. A 9-year-old child with a postauricular mass and dermoid. Axial T1WI (*A*) and trace diffusion-weighted (*B*) image demonstrates a T1 hyperintense mass with increased signal on trace diffusion image and ADC values = 0.75×10^{-3} mm²/s (*arrows*). Signal suppression and no enhancement is present on postgadolinium fat-saturated T1WI (*C*) (*arrow*). Coronal fat-saturated T2WI (*D*) shows the cyst to be homogenously hyperintense (*arrow*).

Dermoid cyst

These likely result from a similar mechanism to first BCC formation and are due to defective closure of the first branchial cleft. They will have a similar appearance to dermoid cysts elsewhere. These tend to be postauricular as opposed to first BCCs being anterior. Diffusion weighted images are helpful in the diagnosis (Fig. 25).[11]

SUMMARY

Congenital cystic masses are encountered frequently when a child is referred for imaging of a neck mass and while congenital in origin these can present throughout childhood. An understanding of embryology related to common congenital cyst within the pediatric neck is necessary for diagnosis and formulating a narrow differential diagnosis. The thyroglossal duct, thymopharyngeal duct, as well as expected location of the different types of branchial anomalies are of paramount importance.

CLINICS CARE POINTS

- Congenital cystic neck masses are a commonly diagnosed in children with neck masses found on clinical examination.
- It is important to differentiate cystic from solid masses in the pediatric population.
- Location is critical in narrowing the differential diagnosis and knowledge of expected location of embryologic remnants is key to an appropriate diagnosis.
- Cystic masses such as LM and dermoid may occur in multiple locations with LMs commonly trans-spacial.

DISCLOSURE

The author has no disclosures.

REFERENCES

1. Bansal AG, Oudsema R, Masseaux JA, et al. US of pediatric superficial masses of the head and neck. Radiographics 2018;38:1239–63.
2. Sidell DR, Shapiro NL. Diagnostic accuracy of ultra-sonography for midline neck masses in children. Otolaryngol Head Neck Surg 2011;144(3):431–4.
3. Siegel MJ, Ramirez-Giraldo JC. Dual-energy CT in children: imaging algorithms and clinical applications. Radiology 2019;291:286–97.
4. Ho ML. Pediatric neck masses imaging guidelines and recommendations. Radiol Clin North Am 2022; 60:1–14.
5. Razek AA, Gaballa G, Elhawarey G, et al. Characterization of pediatric head and neck masses with diffusion-weighted MR imaging. Eur Radiol 2009;19. 210-208.
6. Buch K, Reinshagen KL, Juliano AF. MR imaging evaluation of pediatric neck masses: review and update. Magn Reason Imaging Clin N Am 2019;27:173–99.
7. Zander DA, Smoker WK. Imaging of ectopic thyroid tissue and thyroglossal duct cysts. Radiographics 2014;34:37–50.
8. Glastonbury CM, Davidson HC, Haller JR, et al. The CT and MR imaging features of carcinoma arising in thyroglossal duct remnants. AJNR Am J Neuroradiol 2000;21:770–4.
9. Corvino A, Pignata S, Campanino MR, et al. Thyroglossal duct cysts and site-specific differential diagnoses: imaging findings with emphasis on ultrasound assessment. J Ultrasound 2020;23(2):139–49.
10. Oomen K, Modi VK, Maddalozzo J. Thyroglossal duct cyst and ectopic thyroid. Otolaryngol Clin North Am 2015;48:15–27.
11. Orozco-Cocarrubias L, Lara-Carpio R, Saez-De-Ocariz M, et al. Dermoid cysts: a report of 75 pediatric patients. Pediatr Dermatol 2013;30(6):706–11.
12. Wong KT, Lee YP, King AD, et al. Imaging of cystic or cyst-like neck masses. Clin Radiol 2008;63:613–22.
13. Abdel Razek AAK, Sherif FM. Differentiation of sublingual thyroglossal duct cyst from midline dermoid cyst with diffusion weighted imaging. Int J Pediatr Otorhinolaryngol 2019;126:109623.
14. Kieran SM, Robson CD, Nose V, et al. Foregut duplication cysts in the head and neck. Arch Otolaryngol Head Neck Surg 2010;136(8):778–82.
15. Eaton D, Billings K, Timmons C, et al. Congenital foregut duplication cysts of the anterior tongue. Arch Otolaryngol Head Neck Surg 2001;127(12):1484–7.
16. Koch BL. Cystic malformations of the neck in children. Pediatr Radiol 2005;35:463–77.
17. Dallan I, Seccia V, Bruschini L, et al. Parapharyngeal cyst: considerations on embryology, clinical evaluation, and surgical management. J Craniofac Surg 2008;19(6):1487–90.
18. Smith PG, Dyches TJ, Loomis RA. Clinical aspects of branchio-oto-renal syndrome. Otolaryngol Head Neck Surg 1984;92(4):468–75.
19. Hudgins PA, Gillison M. Second branchial cleft cyst: not. AJNR Am J Neuroradiol 2009;30(9):1628–9.
20. Thomas B, Shroff M, Forte V, et al. Revisiting imaging features and the embryologic basis of third and fourth branchial anomalies. AJNR Am J Neuroradiol 2010;31(4):755–60.
21. Li Y, Mashhood A, Mamlouk MD, et al. Prenatal diagnosis of third and fourth branchial apparatus anomalies: case series and comparison with lymphatic malformation. AJNR Am J Neuroradiol 2021;42(11):2094–100.
22. Gezer HO, Oguzkurt P, Temiz A, et al. Huge neck masses causing respiratory distress in neonates: two cases of congenital cervical teratoma. Pediatr Neonatol 2014;57:526–30.
23. Kulungowski AM, Patel M. Lymphatic malformations. Semin Pediatr Surg 2020;29(5):150971.
24. Griauzde J, Srinivasan A. Imaging of vascular lesions of the head and neck. Radiol Cin N Am 2015;53:197–213.
25. De Leacy R, Bageac DV, Manna S, et al. A radiologic grading system for assessing the radiographic outcome of treatment in lymphatic and lymphatic-venous malformations of the head and neck. AJNR Am J Neuroradiol 2021;42:1859–64.
26. Adams A, Mankad K, Offiah C, et al. Branchial cleft anomalies: a pictorial review of embryologic development and spectrum of imaging findings. Insights Imaging 2016;7:69–76.
27. Liao EN, Chan DK. Congenital aural atresia and first branchial cleft anomalies: cholesteatoma and surgical management. Laryngoscope Investig Otolaryngol 2022;7:863–9.
28. Barkdull GC, Carvalho D. Goldenhar syndrome with external auditory canal stenosis complicated by canal cholesteatoma and first branchial cleft cyst. Int J Pediatr Otorhinolaryngol 2007;2(2):128–32.
29. Wilson J, Jaju A, Wadhwani N, et al. Reworking Classification of First Branchial Cleft Anomalies. Laryngoscope 2023. https://doi.org/10.1002/lary.30783.
30. Yang R, Dong C, Chen Y, et al. Analysis of the clinical features and surgical outcomes of first branchial cleft anomalies. Laryngoscope 2022;132(5):1008–14.
31. Pupic-Bakrac J, Skitarelic N, Novakovic J, et al. Patho-anatomic spectrum of branchial cleft anomalies: proposal of novel classification system. J Oral Maxillofac Surg 2022;80(2):341–8.
32. Mahore D, Mangalgiri AS, Namdev LN, et al. Variations of retromandibular vein and its relation to facial nerve within parotid gland. Indian J Otolaryngol Head Neck Surg 2018;70(3):395–7.
33. Kato H, Kawaguchi M, Ando T, et al. CT and MR imaging findings of non-neoplastic cystic lesions of the parotid gland. Jpn J Radiol 2019;37(9):627–35.

Solid and Vascular Neck Masses in Children

Mark D. Mamlouk, MD[a,b,*]

KEYWORDS

- Pediatric neck mass • Rhabdomyosarcoma • Neuroblastoma • Esthesioneuroblastoma
- Nasopharyngeal carcinoma • Juvenile nasal angiofibroma • Infantile hemangioma
- Venous malformation

KEY POINTS

- Neck masses are common in children, and solid and vascular lesions can have overlapping imaging patterns.
- The combination of the clinical presentation and imaging patterns can usually lead toward the diagnosis.
- Pediatric neck lesions with reduced diffusion reflect high cellularity and are an imaging feature that suggests malignant disease.

MALIGNANT TUMORS

Rhabdomyosarcoma

These malignant tumors are the most common soft tissue sarcoma of childhood and most commonly occur in the head and neck (Table 1).[1] There are four histologic subtypes: embryonal, alveolar, anaplastic, and mixed-type, and the embryonal subtype is the most common in children. Tumor locations in the head and neck are divided into parameningeal, non-parameningeal, and non-parameningeal orbital locations. Parameningeal locations consist of the paranasal sinuses, nasal cavity, nasopharynx, skull base area, mastoid process, infratemporal and pterygopalatine fossae, and the middle ear. Non-parameningeal sites consist of all other regions in the head and neck except the orbit, which is a separate category.[2] The clinical presentation is based on the tumor's location. Most rhabdomyosarcoma occur before 6 years of age but are uncommon in the first year of life,[3] and this time point can help differentiate between infantile hemangiomas which can occasionally be a mimicker on imaging.

At MR imaging, rhabdomyosarcomas demonstrate mild-to-intermediate T2 signal relative to muscle, variable enhancement, and occasionally have necrosis or flow voids. In addition, these masses can show hyperintense signal on arterial spin-labeled imaging (ASL) (Fig. 1). These imaging findings are similar to infantile hemangiomas; however, rhabdomyosarcomas typically show reduced diffusion, whereas infantile hemangiomas show facilitated diffusion.[4,5]

Neuroblastoma

Neuroblastoma is an embryonic tumor of the peripheral nervous system and is the most common extracranial solid tumor of childhood, although primary tumors of the neck are uncommon. The superior cervical sympathetic chain is where cervical tumors originate, and the clinical manifestations include a palpable mass, Horner syndrome, and pain.[6]

Imaging of cervical neuroblastomas reveals a mass in the posterior carotid space with variable adjacent lymphadenopathy. The lesions show intermediate T2 signal, marked enhancement, and

[a] Department of Radiology, The Permanente Medical Group, Kaiser Permanente Medical Center, 700 Lawrence Expy, Santa Clara, CA 95051, USA; [b] Department of Radiology and Biomedical Imaging, University of California, San Francisco, 505 Parnassus Avenue, L371, San Francisco, CA 94143, USA
* Department of Radiology, The Permanente Medical Group, Kaiser Permanente Medical Center, 700 Lawrence Expy, Santa Clara, CA 95051.
E-mail addresses: mark.d.mamlouk@kp.org; mark.mamlouk@ucsf.edu
Twitter: @MarkMamloukMD (M.D.M.)

Neuroimag Clin N Am 33 (2023) 607–621
https://doi.org/10.1016/j.nic.2023.05.010
1052-5149/23/© 2023 Elsevier Inc. All rights reserved.

Table 1
Clinical presentation and imaging patterns of pediatric solid and vascular neck masses

Lesion	General Info	Clinical Presentation	Head/Neck Location	Imaging Findings
Rhabdomyosarcoma	• Most common soft tissue sarcoma of childhood • Most commonly occur in the head and neck	• Based on tumor's location	• Parameningeal • Non-parameningeal • Orbital	• MR imaging: Intermediate T2 signal, variable enhancement, occasional necrosis or flow voids. In addition, high ASL signal
Neuroblastoma	• Primary tumors of the neck are uncommon • Metastases are relatively more common	• Palpable mass • Horner syndrome • Pain	• Cervical tumors: posterior carotid space • Metastases: skull base, calvarium, orbit	• MR imaging: Intermediate T2 signal, marked enhancement, reduced diffusion
Esthesioneuroblastoma	• Malignant tumor of neural crest cells of olfactory mucosa	• Nasal obstruction • Epistaxis	• Nasal cavity, cribriform plate, intracranial extension	• Dumbbell-shaped mass with a "waist" at the cribriform plate • CT: Osseous remodeling and erosion; calcifications uncommonly • MR imaging: Intermediate to hyperintense T2 signal, avid enhancement, mild reduced diffusion
Nasopharyngeal carcinoma	• Rare epithelial origin tumor • Epstein–Barr virus and other risk factors	• Usually clinically silent • Headache, nasal obstruction, epistaxis, conductive hearing loss with middle ear effusions, cranial neuropathies	• Lateral pharyngeal recess • Retropharyngeal and cervical nodes	• MR imaging: T2 hyperintense, heterogenous enhancement, reduced diffusion

Juvenile nasal angiofibroma	• Benign aggressive tumor • Highly vascular • Adolescent males	• Originates at sphenopalatine foramen; spreads to pterygopalatine fossa, nasal cavity, infratemporal fossa	• Nasal obstruction • Epistaxis	• CT: Solid mass, osseous remodeling and erosion • MR imaging: Mild T2 hyperintense signal, low signal from fibrous components, avid enhancement, flow voids, internal maxillary artery supply
Pilomatricoma	• Benign skin tumor of hair matrix • Very commonly excised	• Cutaneous and subcutaneous	• Firm, bluish-red	• US: Well-circumscribed, heterogenous, peripheral hypoechoic and hypervascular rim, calcification and posterior acoustic shadowing • MR imaging: Mixed T2 signal, heterogenous enhancement, facilitated diffusion
Pyogenic granuloma	• Also known as lobular capillary hemangioma • Spontaneous or after trauma	• Cheek, forehead, mucous membranes	• Small red exophytic papules	• MR imaging: Small, pedunculated, mixed T2 signal, marked enhancement
Infantile hemangioma	• Most common vascular tumor of infancy	• Cutaneous/subcutaneous • Facial, orbital, internal auditory canals, and airway in PHACE syndrome	• Bright red • Characteristic lifecycle: absent at birth, proliferate, involute	• US: Solid, well-circumscribed, mixed echogenicity, highly vascular • MR imaging: T2 hyperintense, enhancing, flow voids, high ASL signal
Kaposiform hemangioendothelioma	• Locally aggressive tumor	• Superficial and deep spaces	• Infiltrative reddish-purple skin lesion • Kasabach–Merritt phenomenon	• MR imaging: T2 hyperintense, enhancing, ill-defined and infiltrative

(continued on next page)

Table 1
(continued)

Lesion	General Info	Clinical Presentation	Head/Neck Location	Imaging Findings
Venous malformation	• Most common vascular malformation	• Soft with bluish hue • Enlarge with Valsalva • Hard nodules represent phleboliths	• Subcutaneous tissues, muscles, bones	• US: heterogenous or hypoechoic, tubular vascular spaces, minimal vascular flow • MR imaging: spongiform, T2 hyperintense, homogenous vs heterogenous enhancement due to slow flow, fills in on delayed phases, phleboliths
Lymphatic malformation	• Second most common vascular malformation	• Soft, translucent, fluid-filled, bluish hue • Enlarge with underlying infections	• Cervicofacial • Oral cavity and airway	• Macro or microcystic • US: Multiseptated transpatial cysts • MR imaging: T2 hyperintense, no to mild peripheral enhancement

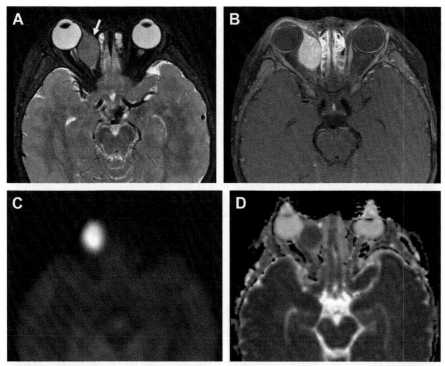

Fig. 1. Orbital rhabdomyosarcoma in a 3-year-old boy. (A) Axial T2-weighted fat-suppressed images show a solid isointense lesion in the right medial orbital soft tissues (arrow). (B) Axial contrast-enhanced T1-weighted fat-suppressed image shows homogenous enhancement. (C) Axial arterial spin-labeled image shows avid hyperintense signal. These imaging characteristics can mimic an infantile hemangioma, but the axial apparent diffusion coefficient image (D) shows low signal related to the high tumor cellularity.

reduced diffusion due to the high cellularity (Fig. 2). Calcification, hemorrhage, and necrosis may also be seen.[7] Tumors can encase vessels and extend to the skull base.

Although cervical neuroblastomas are rare, metastases within the head and neck are relatively more common, particularly the skull base, calvarium, and orbit. Metastases to the orbit can result in "raccoon eyes" due to obstruction of ophthalmic and facial veins and can mimic nonaccidental trauma.[6] CT imaging shows an expansile osteolytic lesion with "hair-on-end" periosteal reaction.[8] I-123 metaiodobenzylguanidine serves as an integral functional imaging test for metastatic disease.

Esthesioneuroblastoma

Esthesioneuroblastoma is a malignant tumor arising from neural crest cells of the olfactory

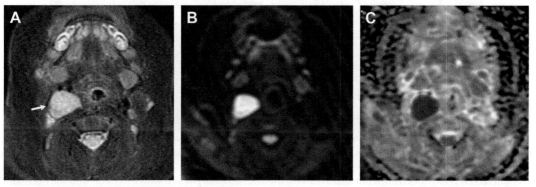

Fig. 2. Cervical neuroblastoma. (A) Axial T2-weighted fat-suppressed image shows an isointense mass in the right retropharyngeal space (arrow). (B, C) Axial diffusion-weighted imaging and apparent diffusion coefficient show marked reduced diffusion within the lesion.

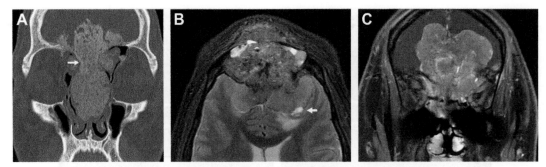

Fig. 3. Esthesioneuroblastoma in a 21-year-old man. (*A*) Coronal CT shows a heavily calcified mass throughout the nasal cavity and frontal lobes with a waist-like appearance at the cribriform plate (*arrow*), which is eroded. The diffuse calcification in this lesion was atypical. (*B*) Axial T2-weighted fat-suppressed image shows a small intratumoral cyst at the periphery of the lesion (*arrow*) with adjacent vasogenic edema. (*C*) Coronal contrast-enhanced T1-weighted image shows diffuse enhancement.

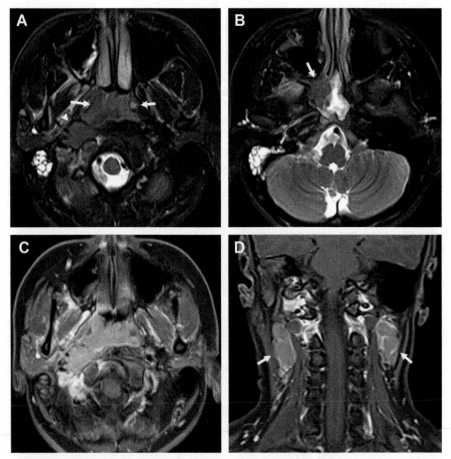

Fig. 4. Nasopharyngeal carcinoma in a 16-year-old girl who presented with right ear pain and effusion and lymphadenopathy. (*A, B*) Axial T2-weighted fat-suppressed images show a solid mass (*arrows, A*) centered in the right lateral pharyngeal recess but also involving the left nasopharynx and with extension into the right sphenoid sinus (*arrow, B*). Right retropharyngeal node present (*arrowhead, A*). (*C, D*) Axial and coronal contrast-enhanced T1-weighted fat-suppressed images show diffuse enhancement of the mass as well as bilateral cervical lymph nodes (*arrows, D*).

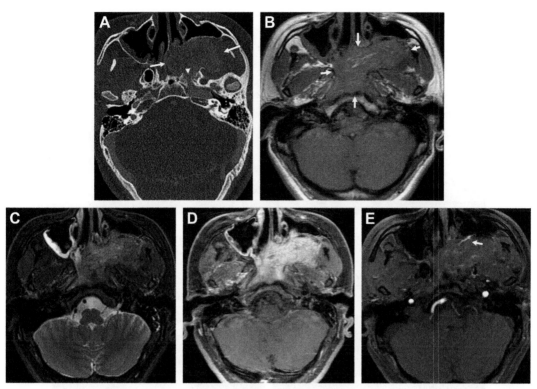

Fig. 5. Juvenile angiofibroma in an 18-year-old man presenting with epistaxis. (A) Axial contrast-enhanced CT shows a solid mass (*arrows*) involving the left sphenopalatine foramen with associated osseous destruction, bowing of the maxillary antrum, and widening of the foramen of rotundum (*arrowhead*). (B) Axial pre-contrast T1-weighted image shows the lesion (*arrows*) is predominantly isointense to muscle. The lesion shows iso to hypointense T2 signal (C) and diffuse enhancement (D). (E) Axial time-of-flight MRA shows the arterial nature of the lesion (*arrow*).

mucosa at the cribriform plate. Lesions are rare in children, but there is a bimodal incidence of disease in the 2nd and 6th decades, and unilateral nasal obstruction and epistaxis are the most common presenting symptoms. Cervical nodal metastases are often present at the time of the discovery.[8]

Esthesioneuroblastomas classically show an expansile dumbbell-shaped nasal cavity mass with a "waist" at the cribriform plate and with intra-cranial tumor extension. CT shows osseous remodeling of the olfactory recess and erosion of the cribriform plate. Scattered calcifications are an uncommon feature. At MR imaging, the mass shows intermediate to hyperintense T2 signal with avid enhancement and mild reduced diffu-sion. Cysts can be present at the tumor–brain interface, a highly suggestive feature of esthesio-neuroblastomas, and there is often vasogenic edema (Fig. 3).[8]

Nasopharyngeal Carcinoma

Pediatric nasopharyngeal carcinoma is a rare epithelial origin tumor but with a predilection for

adolescents and teenagers. Epstein–Barr virus is a well-established risk factor, but human papil-loma virus, genetics, and environmental expo-sures to carcinogens may also be contributory. There are three tumor subtypes: keratinizing squamous cell carcinoma, nonkeratinizing squa-mous cell carcinoma, and undifferentiated carci-noma, with the last subtype most commonly occurring in the pediatric population. Tumors arise from the epithelial mucosa of the pharyngeal recess, and the majority often manifest at a locally advanced stage because they are clinically silent. When symptomatic, headache, nasal obstruc-tion, epistaxis, conductive hearing loss with mid-dle ear effusions, and cranial neuropathies may occur.[9]

At MR imaging, the tumors are T2 hyperin-tense and show heterogenous enhancement (Fig. 4). Reduced diffusion is also commonly pre-sent. Tumor spread may occur to the pterygopa-latine fossa, parapharyngeal and masticator spaces, cavernous sinus and cranial nerves, skull base, and retropharyngeal and cervical lymph nodes.[9]

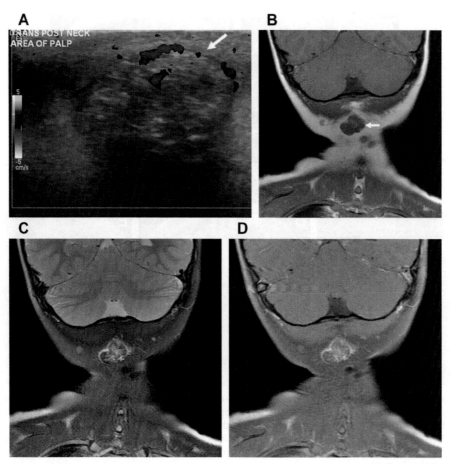

Fig. 6. Pilomatricoma in a 5-year-old boy. (*A*) Transverse sonogram with color Doppler shows a solid heterogenous mass with peripheral border that is hypoechoic and hypervascular (*arrow*). Posterior acoustic shadowing is also observed. (*B*) Coronal precontrast T1-weighted image shows a hypointense lesion (*arrow*). (*C*) Coronal T2-weighted fat suppressed image shows predominantly hypointense signal. (*D*) Coronal contrast-enhanced T1-weighted fat-suppressed image shows mixed enhancement, including the border.

VASCULAR TUMORS
Juvenile Nasal Angiofibroma

These benign aggressive tumors are highly vascular and occur in adolescent males. Clinically, most patients present with nasal obstruction and epistaxis. These lesions are centered in the posterior nasal cavity and arise at the sphenopalatine foramen. The tumors can grow into all directions but frequently extends laterally into the pterygopalatine

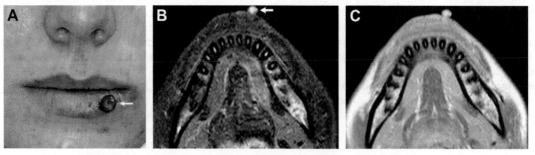

Fig. 7. Pyogenic granuloma in a 16-year-old girl. (*A*) Clinical photograph shows an exophytic red papule of the left lower lip (*arrow*). (*B*) Axial T2-weighted fat-suppressed images show T2 hyperintense signal (*arrow*), and the axial contrast-enhanced T1-weighted image (*C*) shows corresponding enhancement.

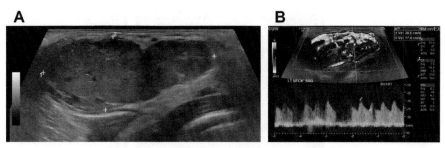

Fig. 8. Infantile hemangioma. (*A*) Grayscale ultrasound shows a solid well-circumscribed lesion (*calipers*) with mixed echogenicity. (*B*) Color Doppler shows high vessel density with high-systolic flow and low-resistance waveforms (*calipers*).

fossa, anteriorly into the nasal cavity, or inferolaterally in the infratemporal fossa via the pterygomaxillary fissure. Intracranial extension can occur.[8]

CT and MR imaging are often complementary for diagnosis and treatment planning. At CT imaging, a destructive soft tissue mass is observed with either osseous remodeling or erosion of the paranasal sinus walls, orbits, and skull base. On MR imaging, lesions show mild T2 hyperintense signal with areas of low signal secondary to fibrous components. Flow voids can be present, and there is avid enhancement after contrast administration (Fig. 5). Owing to the highly vasculature nature of the lesion, digital subtraction angiography is often performed for preoperative embolization, and arterial supply is most commonly from the internal maxillary artery.[8]

Pilomatricoma

Pilomatricomas are benign skin tumors that arise from the hair matrix and are the second most

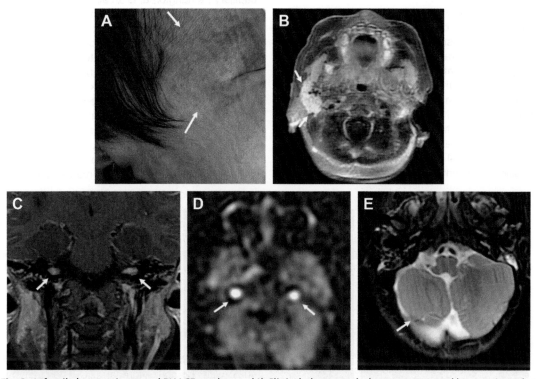

Fig. 9. Infantile hemangioma and PHACE syndrome. (*A*) Clinical photograph shows a segmental hemangioma (*arrows*) in the right S1 distribution. (*B*) Axial contrast-enhanced fat-suppressed T1-weighted image shows a right parotid hemangioma (*arrows*). (*C*) Coronal contrast-enhanced fat-suppressed T1-weighted image shows bilateral internal auditory canal hemangiomas (*arrows*). (*D*) Axial arterial spin-labeled image shows hyperintense signal within the internal auditory canals (*arrows*). (*E*) Axial T2-weighted fat-suppressed image shows right cerebellar hemisphere dysgenesis (*arrow*).

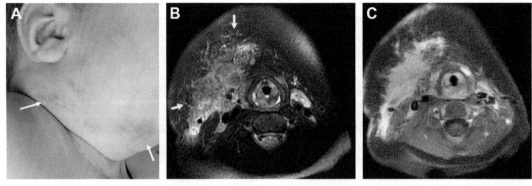

Fig. 10. Kaposiform hemangioendothelioma. (*A*) Clinical photograph shows red macules in the right neck (*arrows*). (*B*) Axial T2-weighted fat-suppressed image shows an ill-defined hyperintense lesion (*arrows*) involving the cutaneous and subcutaneous tissues. The infiltrative pattern is a classical feature of this lesion. (*C*) Axial contrast-enhanced T1-weighted fat-suppressed image shows avid enhancement.

commonly excised pediatric skin mass, after epidermoid cysts. The head and neck are very common sites for pilomatricomas, and on physical examination, these lesions are firm subcutaneous nodules that can contain bluish-red discoloration and mimic a vascular anomaly. Lesions are typically encountered in patients younger than 20 years of age.[10,11]

Imaging uncommonly occurs because the clinical diagnosis is often straightforward or another benign lesion is suspected, but when needed for confirmation, ultrasound is the initial examination. These well-circumscribed lesions show heterogenous echoes with a peripheral hypoechoic and hypervascular rim. Shadowing can be seen from calcifications and mimic a phlebolith in a venous malformation. At MR imaging, there is often mixed T2 signal with areas of low signal, along with peripheral or central enhancement (Fig. 6). Reduced diffusion is absent in these lesions.[10] The low T2

signal within the lesion is another imaging feature to help distinguish from venous malformations, which show high T2 signal.[12]

Pyogenic Granuloma

Pyogenic granuloma, also known as lobular capillary hemangioma, is an acquired benign proliferation of capillaries in the skin or mucous membranes that commonly occur in childhood or pregnancy. They can either occur spontaneously or after trauma and are thought to represent an inflammatory hyperplasia. Within the head and neck, lesions can be seen in the cheek, forehead, and at mucous membranes and are red exophytic papules less than 1 to 2.5 cm in diameter.[13]

Imaging is often unnecessary for pyogenic granulomas based on the distinctive clinical appearance. If imaging is performed, lesions are pedunculated, hypoechoic, and markedly vascular

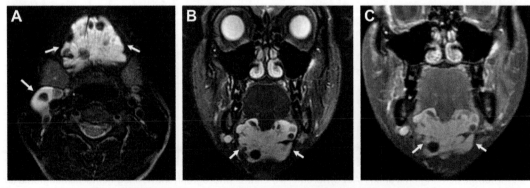

Fig. 11. Venous malformations in an 18-year-old girl. (*A, B*) Axial and coronal T2-weighted fat-suppressed images show spongiform venous malformations in the bilateral floor of mouth and right carotid spaces (*arrows*). Multiple round hypointensities are seen and represent phleboliths. (*C*) Coronal contrast-enhanced T1-weighted fat-suppressed image shows homogenous enhancement of the lesion (*arrows*), with the exception of the phleboliths.

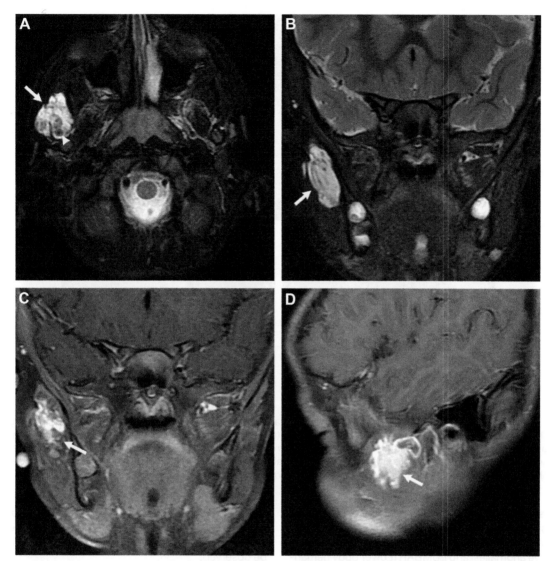

Fig. 12. Intramuscular venous malformation. (*A, B*) Axial and coronal T2-weighted fat-suppressed images show a spongiform intramuscular right masseteric lesion that is predominantly hyperintense (*arrows*). Small phleboliths are seen (*arrowhead, A*). (*C, D*) Coronal and sagittal contrast-enhanced T1-weighted fat-suppressed images show heterogenous enhancement in (*C, arrow*). The later acquired sagittal sequence (*D*) shows increased enhancement within the lesion (*arrow*) and is reflective of the slow filling venous nature of the lesion.

on ultrasound,[14] whereas MR imaging show heterogeneously hyperintense T2 signal and marked enhancement (Fig. 7).[15]

Infantile Hemangiomas

Infantile hemangiomas are the most common vascular tumor of infancy and present clinically as bright red lesions when superficial in location, whereas the deep lesions can have a bluish hue or are skin colored. These lesions have a characteristic life: typically absent at birth, usually present in the first month of life, undergo rapid growth up

to the first year, and regress over multiple years. Deep hemangiomas can manifest slightly later—most often by 2 to 3 months of life—and have a proliferative phase of growth up to 18 months, followed by regression.[16,17] Recognizing hemangioma's lifecycle is important when encountering a new lesion clinically and radiologically to not ascribe this diagnosis in an older patient.

Imaging of infantile hemangiomas is usually unnecessary given their typical clinical and physical examination characteristics. Imaging may help if the diagnosis is uncertain, for deep lesions, to monitor treatment response, or if the hemangioma

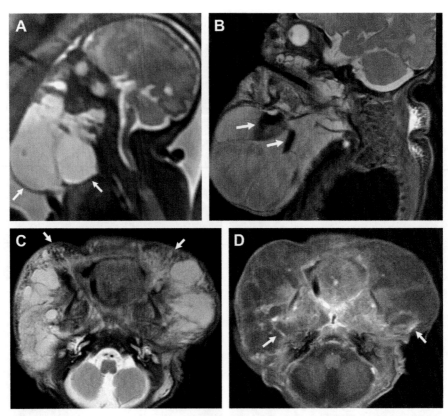

Fig. 13. Lymphatic malformation on fetal and postnatal imaging. (*A*) Sagittal T2-weighted fetal MR imaging shows a large multiseptated cervicofacial mass (*arrows*). (*B*) Sagittal T2-weighted fat-suppressed postnatal MR imaging shows the mass with fluid-hemorrhage levels (*arrows*) within macrocysts, and the axial T2-weighted fat-suppressed image (*C*) shows microcysts (*arrows*). (*D*) Axial contrast-enhanced T1-weighted fat-suppressed images show minimal peripheral enhancement of the lesion (*arrows*).

is segmental and part of an underlying syndrome such as PHACE (Posterior fossa anomalies, Hemangiomas, Arteriopathies, Cardiac abnormalities, Eye anomalies) and LUMBAR (Lower body hemangioma, Urogenital anomalies, Ulceration, Myelopathy, Bony deformities, Anorectal malformations, Arteriopathies, and Renal anomalies). In the context of PHACE syndrome, facial and orbital hemangiomas are most commonly seen; however, intracranial lesions within the auditory canal can be observed. Hemangiomas involving the airway are a less common manifestation but should be scrutinized on the imaging evaluation.

Ultrasound is the preferred first-line imaging modality for hemangiomas, and the lesions usually are subcutaneous, solid, well-circumscribed, and show mixed echogenicity. Vascular interrogation typically shows high vessel density (>5 cm^2), systolic flow greater than 2 kHz, and low-resistance waveforms (Fig. 8).[18] At MR imaging, lesions show T2 hyperintense signal, homogenous contrast enhancement, and flow voids (Fig. 9). Time-resolved contrast-enhanced MR angiography/ venography shows early enhancement, and arterial spin-labeled MR imaging shows avid hyperintense signal.[19] After the hemangioma involutes, fat can be observed.

Kaposiform Hemangioendothelioma

These lesions are locally aggressive tumors that occur throughout the body, and in particular, the neck. Classically, these masses are associated with a consumptive coagulopathy called Kasabach–Merritt phenomenon. Nearly all lesions present in infancy, and the majority present in the first month of life. On physical examination, lesions either manifest as solitary nodules or infiltrating plaques with a reddish-purple hue.[20]

Imaging of kaposiform hemangioendotheliomas characteristically shows an ill-defined and infiltrative lesion that contrasts with the well-defined infantile hemangiomas. At MR imaging, the lesions show T2 hyperintense and enhancing signal that crosses tissues planes (Fig. 10). Differential diagnoses also with an ill-defined pattern include

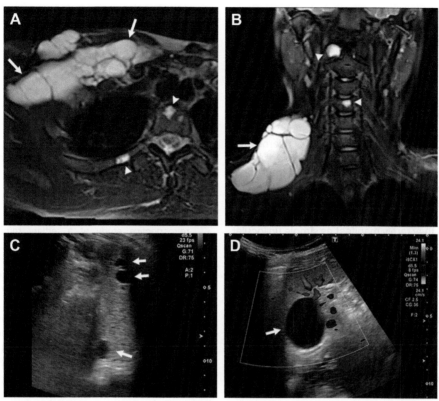

Fig. 14. Lymphatic malformations in generalized lymphatic anomaly. (*A, B*) Axial and coronal T2-weighted fat-suppressed images show a right supraclavicular macrocystic lymphatic malformation (*arrows*). Hyperintense lesions are also present in the ribs and vertebral bodies (*arrowheads*) that are consistent with intraosseous lymphatic malformations. (*C, D*) Gray and color Doppler sonographic images of the spleen show anechoic avascular cysts (*arrows*) that are consistent with visceral lymphatic malformations.

infantile myofibromatosis, microcystic lymphatic malformation, and cellulitis.[12]

VASCULAR MALFORMATIONS
Venous Malformation

Venous malformations are the most common vascular malformation and can occur anywhere in the body, including the head/neck. On physical examination, the lesions are soft and often show a bluish hue, and the masses can enlarge with Valsalva. Hard nodules can be occasionally palpated within venous malformations and represent phleboliths.[13]

Venous malformations may either manifest as ectatic veins or solid masses, which can occur in the subcutaneous tissues, muscles, bones, or solid organs. The sonographic appearance of the solid forms is heterogenous or hypoechoic and often contains tubular vascular spaces with minimal vascular flow. At MR imaging, T2 hyperintense signal is observed in a spongiform-like appearance, and if a phlebolith is present, they demonstrate

low signal on all pulse sequences (Fig. 11). The presence of a phlebolith is essentially pathognomonic for a venous malformation.[13] Fluid-hemorrhage levels may also be present, which are also observed in lymphatic malformations. After contrast administration, venous malformations can show either homogenous or heterogenous enhancement, and the malformation can show progressively increased enhancement on successive MR imaging sequences or dynamic magnetic resonance angiography/magnetic resonance venography (MRA/MRV) due to slow flow (Fig. 12). Because venous malformations may have this incomplete pattern of enhancement, the term "venolymphatic" is sometimes misappropriately used, as most malformations are either venous or lymphatic.[21] Although true mixed malformations can occur, they occur less commonly.

Lymphatic Malformation

These lesions represent the second most common vascular malformation and have a high predilection for the cervicofacial and axillary locations. The oral cavity and airway are frequent sites of disease and may result in obstructive sleep apnea and respiratory compromise. At physical examination, lymphatic malformations are soft, translucent, fluid-filled and can show a bluish hue and enlarge with underlying infections.[13]

On ultrasound, lesions have multiple septations and are often trans-spatial and lack vascular flow. Lesions are referred to macro- or microcystic depending on the cyst. No uniform consensus exists on characterizing these subtypes, but some investigators suggest the term macrocystic to be used if the lesion is large enough to be aspirated or sclerosed.[22] Although lymphatic malformations are cystic, they rarely manifest as simple unilocular cysts, and if present, another diagnosis such as ciliated cyst should be considered.[23] At MR imaging, lesions show T2 hyperintense signal and fluid-hemorrhage levels (Fig. 13). Lesions typically do not enhance, although peripheral enhancement may be observed in macrocysts, and mild diffuse enhancement can be seen in microcysts; however, one tip to accurately evaluate enhancement is to also obtain a pre-contrast T1 sequence with fat suppression to have an accurate comparison with the routine contrast-enhanced T1 fat-suppressed sequence.[24] Misperceiving a lesion as enhancing may incorrectly diagnose a lesion as a venous rather than lymphatic malformation.

If lymphatic malformations also occur systemically throughout the body, they may represent one of the four complex lymphatic anomalies: Gorham-Stout disease, generalized lymphatic anomaly, kaposiform lymphangiomatosis, and central collecting lymphatic anomaly (Fig. 14).[25]

SUMMARY

Solid and vascular neck masses comprise a wide range of congenital and acquired lesions that are either benign or malignant. The clinical presentation and imaging patterns can lead toward the diagnosis in many cases.

CLINICS CARE POINTS

- Neck masses are common in children, and solid and vascular lesions can have overlapping imaging patterns.
- The combination of the clinical presentation and imaging patterns can usually lead toward the diagnosis.

DISCLOSURE

None.

FUNDING

None.

REFERENCES

1. Torsiglieri AJ Jr, Tom LW, Ross AJ 3rd, et al. Pediatric neck masses: guidelines for evaluation. Int J Pediatr Otorhinolaryngol 1988;16:199–210.
2. Häußler SM, Stromberger C, Olze H, et al. Head and neck rhabdomyosarcoma in children: a 20-year retrospective study at a tertiary referral center. J Cancer Res Clin Oncol 2018;144:371–9.
3. Malempati S, Rodeberg DA, Donaldson SS, et al. Rhabdomyosarcoma in infants younger than 1 year: a report from the Children's Oncology Group. Cancer 2011;117:3493–501.
4. Kralik SF, Haider KM, Lobo RR, et al. Orbital infantile hemangioma and rhabdomyosarcoma in children: differentiation using diffusion-weighted magnetic resonance imaging. Journal of AAPOS 2018;22:27–31.
5. Mamlouk MD, Nicholson AD, Cooke DL, et al. Diffusion-weighted imaging for cutaneous vascular anomalies. Clin Imag 2017;46:121–2.
6. Swift CC, Eklund MJ, Kraveka JM, et al. Updates in Diagnosis, Management, and Treatment of Neuroblastoma. Radiographics 2018;38:566–80.
7. Chen AM, Trout AT, Towbin AJ. A review of neuroblastoma image-defined risk factors on magnetic resonance imaging. Pediatr Radiol 2018;48:1337–47.
8. Rodriguez DP, Orscheln ES, Koch BL. Masses of the Nose, Nasal Cavity, and Nasopharynx in Children. Radiographics 2017;37:1704–30.
9. Orman G, Tran BH, Desai N, et al. Neuroimaging Characteristics of Nasopharyngeal Carcinoma in Children. J Neuroimaging 2021;31:137–43.
10. Bulman JC, Ulualp SO, Rajaram V, et al. Pilomatricoma of Childhood: A Common Pathologic Diagnosis Yet a Rare Radiologic One. AJR American journal of roentgenology 2016;206:182–8.
11. Hassanein AH, Alomari AI, Schmidt BA, et al. Pilomatrixoma imitating infantile hemangioma. J Craniofac Surg 2011;22:734–6.
12. Mamlouk MD, Danial C, McCullough WP. Vascular anomaly imaging mimics and differential diagnoses. Pediatr Radiol 2019;49:1088–103.
13. Merrow AC, Gupta A, Patel MN, et al. 2014 Revised Classification of Vascular Lesions from the International Society for the Study of Vascular Anomalies: Radiologic-Pathologic Update. Radiographics 2016;36:1494–516.

14. Lee GK, Suh KJ, Lee JH, et al. Lobular capillary hemangioma in the soft tissue of the finger: sonographic findings. Skeletal Radiol 2010;39:1097–102.

15. Yang BT, Li SP, Wang YZ, et al. Routine and dynamic MR imaging study of lobular capillary hemangioma of the nasal cavity with comparison to inverting papilloma. Am J Neuroradiol 2013;34:2202–7.

16. Frieden IJ, Rogers M, Garzon MC. Conditions masquerading as infantile haemangioma: Part 1. Australas J Dermatol 2009;50:77–97. quiz 8.

17. Smith CJF, Friedlander SF, Guma M, et al. Infantile Hemangiomas: An Updated Review on Risk Factors, Pathogenesis, and Treatment. Birth Defects Research 2017;109:809–15.

18. Dubois J, Patriquin HB, Garel L, et al. Soft-tissue hemangiomas in infants and children: diagnosis using Doppler sonography. Am J Roentgenol 1998;171:247–52.

19. Mamlouk MD, Hess CP. Arterial spin-labeled perfusion for vascular anomalies in the pediatric head and neck. Clin Imag 2016;40:1040–6.

20. Croteau SE, Liang MG, Kozakewich HP, et al. Kaposiform hemangioendothelioma: atypical features and risks of Kasabach-Merritt phenomenon in 107 referrals. J Pediatr 2013;162:142–7.

21. Greene AK. Vascular anomalies: current overview of the field. Clin Plast Surg 2011;38:1–5.

22. Wassef M, Blei F, Adams D, et al. Vascular Anomalies Classification: Recommendations From the International Society for the Study of Vascular Anomalies. Pediatrics 2015;136:e203–14.

23. White CL, Olivieri B, Restrepo R, et al. Low-Flow Vascular Malformation Pitfalls: From Clinical Examination to Practical Imaging Evaluation–Part 1, Lymphatic Malformation Mimickers. AJR American journal of roentgenology 2016;206:940–51.

24. Mamlouk MD, Nicholson AD, Cooke DL, et al. Tips and tricks to optimize MRI protocols for cutaneous vascular anomalies. Clin Imag 2017;45:71–80.

25. Ricci KW, Iacobas I. How we approach the diagnosis and management of complex lymphatic anomalies. Pediatr Blood Cancer 2022;69(Suppl 3):e28985.

Neuroimaging of Ocular Abnormalities in Children

Berna Aygun, MBBS, MRes, FRCR[a,b,*], Asthik Biswas, MBBS, DNB[b],
Ajay Taranath, MBBS, MD, FRANZCR[c], Harun Yildiz, MD[d],
Sri Gore, MBBS, BSc, FRCOphth PGDip Ed[e], Kshitij Mankad, MBBS, FRCR[b,f]

KEYWORDS

- Ocular malignancy • Intraocular lesions • Ocular congenital malformations
- Anterior segment defects • Posterior segment defects • MR imaging • Neuroimaging

KEY POINTS

- Many of the pediatric ocular abnormalities including malignancies and benign tumor mimics have overlapping features at presentation and may coexist. Furthermore, clinical examination may be limited in the presence of associated complications such as retinal detachment, vitreous hemorrhage, or congenital cataracts.
- Radiological evaluation provides additional information to confirm diagnosis and assess the extent of disease, especially in case of retinoblastoma (the most common pediatric ocular malignancy) to plan management.
- Assessment of the complex ocular anatomy especially in pediatrics with ocular abnormalities requires having a tailored approach on imaging and a dedicated protocol for optimizing image quality and increasing sensitivity.

INTRODUCTION

This article deals with congenital lesions involving the pediatric globe. A sizable proportion of children with ocular lesions present with leukocoria, that is, loss of the normal red reflex. Although the diagnosis may be established clinically in a large number, imaging is required for further staging (particularly in retinoblastoma), to delineate the extent of abnormality, and to assess associated anomalies.

Ultrasound (US) and magnetic resonance (MR) imaging constitute supplementary first-line imaging modalities in clinical practice. US A-scan (A = amplitude) forms an amplitude graph of various interfaces helping to identify and characterize some of the masses, whereas US B-scan (B = brightness) transmits sonographic waves at higher frequencies creating an image of the orbit. Indeed, in many instances, the clinical question can be answered with the help of US alone (eg, diagnosis of persistent fetal vasculature). MR imaging offers exquisite soft tissue resolution, and the ability to evaluate the retro-orbital region and intracranial cavity. MR imaging is also superior in evaluating disease spread beyond the ocular margins. Furthermore, it aids with the detection of associated intracranial anomalies that are frequently coexistent with congenital ocular lesions.

The anatomy of the eye is complex and composed of multiple small structures. Optimizing MR imaging protocol is pivotal to increase

[a] Department of Neuroradiology, King's College Hospital NHS Foundation Trust, London, UK; [b] Department of Neuroradiology, Great Ormond Street Hospital for Children NHS Foundation Trust, London, UK; [c] Department of Medical Imaging, Women's and Children's Hospital, South Australia Medical Imaging, University of Adelaide, South Australia, Australia; [d] Department of Radiology, Bursa Dortcelik Children's Hospital, Bursa, Turkey; [e] Department of Ophthalmology, Great Ormond Street Hospital for Children NHS Foundation Trust, London, UK; [f] UCL GOS Institute of Child Health
* Corresponding author. Department of Neuroradiology, King's College Hospital NHS Foundation Trust, Ruskin Wing, Ground Floor, London SE59RS.
E-mail address: berna.aygun2@nhs.net

Neuroimag Clin N Am 33 (2023) 623–641
https://doi.org/10.1016/j.nic.2023.05.011

diagnostic accuracy. We propose an imaging protocol here with justification of sequences used, applicable both to 1.5 T and 3T systems as listed in Table 1.[1] Computed tomography (CT) can offer added advantages because it is readily available and extremely sensitive in the detection of calcification. However, radiation risk limits its use. F-18 fluorodeoxyglucose positron emission tomography has numerous applications in orbital imaging but it is seldom used in ocular disease.

The sections of this review are structured in this manner to enable the reader to understand salient anatomy, embryology, and pathologic conditions affecting the pediatric globe.

Ocular Anatomy

The eye is covered by a membranous conjunctiva and anatomically can be divided into 2 segments: anterior and posterior, separated by the lens (Fig. 1).

The conjunctiva
The conjunctiva is a thin continuous membranous structure that covers the inner most layer of the eyelids as well as the surface of the eye; these are called the palpebral and bulbar layer, respectively.

The key role of the conjunctiva is to protect the eye. It is rich in lymphoid tissue. There is also an abundance of goblet cells in the conjunctiva, which help to secret mucous of the tear film.

The junctions where bulbar and palpebral layers meet are called the fornices. These fornices are important attachment points of the Tenon's capsule (extension of the extraocular muscle sheath) to allow for ocular motion.[2]

Anterior segment
The cornea and sclera comprise the outer fibrous layer of the eye. The cornea is a transparent, avascular, highly innervated, dome-shaped structure, which forms the anterior layer of the outer coat of the eye. In addition to protecting the structures inside the eye, its high refractive index contributes to the overall refractive power of the optical system. The limbus is the transitional zone where the cornea is in continuity with the sclera.

The sclera is an avascular structure that forms the outer most layer of the eye deep to the conjunctiva. Posteriorly, it is contiguous with the insertion of the dura covering the optic nerve sheath complex.

Deep to the sclera is the vascular pigmented layer called the uveal tract. The anterior uveal tract is composed of the ciliary body and the iris. The iris separates the anterior segment into anterior and posterior chambers. These chambers are filled with a transparent fluid called aqueous humor.

The ciliary body is a muscular structure, which anchors and controls the lens curvature. It also has an essential role in secreting the aqueous humor for the anterior and posterior chambers.

Posterior segment
The posterior two-thirds of the eye, including the vitreous humor, retina, choroid, and optic nerve, make up the posterior segment of the eye. It is bounded anteriorly by the lens, is circumscribed

Table 1
MR imaging protocol recommendations for assessment of orbits for assessment of ocular pathology or retinoblastoma.

MR Imaging Sequences for Assessment of Ocular Abnormalities and Malignancies	Plane	Slice Thickness
T2WI TSE (+FS* if orbital extension suspected)	Axial and/or coronal	≤3 mm (≤2 mm for retinoblastoma)
T1WI TSE (+FS if orbital extension suspected)	Axial and/or coronal	≤3 mm (≤2 mm for retinoblastoma)
Post-contrast T1WI FS	Axial and/or coronal Sagittal oblique (ON-affected side only)	≤3 mm (≤2 mm for retinoblastoma)
Additional sequences		
SWI*	Axial	≤3 mm
Brain: T2 TSE/FLAIR and DWI*	Axial	≤3–4 mm
Brain: Postcontrast T1WI TSE	Sagittal	1 mm
Spine: Postcontrast T1WI	Sagittal	≤3 mm

* FS, fat-saturated; SWI, susceptibility weighted imaging; DWI, diffusion-weighted imaging.

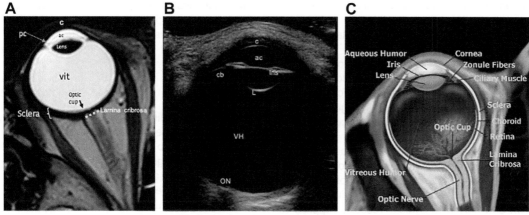

Fig. 1. *Normal anatomy of the eye. (A) Orbital MR imaging T2 sequence thin cross-section. (B) US-B scan of the normal eye. (C) Orbital anatomy.* The anterior chamber (ac) contains the aqueous humor that is T2 hyperintense. The ciliary body and iris are depicted as thin linear structures and difficult to appreciate on routine MR imaging better seen on US-B. The posterior chamber (pc) is the space behind the iris and in front of the lens and ciliary body (cb). Note that normal lens is T2 hypointense on MR imaging and thin echogenic structure on US separating the anterior and posterior segments of the eye. The sclera is seen as thick hypointense structure that is in continuity with the dome-shaped cornea (C). Vitreous is T2 hyperintense jelly-like fluid filling the posterior segment. Note that the inner posterior layers of the eye; the retina and choroid cannot be normally distinguished on routine US and MR imaging and is illustrated on Fig. 1C. The optic nerve exits through a collagenous mesh-like structure named lamina cribrosa that runs between the sclera.

by an outer layer of sclera, followed by an inner choroid and an inner most layer, the retina.

Choroid is the posterior component of the uveal tract and lies between the sclera and the retina. It is highly vascular and its main role is to supply the retina with nutrients. The macula fovea, which is responsible for central vision, lacks a retinal artery. Its only supply comes from the choroidal layer underneath. There are many layers to the choroid. Bruch's membrane runs immediately posterior to the retina and the basement membrane of the retinal pigment epithelium is formed by this layer. Just like the sclera, which is in contiguity with the dura posteriorly, the choroid is in continuity with the arachnoid and pia mater of the optic nerve sheath complex.

The retina is derived from the neuroectoderm and consists of the inner photoreceptors, inner and outer plexiform layers, ganglionic cells, and the outer layer of retinal pigment epithelium.

The macula, which is the main focal point of the retina where the refracted optic arrays from the cornea are focused on, lies approximately 3 mm lateral to the optic nerve head.[2,3]

Development of the Eye

The early signaling for the formation of the eye starts as early as gastrulation (day 22) wherein the bilaminar disc becomes trilaminar (ectoderm, mesoderm, and endoderm). Later the ectoderm reorganizes into two main structures: surface ectoderm and neural ectoderm. This process is controlled by a structure called notochord created during neurulation.

During neurulation, the signals from the notochord instigate a central groove formation within the ectoderm (ie, the neural groove). Adjacent to the central groove, there are neural folds that starts to fold over the neural groove creating a tube-like structure called the neural tube. The neural tube is the primitive central nervous system. It is situated below the surface ectoderm. The neural tube is surrounded by neural crest cells and mesoderm. The neural crest cells are detached lateral cell clusters derived from the ectoderm (also the future derivatives of cranial nerves, peripheral nervous system, and part of meninges).

There are three vesicles that develop from the neural tube. From cranial to caudal, these are the prosencephalon, mesencephalon, and rhombencephalon. The prosencephalon later gives rise to telencephalon and diencephalon.

The optic vesicles and optic stalk evaginate from the diencephalon around days 26 to 27. The optic vesicle remains surrounded by neural crest cells and mesoderm covered by a layer of surface ectoderm just like the rest of the neuroectodermal layers.

Following evagination, there is an invagination of the optic vesicles to form a cup (the future retina, iris, and ciliary body). The surface ectoderm invaginates toward the inner layer of the optic cup, thus becoming the future lens.[4]

Although the surface ectoderm becomes the lens, mesenchyme surrounding the optic stalk and vesicle forms a mesh of vasculature called the hyaloid vessels posteriorly.

The hyaloid vessel extends from posterior lens toward the optic nerve. Later in development, the anterior segment of the hyaloid, which was surrounded by the primary vitreous, regresses, and the remaining segment becomes the central artery of the optic nerve.

Understanding the process of vitreous development is also important. It plays an important part in understanding congenital orbital pathologic condition. The primary vitreous is a derivative of mesoderm and similar to hyaloid vessels, supplies to the anterior and posterior segments. Because it matures and regresses, it becomes acellular and creates a canal between the lens and the optic nerve called the Cloquet canal.[5] Eventually the canal regresses to form the zonular zone of the lens. Failure of this process and failure of regression of the hyaloid vasculature is associated with persistent fetal vasculature (previously known as persistent hyperplastic primary vitreous)—a benign entity and a mimic of retinoblastoma given that both entities present with leukocoria (Fig. 2).

The genes that are paramount to ocular embryogenesis are the RAX gene found on chromosome 18, the PAX6 gene found on chromosome 11p13, the SOX2 gene on chromosome 3, and the OTX2 gene located on chromosome 14q. These genes are expressed in proliferating cells.

The RAX gene is associated with retinal proliferation. Its mutation is associated with anophthalmia, microphthalmia and intracranial structural anomalies. A failure in function or mutation of the PAX6 gene lead to anterior segment anomalies such as congenital cataracts, absence of iris (aniridia), as well as midline fusion defects. Brain abnormalities such as classic commissural agenesis, hypoplasia of the anterior commissure, absence of the pineal gland, auditory processing defects, and anosmia have been described.[6]

SOX2 and OTX2 are transcription factors. SOX2 is essential for maintaining function and pluripotency of neural stem cells and its loss-of-function has been described in association with anophthalmia and microphthalmia, which may coexist with extraocular features such as hippocampal malformations, heterotopias, hamartoma of the tuber cinereum, nonspecific white matter abnormalities, and classic commissural agenesis.[6] The OTX2 gene mutation leads to anophthalmia-microphthalmia in addition to anterior segment defects, congenital amaurosis, hypoplasia of the optic nerves/chiasm, and dysplastic globes. Structural or functional pituitary abnormalities, cerebellar tonsillar ectopia, developmental delay, microcephaly, hypotonia, and abnormalities in other systems have been reported.[6–8]

Genes involved in ocular embryogenesis are listed in table 2.[9]

INTRAOCULAR MASSES AND TUMOR MIMICS

Pediatric ocular diseases are often identified by clinical signs rather than by symptoms because vision is difficult to assess in the early congenital disease. These signs include leukocoria, xanthocoria, strabismus, and periorbital swelling.

Leukocoria is the loss of the normal red-light reflex of the eye on fundoscopy with a white light reflex (Fig. 3). The most common sinister cause of leukocoria is retinoblastoma. Other important causes include persistent fetal vasculature, cataract, Coat's disease, and toxocariasis. Coat's disease may also present with xanthocoria, which is a more yellow variant of leukocoria.

Malignant Ocular Lesions

Retinoblastoma

Retinoblastoma is the most common intraocular malignancy in the pediatric population. Typical presentation is that of leukocoria in a child aged younger than 3 years, with 95% of children presenting before the age of 5 years.[10] The presentation may be unilateral or bilateral. An increased incidence of retinoblastoma is observed in developed countries correlating with increased HPV (Human papillomavirus) prevalence.[11]

Unilateral, unifocal retinoblastoma is associated with nongermline sporadic biallelic mutation of the Rb1 gene on chromosome 13.

In inherited retinoblastoma, there is germline mutation of Rb1 gene on a single allele. Tumor growth occurs subsequent to a sporadic mutation of the second allele. Therefore, the onset of presentation is earlier than its nongermline variant (usually by 2 years of age) and is frequently bilateral. In rare cases, when there is a concurrent intracranial pineoblastoma involving the neuroepithelial cells of the pineal gland, the term used is trilateral disease and when the suprasellar cistern is involved, it is called tetra lateral disease. About 15% of children with unilateral disease have the inherited Rb1 gene.[12]

Based on the spread of the disease and the treatment status, there are three different staging systems. The Reese-Ellsworth Classification system (groups I–IV) or the more commonly used International Intraocular Retinoblastoma Classification system groups A to E are based on intraocular extent at diagnosis.[13,14] The International Retinoblastoma Staging System is based on postsurgical residual disease and is classified from stage 0 to IV.

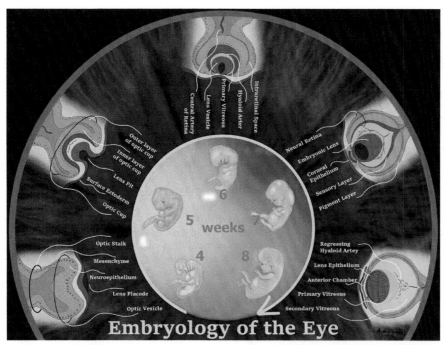

Embryology of the Eye

Fig. 2. *Embryogenesis of the eye.* After gastrulation and neurulation, at day 22, the diencephalon give rise to the optic pits, which evaginates close to the telencephalon to become the optic vesicle and optic stalk, which are the derivatives of the neuroectoderm. The optic stalk and vesicles are surrounded by mesenchyme, which is formed by mesoderm as well as neural crest cells. As the optic vesicle reaches toward the surface ectoderm, the lens placode (derivative of surface ectoderm) starts to invaginate toward the optic vesicle. At week 5, the optic vesicle becomes the optic cup. At the same time, inferiorly and posteriorly the optic cup forms a fissure called the choroidal fissure where the hyaloid vessels pass through. Failure of closure of this fissure can give rise to coloboma. The hyaloid vessels are primitive retinal artery and together with the primary vitreous supply the primitive eye. At weeks 6 and 7 while the optic cup develops further, the outer cell layers become the primitive retinal pigment epithelium while inner cells become the primitive neural retina. At week 8, the mesenchymal cells that form the choroid, sclera and cornea fuses around the optic cup forming the outer layers of the eye while the inner hyaloid and primary vitreous start to regress and becomes acellular. Disruption of this process gives rise to the anomaly called persistent fetal vasculature.

Stage IV disease is characterized by metastases to central nervous system or the body.[12,15]

The clinical presentation is leukocoria, strabismus (commonly esotropia), or reduced vision. Although diagnosis is often made by the clinical examination and B-mode US, MR imaging has a crucial role in staging of disease and planning management. This is critical for eye salvage therapy if diagnosed early and to exclude trilateral/tetra lateral disease and intracranial metastases.

On MR images, the retinal tumor is T2 hypointense and slightly T1 hyperintense relative to the vitreous. The growth pattern may be endophytic (toward the inner aspect of the globe), exophytic (toward the sclera), or a mixed pattern. Endophytic tumors grow into the vitreous and have a higher predilection for vitreous seeding. Exophytic tumors, however, tend to cause subretinal seeding, retinal detachment, and choroidal invasion. Thin high-resolution T2-weighted images are helpful in assessing the

tumor size and its extension (Fig. 4A). The globe may be enlarged (a useful feature separating it from tumor mimics such as persistent fetal vasculature and Coat's disease). Vitreous seeding may be identified as small foci of T2 hypointensity within the vitreous chamber (Fig. 5). It is important to note, however, that ophthalmoscopy is more sensitive than MR imaging for depicting vitreous seeds. Choroidal invasion is well assessed on postcontrast images, where there may be focal thickening or focal thinning with loss of normal enhancement. In scleral involvement, there may be interruption of the normally thin and smooth T2 hypointense outer sclera.[16] Postlaminar involvement is well assessed on contrast-enhanced T1-weighted fat-saturated sequences (FS). (Fig. 4D).

Areas of hypercellularity correlate with high diffusion-weighted imaging (DWI), low ADC, and enhancement (Fig. 4B, C).[17,18] Calcification is present in up to 95% of the cases, and it is the key

Table 2
Genes involved in ocular embryogenesis

Gene Name	Location	Role in Ocular Embryogenesis	Associated Abnormalities
FOXC1 (Forkhead box C1)	Chromosome 6	Expressed by periocular mesenchyma and cornea; role in cornea and iris development	Anterior segment defects, iris hypoplasia, Peters anomaly
OTX2 (Orthodenticle homeobox 2)	Chromosome 14	Expressed by neuroectoderm, optic vesicle, retina and retinal pigment epithelium (RPE); Role in RPE development, retinal neurogenesis	Anophthalmia-microphthalmia, anterior segment defects, congenital amaurosis, hypoplasia of optic nerves/chiasm, and dysplastic globes
PAX6 (Paired box 6)	Chromosome 11	Expressed by surface ectoderm; optic vesicle, lens placode, cornea, RPE, ciliary body, iris; major role in anterior segment development (cornea, iris, ciliary body), retinal neurogenesis; optic cup patterning, and vesicle evagination	Anterior segment anomalies (congenital cataracts, iris hypoplasia) and intracranial midline fusion defects such as agenesis of corpus callosum, hypoplasia of anterior commissure, absent pineal gland
RAX (Retina and anterior neural fold homeobox)	Chromosome 18	Expressed by eye field, optic vesicle, optic cup, neural retinal; major role in the development of the eye	Anophthalmia-microphthalmia
SOX2	Chromosome 3	Expressed by neuroectoderm, lens placode, optic cup, and retina; major role in maintaining function neural stem cells	Anophthalmia-microphthalmia and numerous intracranial congenital abnormalities including hippocampal malformations, heterotopias, intracranial hamartomas, white matter abnormalities, and agenesis of corpus callosum

Adapted from Miesfeld JB, Brown NL. Eye organogenesis: A hierarchical view of ocular development. Curr Top Dev Biol. 2019;132:351-393.

differentiating radiological sign from other congenital ocular tumors and causes of leukocoria. Although CT is the most specific and sensitive modality for identifying calcification, this modality should be used with caution due to an increased risk of secondary tumors with ionizing radiation. US and MR imaging are usually sufficient to confirm the diagnosis.[19,20]

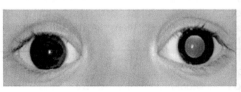
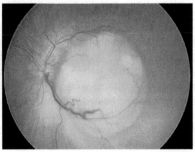

Fig. 3. Left eye leukocoria secondary to retinoblastoma.

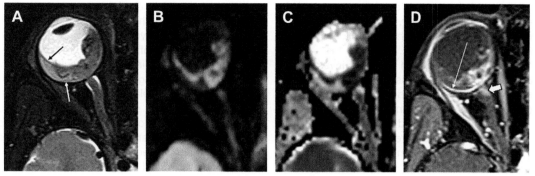

Fig. 4. Typical MR imaging appearances of retinoblastoma demonstrating heterogenous T2 hypointense intraocular mass with predominantly exophytic growth (A) with restricted diffusion (B, C). The lesion demonstrates heterogenous enhancement and postlaminar infiltration of the optic nerve head demonstrated by thick arrow (D). Note retinal detachment (*black arrow, A*).

Treatment is variable depending on disease extension. Ocular disease may be treated by intra-arterial chemotherapy. Extraocular disease is treated by enucleation and radiotherapy or systemic chemotherapy in the presence of intracranial disease or metastases.

Medulloepithelioma

Medulloepithelioma is a rare congenital tumor originating from the nonpigmented epithelial cells of the ciliary body. It can also originate from the retina, optic nerve, and choroid.[21] Majority of cases are diagnosed before 10 years of age, with a mean age of 5 years, and no clear gender predilection has been described. Clinical presentation is often delayed due to its slow growing nature. Symptoms include red eye and reduced vision with leukocoria or cataracs. There may also be lens subluxation or neovascular glaucoma, which are complications of the tumor.[22]

On histology, it has resemblance of an embryonal retina that is derived from the optic cup at 6 weeks gestation surrounded by the mucopolysaccharide-rich matrix. The lesions are classified as teratoid or nonteratoid and further categorized as benign or malignant based on histopathology.[23]

Approximately 5% of the cases are associated with mutations in the with *DICER1* gene. The rare adult manifestation is mostly malignant and thought to be triggered by previous traumatic or inflammatory insult to the ciliary body, which may undergo a hyperplastic change.[24]

The Zimmerman classification is used for the assessment of malignant features that include radiological assessment of invasion of other ocular structures (uvea, lens, sclera, cornea, and optic nerve) and extraocular extension along with histopathological features such as retinoblastoma or sarcoma elements, pleomorphism, and mitotic activity.[23]

US examination demonstrates a hyperechoic mass with multiple cysts. Occasionally, there may be cartilaginous structures or dystrophic

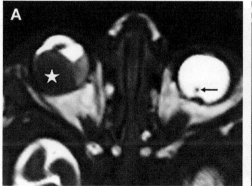
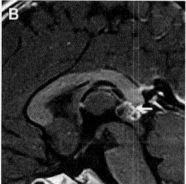

Fig. 5. Case of trilateral retinoblastoma. Growth pattern in the right eye is predominantly exophytic causing retinal detachment (*asterisk, A*), whereas the left eye shows endophytic growth pattern with possible vitreous seeding (*arrow, A*). Note enhancing lesion of the pineal gland in keeping with trilateral disease (*arrow, B*).

calcification in the teratoid subtype that can mimic retinoblastoma. However, retinoblastomas are more posteriorly located than medulloepithelioma and have a younger onset.[24,25]

MR imaging is the gold standard investigation for making the diagnosis and assessment of extension. It reveals a solid cystic mass in the retrolental location that returns slightly hyperintense signal on T1-weighted and hypointense signal on T2-weighted sequences relative to vitreous with post-contrast enhancement (Fig. 6).[26,27]

The treatment of large malignant subtypes is usually enucleation with a high 5-year survival rate of 90% to 95%.[28] If the tumor extends beyond the globe exenteration may be necessary. There are limited cases where intracranial metastases were reported and treated with systemic chemotherapy.[29,30] For smaller tumors, cryotherapy, plaque brachytherapy, and local resection may be considered. Death has only been reported by Broughton and Zimmerman and colleagues in 4 of 33 patients (12%) with malignant tumors and extraocular extension.[23]

Rhabdoid Tumors

Malignant rhabdoid tumors (MRTs) are rare aggressive embryonal tumors. Originally thought to be a type of Wilm's tumor involving the kidneys,[31] they are now identified as a distinct entity. Primary MRTs can be found in the kidneys, in the extrarenal space, and also in the central nervous system.

MRTs affect young children and may present with primary or secondary involvement. It can rarely metastasize intracranially. Some MRTs are associated with rhabdoid tumor predisposition syndrome that is caused by sporadic mutation causing inactivation of tumor suppressor gene *SMARCB1* (hSNF5/INI1) on chromosome 22q11.2.[32,33]

On MR imaging, the lesion shows hypo/isointense signal on T1-weighted and T2-weighted sequences with areas of heterogeneity secondary to

necrosis and hemorrhage (Fig. 7).[34,35] In our experience, they also show reduced ADC values mimicking rhabdomyosarcoma and may also mimic a fulminant inflammatory process potentially misdiagnosed initially as ocular abscess. Close differential diagnoses include medulloepithelioma and retinoblastoma. On immunohistology, the rhabdoid cells have characteristics feature with an eosinophilic cytoplasm, eccentric nuclei and paranuclear globoid, or fibrillar bundles of intermediate filaments.[34]

The pediatric variant is aggressive, and there is no definitive treatment method established yet. Combinations of surgery and systemic chemotherapy with vincristine and doxorubicin have been described in some cases with limited success.[36]

Leukemic Retinopathy

Leukemia is hematological neoplasm that occurs secondary to neoplastic proliferation of hematopoietic stem cells or partially differentiated cells in the bone marrow and can be broadly divided into the acute and chronic subtypes depending on the stem-cell clone involved. Acute types commonly manifest in the pediatric population, where blasts (poorly differentiated immature pluripotent cells) are involved. Ocular manifestations are silent in 90% of the cases and can be asymptomatic for a period.[37] It can directly involve any part of the globe including the retina or the optic nerve. In some cases, ocular invasion may be the only finding indicating relapse or progression and adequate assessment is crucial in disease management.[38] Other ocular manifestations occur subsequent to complications of associated hematological dysfunction presenting with retinal hemorrhages. These retinal appearances are commonly described as "Roth Spots" or cotton wool spots. Opportunistic infection may also develop subsequent to therapy and lymphocytopenia.[39,40]

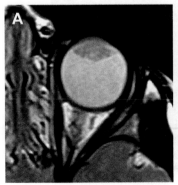 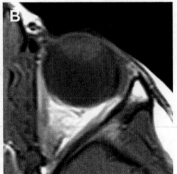 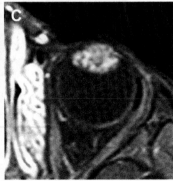

Fig. 6. Medulloepithelioma. T2-weighted sequence (*A*) shows a hypointense solid cystic lesion in the retrolental location. (*A*) The lesion returns slightly hyperintense signal on T1 (*B*) and enhances on the post-contrast FS T1WI (*C*). The mass in this case invades the ciliary body, iris, lens, and anterior chamber.

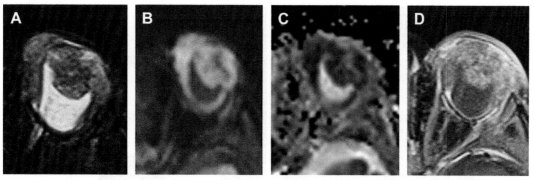

Fig. 7. Malignant rhabdoid tumor. MR imaging shows a heterogenous, predominantly T2 hypointense lesion (*A*) with restricted diffusion (*B, C*), and heterogenous postcontrast enhancement (*D*). These lesions can occasionally mimic an inflammatory process.

Although the role of radiology in the assessment of ocular manifestation is not widely reported, there are cases in which optic nerve infiltration described is associated with leptomeningeal infiltration and may be the only finding of disease progression and metastases.[41]

Melanoma

Ocular melanoma is the most common primary ocular tumor in the adult population. The incidence is low in children. The most common location is the uvea (82.5%) followed by the conjunctiva with increased incidence in those with underlying melanocytosis.

Occasionally, there may be metastases from a cutaneous lesion in particular when this involves the eyelids.[42]

The typical hyperpigmented skin lesion applied to the adult population has been noted in 40% of pediatric skin lesions, where the lesions are most frequently amelanotic (red colored), nodular, and thicker.[43]

Imaging aids in the diagnosis and assessment of extraocular spread. However, a biopsy may be required with the caveat that there is increased risk of seeding in instances with melanocytosis.[44]

Plaque-like lesions (<3 mm thickness) may be difficult to assess on imaging. However, when elevated, it is a sharply margined lesion described as having a collar button shape. Due to the paramagnetic characteristics of melanin, it is intrinsically T1 hyperintense. On T2-weighted images, the lesion is hypointense relative to vitreous but hyperintense to fat. The tumors typically enhance (as opposed to hematomas that may also present as T1 hyperintense masses). Gadolinium-enhanced fat-saturated images are helpful in assessing extraocular extension.[45]

Benign Ocular Lesions

Retinal Astrocytic Hamartoma

Retinal astrocytic hamartomas are benign overgrowths of the retinal nerve fiber layer and composed of several types of glial cells with or without dystrophic calcifications. Morphologically there are 2 types of retinal astrocytic hamartomas; nodular large calcified lesions that have a mulberry shape and small smooth flat noncalcified tumors that are more difficult to detect on imaging.

These lesions are mostly associated with tuberous sclerosis complex (TSC) or neurofibromatosis. However, they can also be sporadic. In cases associated with TSC or neurofibromatosis, the lesions are bilateral and multifocal. In TSC, there is mutation of *TSC1* or *TSC2* suppressor genes, which result in abnormal glial proliferation and maturation derived by the mammalian target of rapamycin (mTOR) pathway. Hamartomas can be found anywhere in the body, particularly, intracranial hamartomas are associated with mental retardation. Similarly, other ocular and orbital abnormalities may coexist. These include chorioretinal and iris colobomata, punched out depigmented retinal pigment epithelial lesions, and adenoma sebaceum of the adnexa.[46,47] In some cases, these lesions are shown to spontaneously regress.[48]

Diagnosis is made by the ophthalmologist. Grossly enlarged lesions that involve the macula may become symptomatic. Investigations with MR imaging and US are not always required, however, lesions may incidentally picked up on these modalities (**Fig. 8**), where one should also exclude TSC as an underlying diagnosis and should not be mistaken for an ocular malignancy.[49] Unlike retinoblastoma or choroidal melanomas, there are no prominent retinal vessels and the lesions are stable in size on follow-up.

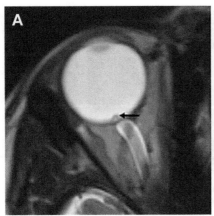
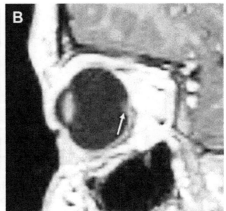

Fig. 8. Astrocytic hamartoma in a patient with tuberous sclerosis. Small nodular lesion is seen involving the right eye at the level of the optic disc insertion (*arrows, A, B*).

Choroidal Capillary Malformation

Choroidal capillary malformations (previously described as choroidal hemangiomas) are rare benign vascular tumors of the choroid and found most commonly associated with Sturge Weber Syndrome (SWS).[50]

In these tumors, there is no disruption to the retinal layers. There are two forms described. The diffuse choroidal capillary malformations are commonly associated with SWS. These have an earlier onset and more common in the pediatric population. The other type is well circumscribed—these are generally sporadic and seen in the adult population. On fundoscopy, these can be easily identified as nonpigmented orange-red lesions near the optic disc.[51]

SWS is a neurocutaneous syndrome with leptomeningeal angiomatosis associated with ipsilateral facial cutaneous vascular. They are also referred to as "Port wine stain or naevus flammeus." Diffuse choroidal capillary malformations are most commonly unilateral (very rarely bilateral) and found in up to half of the cases with no gender predilection. Glaucoma is the most common ocular pathology in this condition, which may be associated with buphthalmos (enlarged globe) (Fig. 9). Children with choroidal capillary malformation usually present with reduced vision that may worsen with age and may have leukocoria on examination. The symptoms occur as a sequela of increased thickness, leakage of the choroidal vasculature that causes exudates and edema complicated by choroidal or retinal detachment.[52]

On fundoscopy, the hypervascular capillary malformation particularly demonstrate avid fluorescent enhancement on angiography. However, an eye examination in the affected children can be extremely difficult particularly if there is a complication such as a retinal or choroidal detachment.

On US, there is increased internal reflectivity and US B demonstrates increased hyperechogenic thickening of the choroid. On MR imaging, the lesion remains T2 isointense to vitreous, T1 hypointense and reveal early avid enhancement. The diffuse type has maximum thickness in the most posterior globe and becomes thinner in the periphery (see Fig. 9). The main differential diagnosis on imaging is a choroidal melanoma. On MR imaging, melanomas are T1 hyperintense and the enhancement pattern is different and less avid than choroidal capillary malformations.[53]

The goal of treatment is to control leakage and hemorrhage, involute the choroidal capillary malformation with an aim to preserve vision and prevent retinal detachment. Treatment options include laser photocoagulation, proton beam therapy, stereotactic radiotherapy, intravitreal anti-VEGF (vascular endothelial growth factor) therapy, and photodynamic therapy, each with various success rates and associated complications.[52]

Choroidal osteoma

Choroidal osteoma is a very rare idiopathic benign bony calcification in the choroid most commonly affecting young girls in their teenage years. It was first described affecting young girls with the description of "lightly and irregularly elevated, yellow-white, juxtapapillary, choroidal tumor and well-defined geographic borders" on fundoscopy. It may be unilateral or bilateral.[54]

Symptoms include gradual visual loss and visual field defects. The overlying retinal pigment epithelium may become atrophied and depigmented over time. In some cases, choroidal neovascularization may occur.

On fluorescein angiography, there are patchy areas of hyperfluorescence with late diffuse staining. On US B-scan, elevated hyperechogenic

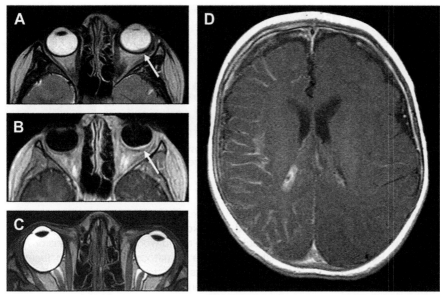

Fig. 9. Diffuse choroidal capillary malformations (*arrows, A, B*) are associated with SWS. SWS is a neurocutaneous syndrome with ipsilateral facial port wine stain. Its ocular manifestation also includes buphthalmos (*C*). Intracranially SWS are associated with leptomeningeal angiomatosis (*D*).

calcification is seen with associated posterior acoustic shadow (referred to as pseudo-optic nerve).[55]

Correlating with calcification bony densities are demonstrated on CT. Ossified lesions demonstrate T1 hyperintensity, in keeping with the presence of fatty marrow.[56]

Tumor Mimics

Persistent Fetal Vasculature

Persistent fetal vasculature (PFV), previously referred to as persistent hyperplastic primary vitreous, is a benign congenital malformation in neonates resulting from failure of regression of the hyaloid system that is a primitive channel between the lens and the optic nerve. It is a benign mimic of retinoblastoma and the second most common cause of leukocoria. The presence of microphthalmia may help differentiate it from retinoblastoma.[17] Presentation is unilateral although bilateral presentations have been documented in the rare Norrie disease, Walker-Warburg syndrome, and trisomy 13.[57,58]

The appearances of this entity have been described as a "martini glass" with a hypervascular stalk remnant connecting the lens to the optic nerve (Fig. 10). The rarer anterior and posterior variants have been described where the stalk may be interrupted and not fully extend between the optic nerve and the lens.[16,59]

Secondary congenital cataract, microphthalmia, glaucoma, retinal detachment, atrophy of the optic

nerve and in severe cases phthisis bulbi may be present.

On CT, a hyperdense vitreous body with soft tissue replacement is observed. On MR imaging, the vitreous is T1 and T2 hyperintense and the fibrovascular hyaloid remnant is often T2 hypointense with enhancement due to hypervascular residual elements.[58]

Treatment is variable based on anterior or posterior disease. The main goal is to preserve vision and prevent secondary complications. Early intervention is recommended, thereby increasing the likelihood of preserving visual outcome and treatments include lensectomy, anterior or total vitrectomy, and trabeculectomy.[60]

Coat's Disease

Coat's disease is an idiopathic telangiectasia of the retina characterized by subretinal exudates. The telangiectatic retinal capillaries are leaky and prone to hemorrhage, leading to proteinaceous subretinal exudates. The most common presentation is unilateral xanthocoria (yellow light reflex on fundoscopy) and reduced vision in young boys aged up to 10 years. Other cases can be associated with strabismus and retinal detachment.[61]

The disease manifestations range from mild to severe. Only a few foci of telangiectasia may be seen on examination that are highly sensitive to fluorescein angiography.

MR imaging and CT may be useful to exclude calcification. On MR imaging, both the

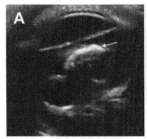 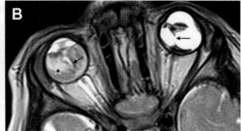 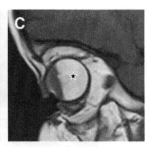

Fig. 10. US image shows right retrolental echogenicity with posterior acoustic shadowing (*arrow, A*). MR imaging shows retrolental lesion with stalk-like extension lens to the retina (*arrows, B*) with complicating vitreous hemorrhage (*asterisks, B, C*).

proteinaceous exudates and intraretinal/subretinal hemorrhages are expected to demonstrate T1 and T2 hyperintensity with or without retinal detachment (Fig. 11A, B). Reports have demonstrated elevated peak between 1 and 1.6 ppm on MR spectroscopy, attributed to lipid rich exudates.[62]

Coat's plus disease is a multisystem small vessel angiopathy involving the eyes, skeletal system, brain, and gastrointestinal tract. In addition to intraocular findings, there is typical asymmetrical confluent calcifications seen intracranially (Fig. 11C).[63] Other associations include Turner syndrome (XO), Senior-Loken syndrome, Norrie disease, Retinitis pigmentosa, and Linear scleroderma. Bilateral Coats presentation in girls should also raise the suspicion for facioscapulohumeral dystrophy.

Treatment depends on exudative state, foveal involvement, and retinal detachment and varies from laser therapy, anti-VEGF treatment, cryotherapy, and vitreoretinal surgery.[64,65]

Toxocariasis

Toxocariasis is a rare ocular infection caused by the round worm *Toxocara canis* or *Toxocara catis*. The nematodes are found in feces of domestic cats and dogs—particularly in the puppies. Children can be exposed to the contaminated soil or sand box. Ingested nematode eggs turn into larvae in the gut and are then absorbed into the systemic circulation and enter the liver enroute to a location anywhere in the body leading to systemic and ocular toxocariasis. The larvae may be present in body for months or even years before causing a systemic reaction. There is a reactive eosinophilic inflammation in the loci and hence the development of eosinophilic granulomata in the affected organs.[66]

The ocular presentation is that of a unilateral visual change, red eye, and pain. The vitreous inflammatory change creates a mass-like appearance, which can cause leukocoria on examination. Coat's disease and retinoblastoma

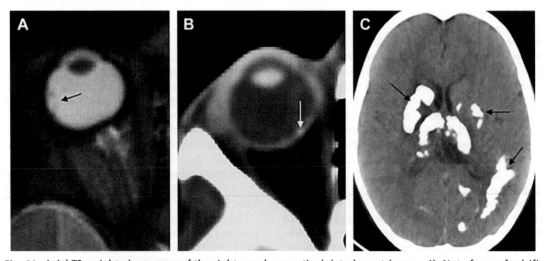

Fig. 11. Axial T2-weighted sequence of the right eye shows retinal detachment (*arrow, A*). Note focus of calcification on CT (*arrow, B*). CT of the brain shows extensive calcification involving the deep gray nuclei and white matter (*arrows, C*) in keeping with Coat's plus disease.

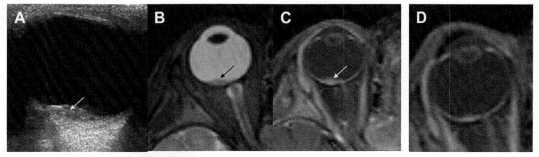

Before Treatment   After treatment

Fig. 12. Toxocariasis. US image shows an echogenic lesion lateral to the optic nerve head insertion (*arrow, A*). Axial T2 and contrast-enhanced fat-saturated axial T1 images show a T2 dark, enhancing lesion abutting the retina lateral to the optic nerve head insertion (*arrows, B, C*). Follow-up MR imaging (*D*) following treatment shows resolution of the lesion.

are the 2 main differential diagnoses. However, there is generally no calcification in ocular toxocariasis. Subsequent to the eosinophilic inflammation, subretinal exudates can mimic Coat's disease. The diagnosis is made on enzyme-linked immunosorbent essay (ELISA) test on blood or vitreous aspirate.[67]

US demonstrates an echogenic mass in the vitreous with or without retinal detachment. The larvae are usually too small to be seen under slit lamp. On CT, a dense mass may be noted with or without calcification. On MR imaging, the vitreous mass may be isointense on T1 and hypointense on T2 relative to the vitreous (Fig. 12).[68]

Congenital Lesions

Congenital cataracts

Congenital cataract (dense lens) occurs 1 in 4000 to 10000 newborns and can be due to a heritable (usually bilateral) or a nonheritable (unilateral) cause and is a major differential for leukocoria. It is responsible for nearly 20% of blindness in children, and therefore, early diagnosis is crucial.[69,70]

Bilateral disease is most likely due to chromosomal disorder (trisomy 21, trisomy 13, Lowe syndrome) or systemic metabolic abnormality such as galactosemia and Wilson disease or intrauterine infections such as cytomegalovirus, rubella, and toxoplasmosis. Unilateral cataracts are often a result of local dysgenesis and can be associated with other orbital dysgenesis such as persistent fetal vasculature as seen in the case of rare X-linked genetic condition called Norrie disease causing congenital retinopathy and blindness in boys.

It is recommended as part of US screening during second trimester anomaly scan, and if positive, the lens will appear hyperechogenic.[71]

Depending on the cause, the MR imaging conspicuity may vary. However, the lens thickness is expected to increase measuring greater than 4 mm. If the cataract is due to an acquired cause, there is increased influx of sodium and water into the lens matter, giving rise to T2 hyperintensity associated with T1 hypointensity[72] (Fig. 13).

Treatment is surgery in a timely manner, without which there is a risk of aphakic glaucoma, amblyopia, and blindness.[73]

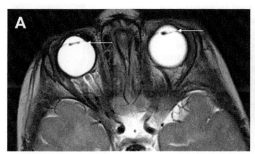
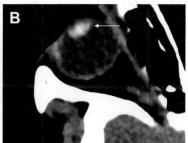

Fig. 13. Lowe syndrome. Axial T2-weighted image shows bilateral cataracts (*arrows, A*). Note dense lens with early central calcification on CT (*arrow, B*).

Congenital Malformation	Definition	Example
Buphthalmos	Enlarged globe Common Associations: Sturge Weber and Walker Walburg Syndromes	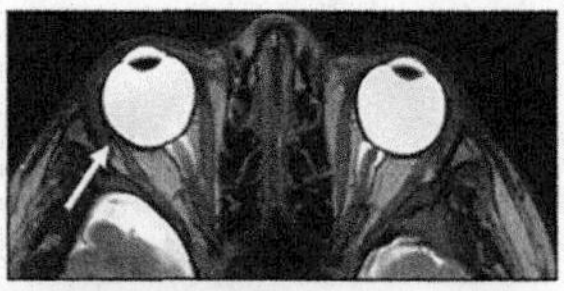
Anophthalmia	Complete Absence of the globe Common Associations: CHARGE syndrome, Aicardi syndrome	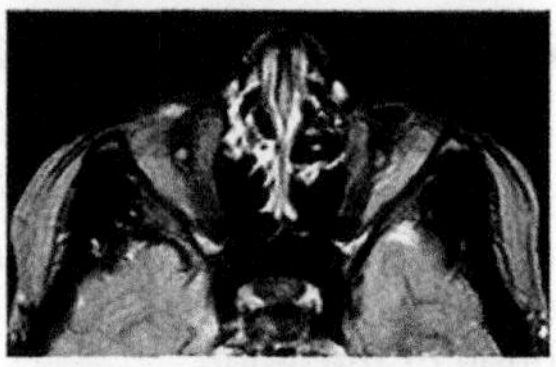
Microphthalmia	Small eyes (less than two standard deviations from the mean for age) Common Associations: CHARGE syndrome, Aicardi syndrome, Walker Walburg Syndrome	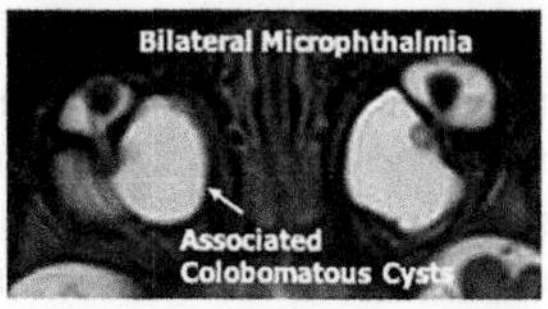
Coloboma	Ocular defect due to failure of closure of the optic fissure during embryogenesis. There is deficiency in the choroidal-scleral layer	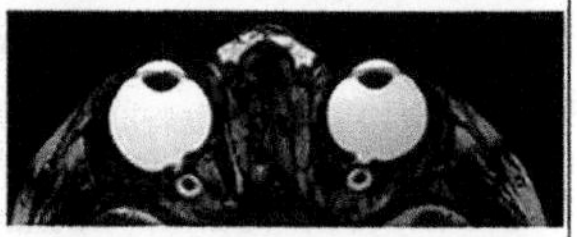
Staphyloma	Acquired outpouching due to weakening of the uveal-scleral layer, the weakened layers remain intact.	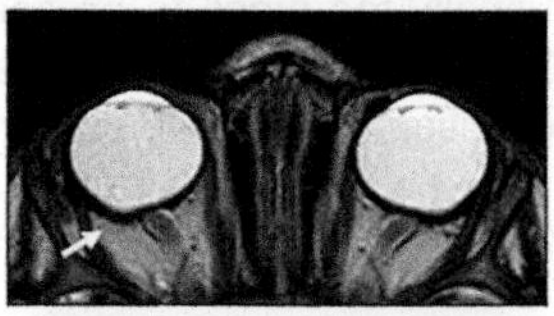
Ectopia Lentis	Dislocation or subluxation of the lens.	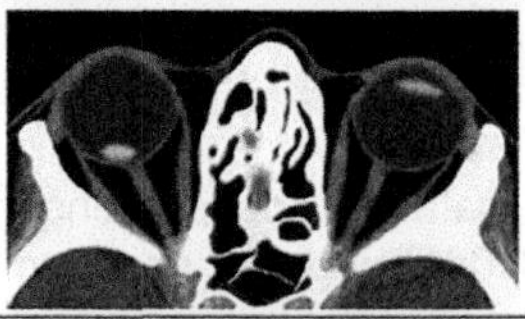
High Myopia	Pathological myopia with refractive error >6 Dioptres (D) Can be associated with staphyloma, Marfan syndrome and at high risk of lens dislocation	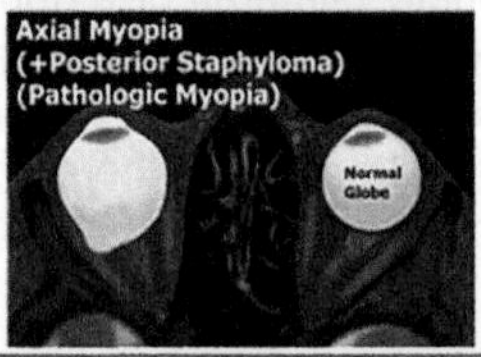
Morning Glory	Funnel shaped excavation of the optic nerve (A) associated PHACE Syndrome demonstrating posterior cranial fossa malformation and arterial abnormalities (B)	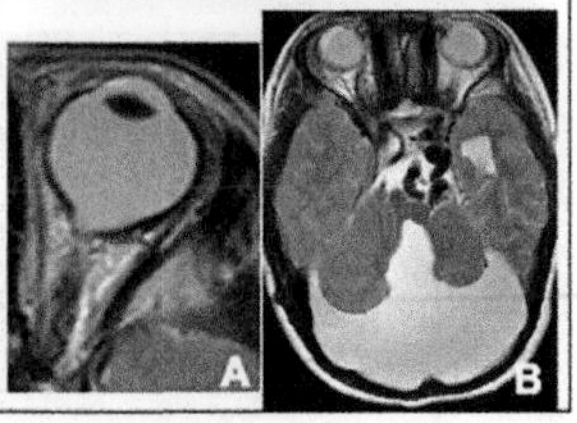

Fig. 14. Summary of congenital malformations with clinical examples and radiological illustrations.

Congenital Malformations

Anophthalmia and microphthalmia and coloboma

Anophthalmia, microphthalmia, and coloboma are a spectrum of related congenital eye malformations and are highly associated with other ocular abnormalities such as cataracts, posterior segment anomalies as well as extraocular abnormalities including brain malformations, craniofacial malformations, cardiac, musculoskeletal system, and uro-genital tract abnormalities (Fig. 14, Table 3).[74]

Both anophthalmia and microphthalmia have been described in association with Aicardi syndrome, CHARGE syndrome, Goltz syndrome, septo-optic dysplasia, short rib–polydactyly dysplasia syndrome, and Werdnig-Hoffmann disease.

Anophthalmia Anophthalmia is described as the complete absence of the eye, although, there may be a small pocket with a small underdeveloped eye and can be unilateral or bilateral.[75] It is very rare affecting 3% of 10,000 live births.

Microphthalmia Microphthalmia refers to small eyes with reduced axial length that is at least 2 standard deviations below the mean for the age.

Coloboma Coloboma occurs due to failure of closure of the optic fissure during embryogenesis. The optic fissure is the cleft situated at the inferior aspect of the optic vesicle when the surface ectoderm migrates in to form the lens. It has many syndromic associations including CHARGE syndrome, Aicardi syndrome, trisomies 13 and 18, and Walker-Warburg syndrome. On cross-sectional imaging, it is described as a cone-like elongation of the inferonasal retina. Often the underlying choroid is involved leaving the sclera visible during fundoscopic examination. Vision may be impaired if the macula or optic nerve are involved.

One differential diagnosis to coloboma is a staphyloma, which is an acquired weakening of the uveal-scleral layer causing a small outpouching usually in the infero-temporal region of the optic disc, however, may involve the anterior segment also. Unlike the coloboma, there is no discontinuity to the choroidal layer. Myopia is the commonest cause of posterior staphyloma followed by other causes such as glaucoma, trauma, infection, and inflammation. With staphyloma, the globe is often enlarged, whereas colobomata are associated with microphthalmia and cystic

Table 3
Systemic syndromes associated with ocular lesions and malformations

Walker-Warburg Syndrome	Sturge Weber Syndrome	Tuberous Sclerosis Complex	PHACE(S)	CHARGE Syndrome
• Inherited autosomal recessive • Ocular abnormalities (colobomas, microphthalmia, unilateral buphthalmos, congenital cataracts, retinal dysplasias) • Fetal hydrocephalus • Neuronal migrational anomalies • Dorsal kink at the mesencephalic-pontine junction	• Choroidal capillary malformations • Buphthalmos • Leptomeningeal angiomatosis • Cutaneous malformations (involving the ophthalmic division of trigeminal nerve)	• Retinal astrocytic hamartoma • Iris colobomas • Punched out de-pigmented lesions • Cortical/subcortical tubers • Subependymoma and subependymal giant cell astrocytoma • Renal angiomyolipomas • Cardiac rhabdomyomas • Sporadic mutation or autosomal dominant inheritance of tumor suppressor genes (TSC1 or TSC2) involved in mTOR pathway	• Posterior cranial fossa malformations (Dandy-Walker malformation, cerebellar dysplasia/hypoplasia) • H: Hemangiomas • A: Arterial anomalies • C: Coarctation of the aorta, cardiac anomalies • E: Ocular anomalies (Persistent fetal vasculature, Morning Glory Disc Anomaly, peripapillary staphyloma, coloboma, retinal vascular Anomaly)	• C: Coloboma • H: Heart Defects • A: Atresia Choanae • R: Retarded growth • G: Genital hypoplasia • E: Ear abnormalities • Other associated ocular abnormalities include microphthalmia and anophthalmia

malformations. Occasionally, the iris may be involved giving the typical keyhole-shaped pupil.[7,8,76]

Ectopia Lentis

Ectopia lentis occurs secondary to dislocation or subluxation of the lens due to damage to the zonular fibers usually secondary to trauma and is unilateral; however, with syndromic associations (Marfan syndrome or homocystinuria), the presentation is commonly bilateral and spontaneous. In Marfan syndrome, the lens displacement is superolateral, whereas in homocystinuria, the displacement is inferonasal. Congenital myopia is any myopia before the age of 6 years. High myopia (pathological >6 diopters (D)) can occur with Marfan syndrome or staphyloma and are at an increased risk of lens ectopia.[77,78]

Morning Glory Disc Anomaly

Morning glory disc anomaly (MGDA) is described as funnel-shaped excavation of the optic nerve and first described by Kindler and colleagues[79] due to its resemblance to a morning glory flower. Pathology is described as failure of maturation of the posterior sclera leading to herniation of the optic disc along with peripapillary retina and choroid.

On fundoscopy, the optic disc is typically enlarged with funnel-shaped excavation, there is central glial tuft making the optic disc blurry and white with halo of pigmentation changes to the choroid. Finally, the orientation of the retinal branches is altered emanating radially rather than branching toward the center of the optic disc.

MGDA can be associated with skull base defects and encephaloceles, callosal dysgenesis, vascular abnormalities such as Moya Moya disease, midline craniofacial malformations, and PHACE syndrome.[8]

In a study on MR imaging features of MGDA, all cases demonstrated funnel-shaped morphology of the posterior sclera with elevation of adjacent retinal surface and discontinuous uveoscleral coat. In addition, the distal ipsilateral optic nerve near the optic disc demonstrated an abnormality with effacement of subarachnoid spaces and T1 hyperintensity, which demonstrated enhancement and fat suppression correlating with the histopathology. Although imaging appearances may be similar to posterior coloboma, the absence of the outpouching inferior to the optic nerve head, optic nerve and adjacent retinal layer elevation and effacemet of the subarachnoid space can be used to distinguishing these two entities.[80]

CLINICS CARE POINTS

- Common retinoblastoma mimics include PFV and Coat's disease, with all these entities presenting with loss of normal red reflex.

- Imaging of the orbits should be tailored to the pathology. Lesions such as PFV are well depicted by US, whereas tumors such as retinoblastoma require dedicated high-resolution MR imaging.

- A precontrast non–fat-saturated T1-weighted sequence is important, in order to maximize the contrast provided by the intrinsic T1 hyperintense signal of retro-orbital fat.

- Congenital ocular malformations are frequently associated with associated intracranial abnormalities and may be syndromic. Therefore, imaging of the brain should also be performed routinely while evaluating these disorders.

DISCLOSURE

Authors have nothing to disclose.

REFERENCES

1. D'Arco F, Mertiri L, de Graaf P, et al. Guidelines for magnetic resonance imaging in pediatric head and neck pathologies: a multicentre international consensus paper. Neuroradiology 2022;64(6):1081–100.

2. Bye L, Modi N, Stanford M. Basic sciences for ophthalmology. Oxford: Oxford University Press; 2013. https://doi.org/10.1093/med/9780199584994.001.0001.

3. Snell RS, Lemp MA. Clinical anatomy of the eye. Hoboken, NJ, USA: Wiley; 1997.

4. Fuhrmann S. Eye morphogenesis and patterning of the optic vesicle. Curr Top Dev Biol 2010;93:61–84.

5. Cvekl A, Tamm ER. Anterior eye development and ocular mesenchyme: new insights from mouse models and human diseases. Bioessays 2004;26(4):374–86.

6. Slavotinek AM. Eye development genes and known syndromes. Mol Genet Metabol 2011;104(4):448–56.

7. FitzPatrick DR, Heyningen V van. Developmental eye disorders. Curr Opin Genet Dev 2005;15(3):348–53.

8. Guercio JR, Martyn LJ. Congenital Malformations of the Eye and Orbit. Otolaryngol Clin 2007;40(1):113–40.

9. Miesfeld JB, Brown NL. Eye organogenesis: A hierarchical view of ocular development. Curr Top Dev Biol 2019;132:351–93.

10. Broaddus E, Topham A, Singh AD. Incidence of retinoblastoma in the USA: 1975-2004. Br J Ophthalmol
2009;93(1):21–3.

11. Javanmard D, Moein M, Esghaei M, et al. Molecular
evidence of human papillomaviruses in the retinoblastoma tumor. Virusdisease 2019;30(3):360–6.

12. Abramson DH, Shields CL, Munier FL, et al. Treatment of Retinoblastoma in 2015: Agreement and
Disagreement. JAMA Ophthalmol 2015;133(11):
1341.

13. Tomar AS, Finger PT, Gallie B, et al. A Multicenter, International Collaborative Study for American Joint
Committee on Cancer Staging of Retinoblastoma:
Part I: Metastasis-Associated Mortality. Ophthalmology 2020;127(12):1719–32.

14. Tomar AS, Finger PT, Gallie B, et al. A Multicenter, In-
ternational Collaborative Study for American Joint
Committee on Cancer Staging of Retinoblastoma:
Part II: Treatment Success and Globe Salvage.
Ophthalmology 2020;127(12):1733–46.

15. Chantada G, Doz F, Antoneli CBG, et al. A proposal
for an international retinoblastoma staging system.
Pediatr Blood Cancer 2006;47(6):801–5.

16. Joseph AK, Guerin JB, Eckel LJ, et al. Imaging Findings of Pediatric Orbital Masses and Tumor Mimics.
Radiographics 2022;42(3):880–97.

17. Balmer A, Munier F. Differential diagnosis of leukocoria and strabismus, first presenting signs of retinoblastoma. Clin Ophthalmol 2007;1(4):431–9.

18. de Graaf P, Pouwels PJW, Rodjan F, et al. Single-
shot turbo spin-echo diffusion-weighted imaging
for retinoblastoma: initial experience. AJNR Am J
Neuroradiol 2012;33(1):110–8.

19. Galluzzi P, Hadjistilianou T, Cerase A, et al. Is CT Still
Useful in the Study Protocol of Retinoblastoma?
AJNR Am J Neuroradiol 2009;30(9):1760–5.

20. Wong JR, Morton LM, Tucker MA, et al. Risk of subsequent malignant neoplasms in long-term hereditary retinoblastoma survivors after chemotherapy
and radiotherapy. J Clin Oncol 2014;32(29):
3284–90.

21. Shields JA, Eagle RC, Shields CL, et al. Congenital
Neoplasms of the Nonpigmented Ciliary Epithelium
(medulloepithelioma). Ophthalmology 1996;
103(12):1998–2006.

22. Kaliki S, Shields CL, Eagle RC, et al. Ciliary body
medulloepithelioma: analysis of 41 cases. Ophthalmology 2013;120(12):2552–9.

23. Broughton WL, Zimmerman LE. A clinicopathologic
study of 56 cases of intraocular medulloepithelio-
mas. Am J Ophthalmol 1978;85(3):407–18.

24. Tadepalli SH, Shields CL, Shields JA, et al. Intraocular medulloepithelioma – A review of clinical features, DICER 1 mutation, and management. Indian
J Ophthalmol 2019;67(6):755–62.

25. Shields CL, Schoenberg E, Kocher K, et al. Lesions
simulating retinoblastoma (pseudoretinoblastoma)

in 604 cases: results based on age at presentation.
Ophthalmology 2013;120(2):311–6.

26. De Potter P, Shield CL, Shields JA, et al. The Role of
Magnetic Resonance Imaging in Children with Intraocular Tumors and Simulating Lesions. Ophthalmology 1996;103(11):1774–83.

27. Sansgiri RK, Wilson M, McCarville MB, et al. Imaging
features of medulloepithelioma: report of four cases
and review of the literature. Pediatr Radiol 2013;
43(10):1344–56.

28. Ang SM, Dalvin LA, Emrich J, et al. Plaque Radiotherapy for Medulloepithelioma in 6 Cases From a
Single Center. Asia Pac J Ophthalmol (Phila).
2019;8(1):30–5.

29. Chidambaram B, Santosh V, Balasubramaniam V.
Medulloepithelioma of the optic nerve with intradural
extension–report of two cases and a review of the
literature. Childs Nerv Syst 2000;16(6):329–33.

30. Lindegaard J, Heegaard S, Toft PB, et al. Malignant
transformation of a medulloepithelioma of the optic
nerve. Orbit 2010;29(3):161–4.

31. Beckwith JB, Palmer NF. Histopathology and prognosis of Wilms tumor Results from the first national
wilms' tumor study. Cancer 1978;41(5):1937–48.

32. Gottlieb C, Nijhawan N, Chorneyko K, et al. Congenital orbital and disseminated extrarenal malignant
rhabdoid tumor. Ophthalmic Plast Reconstr Surg
2005;21(1):76–9.

33. Shah SJ, Ali MJ, Mulay K, et al. Primary intraocular
malignant extrarenal rhabdoid tumor: a clinicopathological correlation. J Pediatr Ophthalmol Strabismus
2013;50:e18–20.

34. Kasturi N, Gera P, Panicker G, et al. Primary Intraocular Malignant Rhabdoid Tumor Mimicking Retinoblastoma in a Child. Ocul Oncol Pathol 2020;6(6):
438–41.

35. Parmar H, Hawkins C, Bouffet E, et al. Imaging findings in primary intracranial atypical teratoid/rhab-
doid tumors. Pediatr Radiol 2006;36(2):126–32.

36. Seeringer A, Reinhard H, Hasselblatt M, et al. Syn-
chronous congenital malignant rhabdoid tumor of
the orbit and atypical teratoid/rhabdoid tumor—feasibility and efficacy of multimodal therapy in a long-
term survivor. Cancer Genetics 2014;207(9):429–33.

37. de Queiroz Mendonca C, Freire MV, Viana SS, et al.
Ocular manifestations in acute lymphoblastic leuke-
mia: A five-year cohort study of pediatric patients.
Leuk Res 2019;76:24–8.

38. Talcott KE, Garg RJ, Garg SJ. Ophthalmic manifestations of leukemia. Curr Opin Ophthalmol 2016;
27(6):545–51.

39. Kincaid MC, Green WR. Ocular and orbital involvement
in leukemia. Surv Ophthalmol 1983;27(4):211–32.

40. Ginsberg LE, Leeds NE. Neuroradiology of leukemia. Am J Roentgenol 1995;165(3):525–34.

41. Vázquez E, Lucaya J, Castellote A, et al. Neuroimaging in Pediatric Leukemia and Lymphoma:

Differential Diagnosis1. Radiographics 2002. https://doi.org/10.1148/rg.226025029.

42. Jovanovic P, Mihajlovic M, Djordjevic-Jocic J, et al. Ocular melanoma: an overview of the current status. Int J Clin Exp Pathol 2013;6(7):1230–44.

43. Cordoro KM, Gupta D, Frieden IJ, et al. Pediatric melanoma: Results of a large cohort study and proposal for modified ABCD detection criteria for children. J Am Acad Dermatol 2013;68(6):913–25.

44. Szervat JJ, Black EH, Nesi FA, et al, editors. Smith and Nesi's ophthalmic Plastic and Reconstructive surgery. 4th edition. New York, NY: Springer; 2021. https://doi.org/10.1007/978-3-030-41720-8.

45. Bond JB, Haik BG, Mihara F, et al. Magnetic Resonance Imaging of Choroidal Melanoma with and without Gadolinium Contrast Enhancement. Ophthalmology 1991;98(4):459–66.

46. Rowley S, O'Callaghan F, Osborne J. Ophthalmic manifestations of tuberous sclerosis: a population based study. Br J Ophthalmol 2001;85(4):420–3.

47. Martin K, Rossi V, Ferrucci S, et al. Retinal astrocytic hamartoma. Optometry - Journal of the American Optometric Association. 2010;81(5):221–33.

48. Kiratli H, Bilgiç S. Spontaneous regression of retinal astrocytic hamartoma in a patient with tuberous sclerosis. Am J Ophthalmol 2002;133(5):715–6.

49. Rao AA, Naheedy JH, Chen JYY, et al. A Clinical Update and Radiologic Review of Pediatric Orbital and Ocular Tumors. J Oncol 2013;2013:975908.

50. Warne RR, Carney OM, Wang G, et al. The Bone Does Not Predict the Brain in Sturge-Weber Syndrome. AJNR Am J Neuroradiol 2018;39(8):1543–9.

51. Heimann H, Jmor F, Damato B. Imaging of retinal and choroidal vascular tumours. Eye (Lond). 2013; 27(2):208–16.

52. Formisano M, Abdolrahimzadeh B, Mollo R, et al. Bilateral diffuse choroidal hemangioma in Sturge Weber syndrome: A case report highlighting the role of multimodal imaging and a brief review of the literature. J Curr Ophthalmol 2018;31(2):242–9.

53. Stroszczynski C, Hosten N, Bornfeld N, et al. Choroidal hemangioma: MR findings and differentiation from uveal melanoma. AJNR American journal of neuroradiology 1998;19:1441–7.

54. Gass JD, Guerry RK, Jack RL, et al. Choroidal Osteoma. Arch Ophthalmol 1978;96(3):428–35.

55. Shields CL, Shields JA, Augsburger JJ. Choroidal osteoma. Surv Ophthalmol 1988;33(1):17–27.

56. DePotter P, Shields JA, Shields CL, et al. Magnetic resonance imaging in choroidal osteoma. Retina 1991;11(2):221–3.

57. Payabvash S, Anderson JS, Nascene DR. Bilateral persistent fetal vasculature due to a mutation in the Norrie disease protein gene. NeuroRadiol J 2015; 28(6):623–7.

58. Kaste SC, Jenkins JJ, Meyer D, et al. Persistent hyperplastic primary vitreous of the eye: imaging findings with pathologic correlation. AJR Am J Roentgenol 1994;162(2):437–40. https://doi.org/10.2214/ajr.162.2.8310942.

59. Castillo M, Wallace DK, Mukherji SK. Persistent hyperplastic primary vitreous involving the anterior eye. AJNR Am J Neuroradiol 1997;18(8): 1526–8.

60. Hunt A, Rowe N, Lam A, et al. Outcomes in persistent hyperplastic primary vitreous. Br J Ophthalmol 2005;89(7):859–63.

61. Sen M, Shields CL, Honavar SG, et al. Coats disease: An overview of classification, management and outcomes. Indian J Ophthalmol 2019;67(6): 763–71.

62. Eisenberg L, Castillo M, Kwock L, et al. Proton MR spectroscopy in Coats disease. AJNR Am J Neuroradiol 1997;18(4):727–9.

63. Maia C, Batista M, Palavra F, et al. Coats-plus syndrome: when imaging leads to genetic diagnosis. BMJ Case Reports CP 2022;15(5):e249702.

64. Shields JA, Shields CL, Honavar SG, et al. Clinical variations and complications of Coats disease in 150 cases: the 2000 Sanford Gifford Memorial Lecture. Am J Ophthalmol 2001; 131(5):561–71.

65. Sigler EJ, Randolph JC, Calzada JI, et al. Current management of Coats disease. Surv Ophthalmol 2014;59(1):30–46.

66. Schneier AJ, Durand ML. Ocular Toxocariasis: Advances in Diagnosis and Treatment. Int Ophthalmol Clin 2011;51(4):135–44.

67. Edwards MG, Pordell GR. Ocular toxocariasis studied by CT scanning. Radiology 1985. https://doi.org/10.1148/radiology.157.3.4059556.

68. Chung EM, Specht CS, Schroeder JW. Pediatric Orbit Tumors and Tumorlike Lesions: Neuroepithelial Lesions of the Ocular Globe and Optic Nerve. Radiographics 2007;27(4):1159–86.

69. Birth prevalence of visually significant infantile cataract in a defined U.S. population: Ophthalmic Epidemiology: Vol 10, No 2. Available at: https://www.tandfonline.com/doi/abs/10.1076/opep.10.2.67.13894. Accessed January 7, 2023.

70. Rahi J, Dezateux C. Measuring and Interpreting the Incidence of Congenital Ocular Anomalies: Lessons from a National Study of Congenital Cataract in the UK. Investigative ophthalmology & visual science 2001;42:1444–8.

71. Bethune M, Alibrahim E, Davies B, et al. A pictorial guide for the second trimester ultrasound. Australas J Ultrasound Med 2013;16(3):98–113.

72. Barakat E, Ginat DT. Magnetic resonance imaging (MRI) features of cataracts in pediatric and young adult patients. Quant Imaging Med Surg 2020; 10(2):428–31.

73. Infant Aphakia Treatment Study Group, Lambert SR, Buckley EG, et al. The infant aphakia treatment

study: design and clinical measures at enrollment. Arch Ophthalmol 2010;128(1):21–7.

74. Skalicky SE, White AJR, Grigg JR, et al. Microphthalmia, anophthalmia, and coloboma and associated ocular and systemic features: understanding the spectrum. JAMA Ophthalmol 2013;131(12): 1517–24.

75. El Essawy RA, Abdelbaky SH. Successful conjunctival socket expansion in anophthalmic patients until the age of 2 years: an outpatient procedure. Clin Ophthalmol 2016;10:1743–8.

76. George A, Cogliati T, Brooks BP. Genetics of syndromic ocular coloboma: CHARGE and COACH syndromes. Exp Eye Res 2020;193:107940.

77. Lorente-Ramos RM, Armán JA, Muñoz-Hernández A, et al. US of the Eye Made Easy: A Comprehensive How-to Review with Ophthalmoscopic Correlation. Radiographics 2012;32(5):E175–200.

78. Kaur K, Gurnani B. Ectopia Lentis. In: StatPearls. StatPearls Publishing; 2022. Available at: http://www.ncbi.nlm.nih.gov/books/NBK578193/. Accessed February 14, 2023.

79. Kindler P. Morning glory syndrome: unusual congenital optic disk anomaly. Am J Ophthalmol 1970;69(3): 376–84.

80. Ellika S, Robson CD, Heidary G, et al. Morning Glory Disc Anomaly: Characteristic MR Imaging Findings. AJNR Am J Neuroradiol 2013;34(10):2010–4.

Extraocular Orbital and Peri-Orbital Masses

Asthik Biswas, MBBS, DNB[a],[*], Oi Yean Wong, MBBS, FRCR[a], Berna Aygun, MBBS, MRes, FRCR[b], Sri Gore, MBBS, BSc FRCOphth, PGDip Ed[c], Kshitij Mankad, MBBS, FRCR[a],[d]

KEYWORDS

- Orbit • Intraconal • Extraconal • Masses • Pediatric • Hemangioma • Rhabdomyosarcoma
- MR imaging

KEY POINTS

- Orbital masses can involve the intraconal, conal, and extraconal compartments. The concept of *cell of origin* along with knowledge of orbital anatomy is useful when encountering challenging cases.
- Orbital infantile hemangiomas are benign vascular tumors of infancy and are distinct from vascular malformations. The major differential diagnosis on imaging is rhabdomyosarcoma.
- Ectodermal inclusion cysts are benign, form close to suture lines, and cause remodeling of the adjacent bone. Aggressive lesions such as neuroblastoma metastases, and Langerhans cell histiocytosis, however, cause osseous destruction.

INTRODUCTION

A practical approach to imaging interpretation of extraocular orbital masses is by studying their origin based on location. Although large masses can occupy multiple compartments, the concept of *cell of origin* is useful when encountering difficult cases. A working knowledge of orbital anatomy, its compartments, and normal contents within each compartment is therefore essential to reach a meaningful list of differentials. Once this is achieved, intrinsic imaging characteristics can help further narrow down the differential diagnoses. We begin this article with a brief recollection of orbital anatomy, and follow it up with discussion of common disorders.

ANATOMY OF THE BONY ORBIT

The orbit is a pyramidal structure with the apex formed by the optic foramen. The orbital roof is formed by the orbital plate of the frontal bone and the lesser wing of the sphenoid. The roof separates the bony orbit from the anterior cranial fossa. The medial wall is composed of, anterior to posterior, the lacrimal bone, frontal process of the maxillary bone, orbital plate of the ethmoid bone and the lesser wing of sphenoid. The major component of the medial wall is the ethmoid bone, a thin structure known as the lamina papyracea, which separates the orbit from the ethmoid air cells. The lateral wall of the orbit is the strongest and is formed by the zygomatic bone and the greater wing of sphenoid bone. The floor of the orbit is formed by the maxillary bone, palatine bone, and orbital plate of the zygomatic bone. The orbital floor constitutes the roof of the maxillary sinus.[1]

The orbital rim refers to the base of the orbit, which opens out into the face. The osseous structures forming the rim are depicted in **Fig. 1**.

The orbital apex refers to the posterior confluence of the orbital walls. It forms an important landmark separating the intracranial cavity from the orbit and is a major conduit for several nerves and vessels. The orbital apex is composed of the following bony apertures:

---

[a] Department of Neuroradiology, Great Ormond Street Hospital for Children NHS Foundation Trust, Great Ormond Street, London WC1N 3JH, UK; [b] Department of Neuroradiology, UK Kings College Hospital NHS Foundation Trust, Denmark Hill, London SE5 9RS, UK; [c] Department of Ophthalmology, Great Ormond Street Hospital for Children NHS Foundation Trust, London, UK; [d] UCL GOS Institute of Child Health, 30 Guilford Street, London WC1N 1EH, UK
* Corresponding author.
E-mail address: asthikbiswas@gmail.com

Neuroimag Clin N Am 33 (2023) 643–659
https://doi.org/10.1016/j.nic.2023.05.012
1052-5149/23/© 2023 Elsevier Inc. All rights reserved.

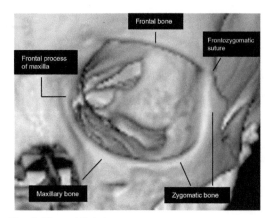

Fig. 1. The orbital rim.

The optic canal transmits the optic nerve and ophthalmic artery. It is bounded medially by the body of the sphenoid bone, and laterally by the lesser wing of the sphenoid, and is situated medial to the superior orbital fissure (Fig. 2).

The superior orbital fissure is bounded inferolaterally by the greater wing of sphenoid and superomedially by the lesser wing of sphenoid. It transmits the superior ophthalmic vein, a branch of the inferior ophthalmic vein and several cranial nerves and their branches (superior and inferior divisions of the oculomotor nerve, branches of the ophthalmic division of trigeminal nerve, the trochlear and abducens nerves) (see Fig. 2).[1]

The inferior orbital fissure is located lateral to the orbital floor and transmits the inferior ophthalmic vein, infraorbital artery, branches of the maxillary division of trigeminal nerve (infraorbital nerve and zygomatic nerve) and orbital branches of the pterygopalatine ganglion (see Fig. 2).[1]

Orbital Compartments

The extraocular orbit can be anatomically divided by the orbital muscle cone into the intraconal, conal, and extraconal compartments (Fig. 3). The orbital muscle cone is a myofascial structure composed of the recti muscles and their fasciae. The base of the cone is limited by the globe, and its apex is at the level of the optic canal.

The *intraconal compartment* is limited on either side by the musculofascial cone. It contains fat, nerves including the optic nerve surrounded by meninges, and blood vessels.[1]

The *conal compartment* is constituted by recti muscles and fasciae. The 4 recti muscles share a common origin from the annulus of Zinn—a tendinous ring of fibrous tissue at the orbital apex. The muscles insert into the globe at various positions behind the limbus.[2]

The *extraconal compartment* is limited anteriorly by the orbital septum, laterally by the orbital wall and its periosteum, and medially by the recti muscles. It contains fat, nerves, vessels, nonrectus extraocular muscles (superior oblique, inferior oblique, and levator palpebrae superioris), and the lacrimal gland.[1]

Knowledge of the contents of the orbital compartments aid in narrowing down the differential diagnoses. For instance, important intraconal masses include optic nerve glioma, optic nerve sheath meningioma (ONSM), schwannomas, and vascular malformations; the myofascial cone is often the primary site of orbital rhabdomyosarcoma; lacrimal gland pathologies occur in the extraconal space, and idiopathic orbital inflammation (IOI) can affect any of the spaces. It is important, however, to understand that most lesions are commonly transcompartmental (eg, vascular malformations, lymphoma, rhabdomyosarcoma). It can be difficult to ascertain the compartment of origin of large tumors, which tend to distort the anatomy. Furthermore, conal and orbital rim masses often involve the extraconal space. The relationship of the lesion and its effect on surrounding structures should therefore be carefully assessed.

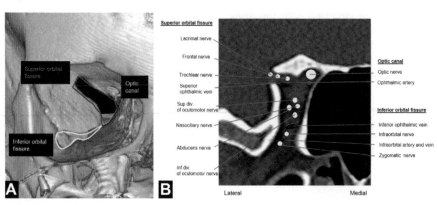

Fig. 2. The orbital apex. (*A*) 3D volume rendered, and (*B*) Coronal CT of the orbit in bone window.

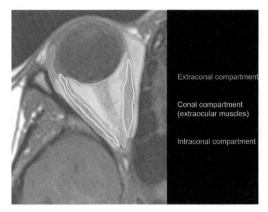

Fig. 3. The orbital compartments.

INTRACONAL MASSES
Optic Pathway Glioma

Optic pathway gliomas (OPGs) are low-grade astroglial neoplasms, with pilocytic astrocytoma comprising the most common histopathological subtype.[3] OPGs may involve the anterior visual pathway (optic nerves), the posterior visual pathway (optic chiasm, tracts, hypothalamus), or both.[4] OPGs may occur sporadically or in association with neurofibromatosis type 1 (NF1). Sporadic OPGs more commonly involve the posterior visual pathway, whereas NF1-associated (syndromic) OPGs have a predilection for the anterior visual pathway (although about half of these lesions also extend posteriorly). Syndromic OPGs are frequently but not always bilateral.[3,4]

On MR imaging, OPGs are typically T2 hyperintense and cause expansion of the optic nerves (Fig. 4). Associated optic nerve tortuosity is also common, especially with larger tumors. Sporadic tumors tend to be more nodular, with cystic components.[4,5] The extent of the lesion should be carefully studied on T2 and fluid attenuated inversion recovery (FLAIR) sequences. Enhancement is variable, can wax and wane over time, and varies according to the chemotherapy regimen—for this reason, T2 and FLAIR sequence are preferable to contrast-enhanced imaging for tumor surveillance.[6] Table 1 lists differential features of syndromic and sporadic OPGs.

Optic Nerve Sheath Meningioma

ONSMs are benign, slowly growing tumors that originate from the arachnoid cap cells of the optic nerve sheath.[7] The most common site of origin is the intraorbital segment of the optic nerve, and majority are unilateral. These are rare tumors, especially in the pediatric population, with about 30% of ONSM occurring in children with type 2

neurofibromatosis.[7] Presentation is with slow, progressive, visual loss.[8] The lesion most commonly grows circumferentially around the optic nerve, compromising its pial vascular supply, and eventually leads to optic atrophy.[9] Occasionally, eccentric and pedunculated patterns of growth may occur.[10]

MR imaging is the modality of choice to demonstrate the extent of disease and its relationship to surrounding structures. On imaging, ONSM is typically uniformly enhancing and surrounds the intraorbital segment of the optic nerve (Fig. 5).[10] Calcification has been described in one-third to one-half of cases, best appreciated on computed tomography (CT), with linear or punctate appearance.[11] On MR imaging, the lesions have variable T2 signal intensity depending on the degree of calcification. A peculiar feature is the presence of perioptic cysts that lie between the lesion and the globe, due to trapped cerebrospinal fluid (CSF) within the optic nerve sheath[12]; these are best demonstrated on fat-suppressed T2-weighted sequences. Contrast-enhanced images show moderate to marked enhancement of the tumor surrounding the centrally nonenhancing optic nerve (see Fig. 5).[13] The tram-track sign refers to circumferentially growing tumors that show calcification and/or postcontrast enhancement (see Fig. 5).[13]

INTRACONAL, EXTRACONAL, AND TRANSCONAL MASSES
Infantile Hemangioma

Infantile hemangiomas are benign vascular tumors (not malformations) that occur due to clonal proliferation of endothelial cells resulting from vasculogenesis.[14] Unlike congenital hemangiomas, infantile hemangiomas are not fully developed at birth. Instead, these are generally noticeable in the first few days to weeks of life ie, when they are in the proliferative phase.[15,16] The proliferative phase generally lasts for 12 to 24 months followed by an involution phase during which the hemangioma regresses, sometimes with complete regression by 5 years of age or into a residual fibrofatty mass.[15,17] Propanolol is usually commenced during the proliferative phase of these lesions due to the high risk of developing amblyopia.

Infantile hemangiomas are commonly superficial, involving the eyelids, periorbital soft tissue, and superomedial extraconal space. They may also occur in multiple orbital compartments, and occasionally are exclusively intraconal in location. An infantile hemangioma can have eyelid and orbital components that hide the presence of proptosis and/or globe displacement. Presence of

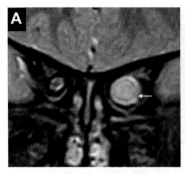 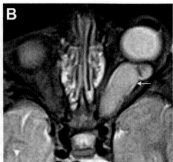 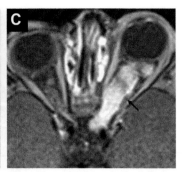

Fig. 4. Optic nerve glioma. (*A*) Coronal and (*B*) axial T2-STIR MR imaging sequences demonstrate a mass expanding the left optic nerve in a 2-year-old girl with known NF1 (*arrows*). (*C*) The mass demonstrates postcontrast enhancement (*arrow*).

multiple or bilateral facial infantile hemangiomas should raise the possibility of PHACES syndrome.[18]

Infantile hemangiomas may have lobular and infiltrative growth patterns. They demonstrate increased vascularity on ultrasound, with high vessel density demonstrating arterial tracing and low-resistive indices on Doppler examination.[19] On MR imaging, relative to muscle signal intensity, hemangiomas are T1 iso-hyperintense and T2 hyperintense, often with flow voids. Enhancement is typically diffuse and avid (Fig. 6).[19] Typically, there is no calcification unlike venous malformations, which commonly have phleboliths. In the involuting phase, the enhancement characteristics tend to become heterogeneous due to fatty infiltration.[16]

The main differential diagnosis to consider is rhabdomyosarcoma. A useful differentiating feature is lower mean apparent diffusion coefficient (ADC) values in rhabdomyosarcomas (RMS) compared with hemangiomas.[20] Other features include osseous destruction in RMS (when large), and rapid progression (although proliferating hemangiomas can also rapidly grow). In equivocal cases, tissue is required for final diagnosis.[21]

Rhabdomyosarcoma

RMS are the most common soft tissue sarcomas in children. Given its origin from extraocular muscles or the eyelid, orbital RMS are generally extraconal, although involvement of the orbital wall and intraconal extension are not uncommon.

Table 1
Syndromic versus nonsyndromic optic pathway glioma

Parameter	Syndromic (NF-1)	Sporadic
Location	Predilection for anterior visual pathway, ie, optic nerve	Predilection for posterior visual pathway, ie, optic chiasm, hypothalamus, optic tracts
Macroscopic appearance or MR imaging feature	More commonly present as tubular and tortuous enlargement of optic nerve	More commonly have nodular and cystic changes
Diagnosis	Diagnosis is presumptive, that is, biopsy not required	Biopsy may be suggested but not routinely
Growth pattern	Circumferential growth with relative sparing of the central nerve—hence *frequently asymptomatic*	More likely to be larger with intraneural infiltration, and therefore *more frequently symptomatic*
Growth over time	Tend to progress slowly early on following diagnosis, and then plateau around 6–12 y of life. May spontaneously regress	Less indolent

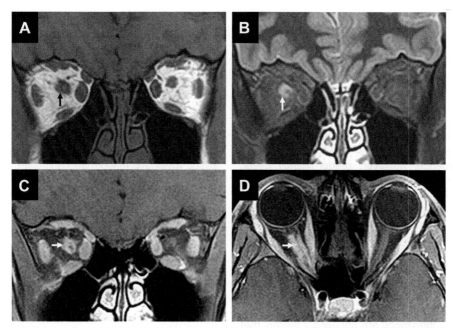

Fig. 5. Optic nerve sheath meningioma. (*A*) Coronal T1 and (*B*) T2-STIR MR imaging sequences demonstrate thickening of the right optic nerve sheath characterized by T1 hypointensity and T2 hyperintensity (*arrows*). (*C, D*) The right ONSM demonstrates postcontrast enhancement. Note sparing of the optic nerve, with tram track thickening and enhancement of the optic nerve sheath (*arrows, C, D*).

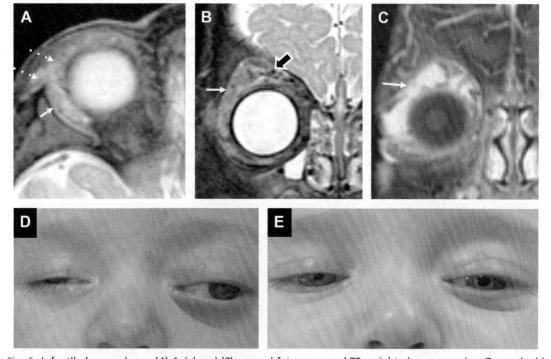

Fig. 6. Infantile hemangioma. (*A*) Axial and (*B*) coronal fat-suppressed T2-weighted sequences in a 7-month-old boy shows right periorbital hemangioma (*dash arrows, A*) extending into the superior and lateral extraconal compartments of the right orbit (*arrows, A and B*). Note numerous vascular flow voids within the lesion (*thick arrow, B*). (*C*) Coronal contrast-enhanced T1 fat-suppressed image shows diffuse avid enhancement of the lesion. Clinical photographs of a different patient at 4 weeks of age (*D*) shows left-sided proptosis with swelling and discoloration of the eyelids and periorbital soft tissue. A diagnosis of infantile hemangioma was made and the infant was treated with propranolol. Follow-up image during propranolol treatment at 7 months of age (*E*) shows resolution of proptosis with decreased periorbital swelling.

Typically, these present with a rapid onset of unilateral eyelid swelling, proptosis, and/or ptosis.[22] On MR imaging, RMS show variable signal intensity on T2-weighted images, reduced diffusivity, and variable enhancement (Fig. 7). Indeed, T2 hyperintense RMS without osseous erosion can mimic hemangiomas, especially when enhancement is marked.[21] ADC values help in differentiating these two entities in most instances.[20] In our experience, however, predominantly cystic RMS is difficult to distinguish from hemangiomas, necessitating biopsy for diagnosis. CT is useful to demonstrate osseous erosion when present. It is important to scan the head, neck, and brain for the evaluation of contiguous tumor spread.

Orbital Lymphatic and Venolymphatic Malformation

Orbital lymphatic (OLM) and venolymphatic (OVLM) malformations are congenital lesions that contain variable lymphatic and venous vascular elements. OLM is composed of embryonic lymphatic sacs, whereas OVLM contains venous and lymphatic elements.[23] In reality, however, it is difficult to distinguish between OLM and OVLM, and the term slow flow venolymphatic malformation is commonly used.

The lesions may be extraconal and/or intraconal, and similar to lymphatic malformations elsewhere in the body, are often trans-spatial. Depending on the size of the cysts, macrocystic (>1 cm), microcystic (< 1 cm), and mixed types are described.[24]

Macrocystic lymphatic malformations usually manifest as septated multilocular lesions. Fluid levels are common due to the presence of lymphatic, hemorrhagic (of varying ages) and proteinaceous content, and these can be depicted on ultrasound, CT and MR imaging as fluid–fluid levels

of mixed echogenicity, density, and signal intensity, respectively (Fig. 8).[25] Purely lymphatic malformations do not demonstrate vascular flow on Doppler ultrasound and do not typically enhance on contrast-enhanced CT and MR imaging except along septations and cyst walls wherein normal vessels may traverse. The presence of enhancement and/or phleboliths suggests the presence of a venous component to the malformation. Microcystic lymphatic malformations are ill-defined and solid appearing and tend to show patchy enhancement because of closely apposed cyst walls.[25]

Orbital Schwannoma

Orbital schwannoma, similar to ONSM, are rare in children. These are benign lesions that most commonly originate from the branches of the ophthalmic division of the trigeminal nerve (CN V).[26,27] About half of the cases involve the superior and medial compartments of the orbit in the extraconal space, suggesting that these lesions most commonly originate from the supraorbital or supratrochlear branches of the frontal nerve (a branch of the ophthalmic division of cranial nerve V [CN V]).[28] Appearances on MR imaging vary depending on histology ie, the relative proportion of Antoni A versus Antoni B cells.[28] Regions rich in Antoni A cells tend to be T2 hypointense with greater degree of enhancement compared with Antoni B rich areas. Areas of hemorrhage, cysts, and calcifications are well described.[28] The overall appearance of the tumor is, therefore, typically heterogeneous on T2-weighted images, with heterogeneous enhancement.

Orbital and Periorbital Plexiform Neurofibroma

Plexiform neurofibromas involving the orbit and periorbital soft tissues are commonly trans-spatial,

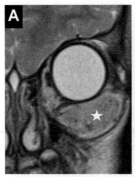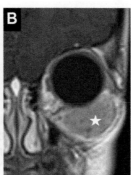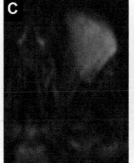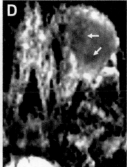

Fig. 7. Rhabdomyosarcoma. (A) Coronal T2 and (B) contrast-enhanced coronal T1-weighted images show a well-defined mass in the inferior rectus muscle extending into the extraconal compartment. The lesion is T2 hyperintense (*asterisk, A*) and shows moderate homogenous enhancement (*asterisk, B*). Axial DWI (C) and ADC (D) images show foci of reduced diffusivity (*arrows, D*).

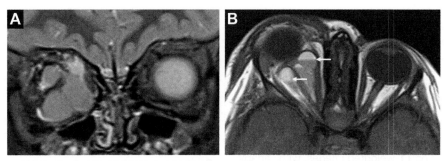

Fig. 8. Lymphatic malformation. (*A*) Coronal T2 STIR and (*B*) Axial T1 MR imaging sequences in a 2-year-old boy demonstrate a predominantly intraconal multilocular lesion with internal septations and fluid–fluid levels (*arrows, B*) in keeping with a lymphatic malformation.

involving the orbital, cranial, and peripheral nerve branches. These are almost exclusively seen in children with NF-1. On imaging, these appear as infiltrative, often serpentine soft tissue masses (**Figs. 9**A, B).[29] The target sign refers to central T2 hypointensity within T2 hyperintense nodular masses and is characteristic of plexiform neurofibromas.[30] Enhancement is variable. Secondary osseous changes may occur such as sphenoid wing dysplasia (see **Fig. 9**A), expansion of the orbital rim, and widened foramina.[31] These can cause an array of anatomical and functional disruption including features such as S-shaped ptosis, progressive proptosis, and vision loss (**Fig. 9**C).

Idiopathic Orbital Inflammation

IOI is an uncommon but important cause of acute orbital symptoms in children.[32] The term IOI refers to nonspecific inflammation that may involve any structure within the orbit. The lacrimal gland is most commonly involved, followed by the extraocular muscles. Less commonly, there may be involvement of the globe, the apex, and also

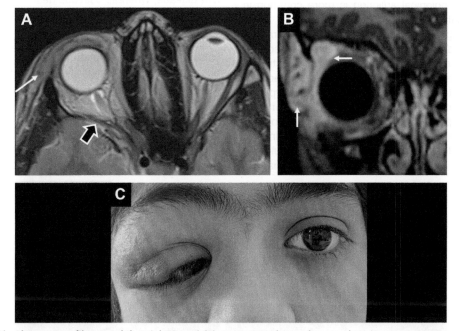

Fig. 9. Plexiform neurofibroma. (*A*) Axial T2 and (*B*) Contrast-enhanced coronal T1 images in a 9-year-old boy with NF-1 shows soft tissue thickening in the right periorbital region, which extends into the extraconal compartment of the orbit (*white arrows, A and B*). Note right sphenoid wing dysplasia (*thick arrow, A*). Clinical photograph (*C*) of a different patient with right orbital and eyelid plexiform neurofibroma and sphenoid wing dysplasia shows S-shaped ptosis, hypoglobus, and mild proptosis.

diffuse multifocal patterns (intraconal and extraconal).[32–34] Presentation may be acute or subacute with episodes of pain, edema, proptosis, diplopia, and restricted eye movements. In a retrospective study, bilateral involvement was reported in 13% of children, and 40% of children had constitutional symptoms.[32]

Imaging shows enlargement of the involved structures with poorly defined, mass-like, enhancing inflammatory soft tissue. These are hypointense on T1-weighted images, with variable signal on T2 fat-saturated images. Relative T2 hypointensity compared with other orbital lesions may occur due to dense cellular infiltrate and fibrosis (Fig. 10).[33,34] Differential diagnoses include other inflammatory processes such as thyroid eye disease, sarcoidosis, granulomatosis with polyangiitis, and neoplasms such as lymphoma. Lymphomatous infiltrates tend to have lower ADC values compared with IOI. However, it can be difficult to accurately differentiate the two based on imaging alone.

Lacrimal Gland Lesions

The lacrimal gland is an extraconal structure located within the lacrimal fossa in the superolateral aspect of the orbit. The levator palpebrae aponeurosis separates the lacrimal gland into an anterior palpebral lobe and a posterior orbital lobe.[1] Pathological affliction is more common in the orbital lobes.

On imaging, normal lacrimal glands are symmetric (unless bilaterally involved in disease), isoattenuating to muscle on CT, and demonstrating intermediate signal intensity on T1-weighted and T2-weighted sequences. Enhancement is typically homogenous. Pathologic conditions of the lacrimal gland with unilateral involvement include pleomorphic adenoma, adenoid cystic carcinoma, mucoepidermoid carcinoma, and leukemia (Fig. 11).[19] Lymphomatous involvement may be unilateral or bilateral.[35] Bilateral involvement is common in inflammatory conditions such as IOI, granulomatosis with angiitis, and sarcoidosis.[19,21]

Orbital Lymphoproliferative Lesions

Orbital lymphoproliferative lesions (OLPLs) are rare in children. These comprise a spectrum ranging from benign lymphoid hyperplasia to malignant lymphoma.[36] Orbital lymphomas are usually low-grade B-cell non-Hodgkin lymphoma. Secondary involvement from systemic disease generally represents diffuse large B cell lymphomas.[36]

OLPLs can involve any part of the orbit and have a predilection for the lacrimal gland. The lesions can be unilateral or bilateral and can present as focal masses or be diffuse and infiltrative in nature. Disease can also be limited to the extraocular musculature simulating thyroid eye disease.[36] On imaging, OLPLs are solid, lobulated masses that may encase and mold orbital structures. Benign hyperplasias tend to have well-defined margins, whereas lymphomas tend to be more irregular in appearance.[37] On CT, OLPLs are isodense to slightly hyperdense (on account of being densely cellular) (Fig. 12). Enhancement is typically moderate and homogeneous. The effect on surrounding structures may provide helpful clues as to the underlying nature of the OLPL—molding favors indolent disease, whereas osseous destruction favors an aggressive cause. On MR imaging, the lesions are mildly hyperintense relative to muscle on T1-weighted and T2-weighted images. Low ADC values are noted in lymphoma (Fig. 13).[37] In practice, differentiating benign hyperplasia from lymphoma is often challenging on imaging, necessitating the need for biopsy.

Orbital Leukemia

Orbital leukemic lesions in the context of acute myeloid leukemia are referred to as granulocytic

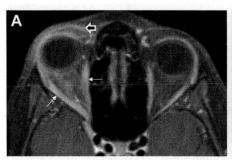
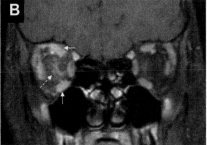

Fig. 10. Idiopathic orbital inflammation. (A) Contrast-enhanced T1 fat-saturated sequences in the axial (A) and coronal (B) planes show thickening and enhancement of the right extraocular muscles (*white arrows*), as well as the preseptal space (*thick arrow, A*). In addition, there is inflammatory fat stranding in the retroorbital region (*dashed arrow, B*). Note normal left-sided extraocular muscles for comparison.

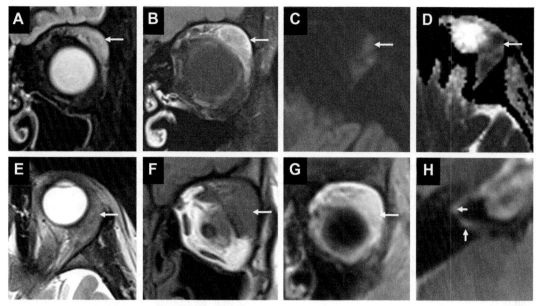

Fig. 11. Lacrimal gland lesions. (A–D): Leukemic infiltrate in a child with known acute lymphoblastic leukemia. Coronal T2 STIR (A), contrast-enhanced coronal T1 fat-saturated (B), axial DWI (C), and axial ADC (D) images show enlargement of the left lacrimal gland with T2 hyperintense signal (arrow, A), homogenous postcontrast enhancement (arrow, B), and restricted diffusion (arrow, C and D). (E–H): Sarcoidosis involving lacrimal gland and right facial nerve. Axial T2 (E), coronal T1 (F), and contrast-enhanced coronal T1 (G) images of the left orbit show enlargement and homogenous enhancement of the left lacrimal gland (arrows, E–G). Contrast-enhanced axial T1-weighted image of the right temporal bone shows enhancement of the meatal and labyrinthine segments of the right facial nerve (arrows, H).

sarcoma due to the presence of primitive granulocyte precursors.[38] Presentation is typically as a rapidly enlarging mass, which may cause pain, eyelid swelling, proptosis, diplopia, and ecchymosis. Indeed, the acute presentation can mimic an inflammatory process such as orbital cellulitis. Granulocytic sarcomas have a predilection for the lateral compartment and tend to encase the lacrimal gland and extraocular muscles. Osseous erosion and periosteal reaction may be seen on CT. On MR imaging, the lesions are usually isointense to hypointense on T1-weighted images,

and heterogenous, predominantly hyperintense on T2-weighted images. Enhancement is generally heterogenous (Fig. 14).[38]

Other Rare Orbital Masses

Intraorbital hemorrhage has been reported in patients with sickle cell disease. This occurs secondary to orbital wall infarction triggered by vaso-occlusive crises. Subsequent necrosis of local vessels leads to extravasation of blood and hematoma formation.[39,40] Presentation is with

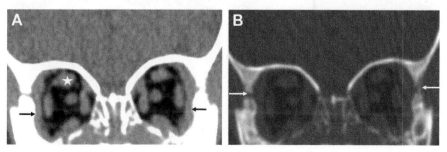

Fig. 12. Orbital lymphoproliferative lesion. Coronal noncontrast CT in soft tissue window (A) and bone window (B) demonstrate bilateral soft tissues in the extraconal space adjacent to the bony orbital rim (black arrows, A) that are isoattenuating with respect to the normal extraocular muscles (asterisk, A). Note permeative texture and suture diastasis of the lateral orbital rims (arrows, B) in keeping with malignant disease.

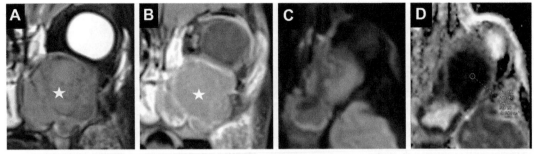

Fig. 13. Lymphoma. (A) Coronal T2 and (B) coronal contrast-enhanced fat-saturated T1-weighted images show a T2 intermediate-to-low signal intensity lesion (*asterisk, A*) with heterogenous enhancement (*asterisk, B*). Note the transcompartmental extent of the lesion with destruction of the inferior and lateral orbital walls. Axial DWI (C) and ADC (D) images show reduced diffusivity (average ADC value = $0.47 \times 10\text{–}3 \text{ mm}^2\text{/s}$) indicating high cellularity typical of lymphoma.

acute periorbital pain and swelling. Imaging helps confirm the presence of extraconal hemorrhage (Fig. 15) and may identify signs of bone infarction.[39]

Glial heterotopia refers to the presence of normal glial tissue (choristoma) without connection to the subarachnoid space.[41] The commonest location for glial heterotopias is in nasal and nasopharyngeal regions.[42] Orbital glial heterotopias are exceedingly rare.[43,44] On imaging, these are generally well-defined lesions that remodel the adjacent osseous structures (Fig. 16). Cystic components may be present.[44] By definition, there should be no communication with the brain.[44,45]

Orbital teratomas are rare congenital tumors that usually contain cells originating from all 3 germ cell layers, that is, ectoderm, endoderm, and mesoderm. On imaging, these are generally multiloculated cystic lesions with varying fat, calcium, and osseous elements (Fig. 17).[46] Majority of orbital teratomas are benign, although a few cases have reported malignancy.[47,48] Treatment

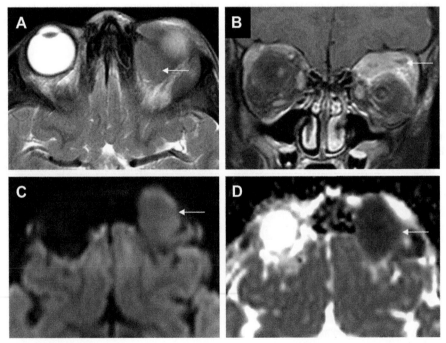

Fig. 14. Acute myeloid leukemia. (A) Axial T2 and (B) coronal contrast-enhanced T1 fat-saturated sequences demonstrate a T2 intermediate signal intensity lesion centered in the superior extraconal space of the left orbit (*arrow, A*) with heterogenous enhancement (*arrow, B*). Axial DWI (C) and ADC (D) images show reduced diffusivity (*arrows, C* and *D*).

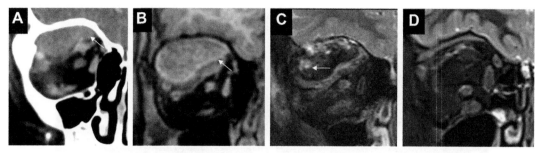

Fig. 15. Sickle cell disease and orbital hemorrhage. (*A*) Coronal noncontrast CT shows a lobulated iso-hyperdense lesion in the extraconal space superiorly (*arrow, A*). The lesion is T1 hyperintense (*arrow, B*), and heterogenous on T2-weighted sequence with layering T2 hypointense contents (*arrow, C*). Follow-up imaging after 3 months (*D*) shows near complete resolution of the lesion.

is complete surgical excision with sparing of vision. Close follow-up is necessary to exclude recurrence and malignant degeneration.

ORBITAL RIM MASSES
Ectodermal Inclusion Lesions (Dermoid and Epidermoid Cysts)

These refer to congenital cystic lesions occurring due to trapped ectodermal elements close to suture lines. Dermoid cyst contains dermal appendages, whereas epidermoid cysts do not.[49] Majority of these lesions are located along the superolateral aspect of the orbital rim (ie, along the fronto-zygomatic suture), whereas the remainder involve the superonasal aspect of the orbit.[49,50] Presentation is with a slowly progressive nontender, well-defined mass. Occasionally, these will present acutely when infected. Imaging shows a well-defined, cystic lesion closely related to a suture (Fig. 18). An ultrasound examination suffices for superficial lesions and may show internal debris within an otherwise cystic avascular lesion. Cross-sectional imaging should be reserved for assessing lesions that extend deep. On CT, the lesions may show fat, fluid, or mixed content depending on whether it represents a dermoid or epidermoid.[21] Typically, the underlying bone is remodeled by way of scalloping and dehiscence. On MR imaging, imaging appearances depend on the contents of the cyst. The presence of fat contributes to T1 hyperintense signal, and fat-saturated sequences can confirm this. Fluid-filled lesions are T1 hypointense and T2 hyperintense. Mixed content lesions will have a more heterogeneous appearance.[19] Thin rim enhancement may be appreciated on postcontrast images. An important finding in epidermoid cysts is restricted diffusion due to the presence of layered keratin minimizing movement of water molecules.[51] Restricted diffusion can also occur if the cyst is secondarily infected. Therefore, care must be taken to look for ancillary signs of infection such as inflammatory stranding in the surrounding soft tissues.

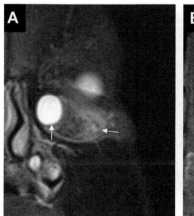
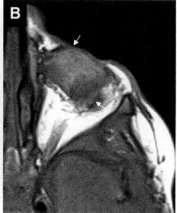
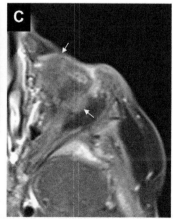

Fig. 16. Glial heterotopia. Coronal T2 STIR (*A*), axial T1 (*B*), and contrast-enhanced axial T1 fat-saturated imaging (*C*) shows a solid and cystic lesion involving the lower eyelid and the inferior extraconal space (*arrows*).

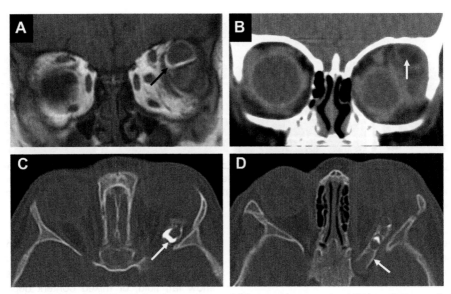

Fig. 17. Teratoma. (A) Coronal T1-weighted sequence and (B) coronal noncontrast CT in soft tissue window show an extraconal lesion deep to the lateral orbital wall with T1 hyperintense (arrow, A), and fat density (arrow, B) contents. (C and D) Axial CT images in bone window show well-matured tooth and bony structure within the lesion (arrows, C and D) in keeping with a teratoma.

Differential diagnoses include orbital dermolipoma, which shows homogeneous fat content without debris or fluid levels.[52] Other differentials include lacrimal gland cysts, frontal and ethmoidal mucocele when encountered in the superonasal region, and occasionally neoplasms (eg, cystic rhabdomyosarcoma, teratoma). A fat-containing lesion that shows rapid growth should raise the possibility of a teratoma (see Fig. 17).

METASTASES

Neuroblastoma (NB) is a malignant tumor originating from embryonal neural crest cell derivatives.[53] The orbit and calvarium are also largely derived from neural crest precursors, perhaps explaining their common involvement in metastatic NB.[54] Ophthalmic involvement has been described in approximately one-third of cases.[54] Typical presentation is with "raccoon eyes" (due to ecchymosis), and proptosis.[55] Osseous involvement is well demonstrated on plain radiographs and CT with a hair-on-end spiculated appearance and periosteal new bone formation (Fig. 19). Tumor cells may also lead to sutural diastasis. The soft tissue components of the lesion are usually iso-hyperattenuating and may mimic acute hemorrhage. On MR imaging,

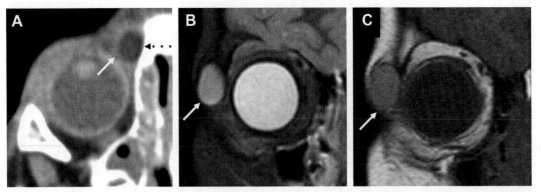

Fig. 18. Dermoid cyst. Axial CT (A) in a patient shows a well-defined cyst in medial periorbital region (arrow). Note subtle remodeling of the adjacent bone (dashed arrow). Coronal T2-weighted (B) and coronal T1-weighted (C) images in a different patient show a well-defined T2 hyperintense and T1 intermediate signal intensity cyst (arrows) closely related to the frontozygomatic suture along the lateral orbital rim.

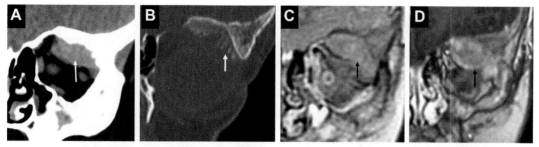

Fig. 19. NB metastases. (*A*) Coronal CT in soft tissue (*A*) and bone (*B*) windows show an extraconal soft tissue mass (*arrow, A*) with osseous involvement with spiculated periosteal new bone formation (also referred to as "hair-on-end" appearance) (*arrow, B*). Coronal T2 (*C*) and contrast-enhanced coronal T1-weighted (*D*) sequences show a heterogeneously enhancing lesion involving the orbital rim and the extraconal space (*arrows, C* and *D*).

the lesions are usually slightly T1 hypointense and T2 hyperintense relative to muscle and show avid or heterogeneous enhancement (see **Fig. 19**).[19,54] Meta-iodobenzylguanidine (MIBG) bone scan, when positive, is highly specific for NB.[56] However, up to a third of NBs may be MIBG negative.[57] Other radiotracers that may be used in these instances are fluorodeoxyglucose (FDG)-positron emission tomography (PET) and Tc-99m methylene diphosphonate.[19] Important differentials include Langerhans cell histiocytosis (LCH), rhabdomyosarcoma and leukemic infiltrates. Orbital LCH usually do not incite the typical hair-on-end periosteal reaction seen in NB. Other pediatric tumors that may metastasize to the orbital rim include Ewing sarcoma (**Fig. 20**).

Langerhans Cell Histiocytosis

LCH is a neoplastic disorder driven by the mitogen-activated protein kinase pathway and is characterized by the proliferation of myeloid dendritic cells.[58,59] Orbital LCH most commonly involves the lateral wall and orbital roof.[60,61] It is usually unilateral and may either be isolated or be as part of disseminated disease. Early in the

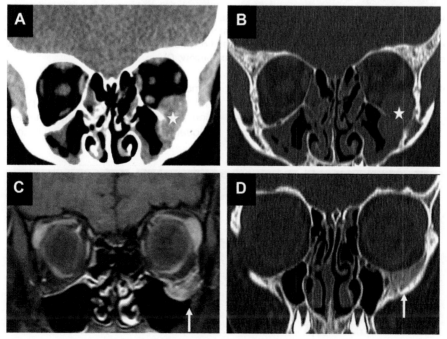

Fig. 20. Ewing sarcoma metastasis. (*A, B*) Coronal CT of a 7-year-old girl with Ewing sarcoma demonstrates an osteolytic lesion with soft tissue mass at the left inferior orbital rim (*asterisks*). (*C*) Coronal postcontrast fat-saturated T1-weighted sequence after 2 months of chemotherapy shows residual enhancing mass along the inferior orbital rim (*arrow, C*). (*D*) Coronal CT in bone window (*D*) after 4 months of therapy shows sclerosis and new bone formation in the inferior orbital rim (*arrow, D*).

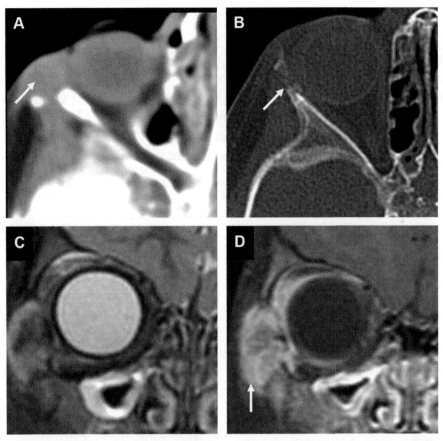

Fig. 21. Langerhans cell histiocytosis. Axial CT in soft tissue (*A*) and bone (*B*) windows show a lesion involving the lateral wall of the right orbit (*arrow, A*), causing permeative destruction of the greater wing of sphenoid (*arrow, B*). Coronal T2 STIR (*C*) and contrast-enhanced fat-saturated coronal T1-weighted (*D*) sequences show the destruction of the lateral orbital wall with enhancing soft tissue (*arrow, D*).

course of the disease, LCH lesions seem as aggressive lesions with a wide transition zone, mimicking osteomyelitis, and other malignant neoplasms (**Fig. 21**). This then evolves into the typical

punched out lytic lesion. LCH lesions generally do not incite the typical hair-on-end periosteal reaction seen in NB. MR imaging with fat-suppressed sequences enables visualization of the soft tissue

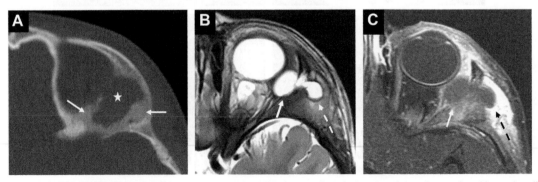

Fig. 22. Orbital myofibroma. Axial CT in bone window (*A*) shows a lytic lesion involving the roof and lateral wall of the left orbit (*asterisk, A*). Note also the presence of sclerosis along the margins of the lesion (*arrows, A*). Axial T2 (*B*) and contrast-enhanced fat-saturated T1-weighted (*C*) sequences show a solid and cystic heterogeneously enhancing lesion causing destruction of the lateral orbital wall (*arrows, B* and *C*). Note extraorbital extension of enhancing soft tissue (*dashed arrows, B* and *C*).

components (see **Fig. 21**).[61] Care must be taken to image the brain adequately to exclude parenchymal disease and pituitary involvement.[62]

Orbital Myofibroma

Myofibroma belongs to the spectrum of myofibromatoses that are nonencapsulated benign fibrous tumors that may be solitary, multicentric, and generalized.[63–65] The solitary form of orbital myofibromas present as benign, slow-growing, and painless masses. Myofibromas are generally well-circumscribed lesions with or without lobulations. On CT, these can mimic an aggressive process due to the presence of osseous destruction. On MR imaging, myofibromas are well-defined T2 hyperintense, T1 hypointense lesions that show enhancement (**Fig. 22**).[63,65]

SUMMARY

The clinical presentation of pediatric orbital masses is often nonspecific. Imaging, therefore, has a crucial role in the workup of these cases. A compartment-based approach is useful in narrowing down the differential diagnoses. MR imaging is the primary imaging modality of choice, with ultrasound and CT playing complimentary roles.

CLINICS CARE POINTS

- OPGs are low-grade neoplasms and can either be syndromic (NF-1) or sporadic.
- Syndromic OPGs are frequently asymptomatic and have an indolent course compared with sporadic OPGs.
- Enhancement characteristics of OPGs can wax and wane over time and, therefore, should not be used as a surrogate marker for disease activity.
- Infantile orbital hemangiomas have a proliferative phase and an involution phase. Majority of these regress by 5 years of age. Most involving the eyelid or orbit require treatment with propanolol.
- Growth of infantile hemangiomas can be rapid during the proliferative phase, and therefore, in lesions that do not have cutaneous findings, RMS is the main differential. A useful differentiating feature is the presence of low ADC values in the latter. However, care must be taken because not all RMS (eg, cystic RMS) have low ADC values.
- Ectodermal inclusion cysts frequently occur close to suture lines. The adjacent bone is typically scalloped and remodeled rather than eroded.
- The main differential diagnoses to consider for lesions that destruct or erode the orbital rim in children are NB metastases, LCH and RMS. The presence of hair-on-end periosteal reaction is characteristic of NB metastasis.

DISCLOSURE

Nothing to disclose.

REFERENCES

1. Reinshagen KL, Massoud TF, Cunnane MB. Anatomy of the Orbit. Neuroimaging Clin N Am 2022; 32(4):699–711.
2. Haładaj R. Normal Anatomy and Anomalies of the Rectus Extraocular Muscles in Human: A Review of the Recent Data and Findings. BioMed Res Int 2019;2019:e8909162.
3. Nicolin G, Parkin P, Mabbott D, et al. Natural history and outcome of optic pathway gliomas in children. Pediatr Blood Cancer 2009;53(7):1231–7.
4. Chateil JF, Soussotte C, Pédespan JM, et al. MRI and clinical differences between optic pathway tumours in children with and without neurofibromatosis. Br J Radiol 2001;74(877):24–31.
5. Kornreich L, Blaser S, Schwarz M, et al. Optic Pathway Glioma: Correlation of Imaging Findings with the Presence of Neurofibromatosis. Am J Neuroradiol 2001;22(10):1963–9.
6. Fangusaro J, Witt O, Hernáiz Driever P, et al. Response assessment in paediatric low-grade glioma: recommendations from the Response Assessment in Pediatric Neuro-Oncology (RAPNO) working group. Lancet Oncol 2020;21(6):e305–16.
7. Parker RT, Ovens CA, Fraser CL, et al. Optic nerve sheath meningiomas: prevalence, impact, and management strategies. Eye Brain 2018;10:85–99.
8. Li P, Wang Z, Zhou Q, et al. A Retrospective Analysis of Vision-Impairing Tumors Among 467 Patients with Neurofibromatosis Type 2. World Neurosurg 2017; 97:557–64.
9. Patel BC, De Jesus O, Margolin E. Optic Nerve Sheath Meningioma. In: StatPearls. Treasure Island, FL: StatPearls Publishing; 2022. Available at: http://www.ncbi.nlm.nih.gov/books/NBK430868/. Accessed March 1, 2023.
10. Mafee MF, Goodwin J, Dorodi S. Optic nerve sheath meningiomas. Role of MR imaging. Radiol Clin North Am 1999;37(1):37–58, ix.
11. Husum YS, Skogen K, Brandal P, et al. Bilateral calcification of the optic nerve sheath: A diagnostic dilemma. Am J Ophthalmol Case Rep 2021;22: 101106.

12. Arnold AC, Lee AG. Dilation of the Perioptic Sub-arachnoid Space Anterior to Optic Nerve Sheath Meningioma. J Neuro Ophthalmol 2021;41(1):e100–2.

13. Jackson A, Patankar T, Laitt RD. Intracanalicular optic nerve meningioma: a serious diagnostic pitfall. AJNR Am J Neuroradiol 2003;24(6):1167–70.

14. Boye E, Yu Y, Paranya G, et al. Clonality and altered behavior of endothelial cells from hemangiomas. J Clin Invest 2001;107(6):745–52.

15. Jacobs AH. Strawberry hemangiomas; the natural history of the untreated lesion. Calif Med 1957; 86(1):8–10.

16. Harter N, Mancini AJ. Diagnosis and Management of Infantile Hemangiomas in the Neonate. Pediatr Clin North Am 2019;66(2):437–59.

17. Briones M, Adams D. Neonatal Vascular Tumors. Clin Perinatol 2021;48(1):181–98.

18. Rotter A, Samorano LP, Rivitti-Machado MC, et al. PHACE syndrome: clinical manifestations, diagnostic criteria, and management. An Bras Dermatol 2018;93(3):405–11.

19. Joseph AK, Guerin JB, Eckel LJ, et al. Imaging Findings of Pediatric Orbital Masses and Tumor Mimics. Radiographics 2022;42(3):880–97.

20. Kralik SF, Haider KM, Lobo RR, et al. Orbital infantile hemangioma and rhabdomyosarcoma in children: differentiation using diffusion-weighted magnetic resonance imaging. J AAPOS 2018;22(1):27–31.

21. Chung EM, Murphey MD, Specht CS, et al. From the Archives of the AFIP Pediatric Orbit Tumors and Tumorlike Lesions: Osseous Lesions of the Orbit. Radiographics 2008;28(4):1193–214.

22. Karcioglu ZA, Hadjistilianou D, Rozans M, et al. Orbital rhabdomyosarcoma. Cancer Control 2004; 11(5):328–33.

23. Kunimoto K, Yamamoto Y, Jinnin M. ISSVA Classification of Vascular Anomalies and Molecular Biology. Int J Mol Sci 2022;23(4):2358.

24. Colletti G, Biglioli F, Poli T, et al. Vascular malformations of the orbit (lymphatic, venous, arteriovenous): Diagnosis, management and results. J Cranio-Maxillo-Fac Surg 2019;47(5):726–40.

25. White CL, Olivieri B, Restrepo R, et al. Low-Flow Vascular Malformation Pitfalls: From Clinical Examination to Practical Imaging Evaluation–Part 1, Lymphatic Malformation Mimickers. AJR Am J Roentgenol 2016;206(5):940–51.

26. Kim KS, Jung JW, Yoon KC, et al. Schwannoma of the Orbit. Arch Craniofac Surg 2015;16(2):67–72.

27. Chaskes MB, Rabinowitz MR. Orbital Schwannoma. J Neurol Surg B Skull Base 2020;81(4):376–80.

28. Wang Y, Xiao LH. Orbital schwannomas: findings from magnetic resonance imaging in 62 cases. Eye (Lond). 2008;22(8):1034–9.

29. Milburn JM, Gimenez CR, Dutweiler E. Clinical Images: Imaging Manifestations of Orbital Neurofibromatosis Type 1. Ochsner J 2016;16(4):431–4.

30. Ghosh PS, Ghosh D. Teaching NeuroImages: MRI "target sign" and neurofibromatosis type 1. Neurology 2012;78(9):e63.

31. Jacquemin C, Bosley TM, Liu D, et al. Reassessment of sphenoid dysplasia associated with neurofibromatosis type 1. AJNR Am J Neuroradiol 2002; 23(4):644–8.

32. Spindle J, Tang SX, Davies B, et al. PediatricIdiopathic Orbital Inflammation: Clinical Features of 30 Cases. Ophthalmic Plast Reconstr Surg 2016; 32(4):270–4.

33. Chen F, Tang J, Zhou Q. Bilateral idiopathic orbital pseudotumour in a child: a case report. BMC Ophthalmol 2020;20(1):449.

34. Yazicioglu T, Kutluturk I. Idiopathic Orbital Myositis in a 9-Year-Old Girl: A Case Report. Iran J Pediatr 2015;25(3):e371.

35. Moustafa GA, Topham AK, Aronow ME, et al. Paediatric ocular adnexal lymphoma: a population-based analysis. BMJ Open Ophthalmology 2020;5(1): e000483.

36. Rao AA, Naheedy JH, Chen JYY, et al. A Clinical Update and Radiologic Review of Pediatric Orbital and Ocular Tumors. J Oncol 2013;2013:975908.

37. Haradome K, Haradome H, Usui Y, et al. Orbital Lymphoproliferative Disorders (OLPDs): Value of MR Imaging for Differentiating Orbital Lymphoma from Benign OPLDs. Am J Neuroradiol 2014; 35(10):1976–82.

38. Noh BW, Park SW, Chun JE, et al. Granulocytic Sarcoma in the Head and Neck: CT and MR Imaging Findings. Clin Exp Otorhinolaryngol 2009;2(2):66–71.

39. Ganesh A, William RR, Mitra S, et al. Orbital involvement in sickle cell disease: A report of five cases and review literature. Eye 2001;15(6):774–80.

40. Andriamiarintsoa H, Ramanandafy H, Andriamiadanalisoa OA, et al. Spontaneous bilateral intraorbital hematoma: A particular form of sickle cell disease complications in children. Clinical Case Reports 2022;10(6):e5994.

41. Patterson K, Kapur S, Chandra RS. "Nasal gliomas" and related brain heterotopias: a pathologist's perspective. Pediatr Pathol 1986;5(3–4):353–62.

42. Julie CP, Sophie B, Frédérique D, et al. Nasal glial heterotopia: Four case reports with a review of literature. Oral and Maxillofacial Surgery Cases 2019; 5(3):100107.

43. Kiratli H, Şekeroğlu MA, Tezel GG. Orbital Heterotopic Glial Tissue Presenting as Exotropia. Orbit 2008;27(3):165–8.

44. Mehta NS, Tenzel PA, Sharfi D, et al. Orbital Glial Heterotopia: A Report of 2 Cases and Review of the Literature. Ophthalmic Plast Reconstr Surg 2020;36(1):2.

45. Sitaula R, Shrestha GB, Paudel N, et al. Glial Heterotopia of the orbit: A rare presentation. BMC Ophthalmol 2011;11:34.

46. Tsoutsanis PA, Charonis GC. Congenital orbital teratoma: a case report with preservation of the globe and 18 years of follow-up. BMC Ophthalmol 2021; 21(1):456.

47. Mahesh L, Krishnakumar S, Subramanian N, et al. Malignant teratoma of the orbit: a clinicopathological study of a case. Orbit 2003;22(4):305–9.

48. Garden JW, McManis JC. Congenital orbital-intracranial teratoma with subsequent malignancy: case report. Br J Ophthalmol 1986;70(2):111–3.

49. Cavazza S, Laffi GL, Lodi L, et al. Orbital dermoid cyst of childhood: clinical pathologic findings, classification and management. Int Ophthalmol 2011; 31(2):93–7.

50. Pushker N, Meel R, Kumar A, et al. Orbital and peri-orbital dermoid/epidermoid cyst: a series of 280 cases and a brief review. Can J Ophthalmol 2020; 55(2):167–71.

51. Ahmed RA, Eltanamly RM. Orbital Epidermoid Cysts: A Diagnosis to Consider. Journal of Ophthalmology 2014;2014:e508425.

52. McNab AA, Wright JE, Caswell AG. Clinical features and surgical management of dermolipomas. Aust N Z J Ophthalmol 1990;18(2):159–62.

53. Tomolonis JA, Agarwal S, Shohet JM. Neuroblastoma pathogenesis: deregulation of embryonic neural crest development. Cell Tissue Res 2018;372(2): 245–62.

54. D'Ambrosio N, Lyo J, Young R, et al. Common and unusual craniofacial manifestations of metastatic neuroblastoma. Neuroradiology 2010;52(6):549–53.

55. Musarella MA, Chan HS, DeBoer G, et al. Ocular involvement in neuroblastoma: prognostic implications. Ophthalmology 1984;91(8):936–40.

56. Sharp SE, Trout AT, Weiss BD, et al. MIBG in Neuroblastoma Diagnostic Imaging and Therapy. Radiographics 2016;36(1):258–78.

57. Bleeker G, Tytgat GA, Adam JA, et al. 123I-MIBG scintigraphy and 18F-FDG-PET imaging for diagnosing neuroblastoma. Cochrane Database Syst Rev 2015;2015(9):CD009263.

58. Allen CE, Li L, Peters TL, et al. Cell-specific gene expression in Langerhans cell histiocytosis lesions reveals a distinct profile compared with epidermal Langerhans cells. J Immunol 2010;184(8):4557–67.

59. Berres ML, Lim KPH, Peters T, et al. BRAF-V600E expression in precursor versus differentiated dendritic cells defines clinically distinct LCH risk groups. J Exp Med 2014;211(4):669–83.

60. Lakatos K, Sterlich K, Pötschger U, et al. Langerhans Cell Histiocytosis of the Orbit: Spectrum of Clinical and Imaging Findings. J Pediatr 2021;230: 174–81.e1.

61. Wu C, Li K, Hei Y, et al. MR imaging features of orbital Langerhans cell Histiocytosis. BMC Ophthalmol 2019;19(1):263.

62. Grois N, Prayer D, Prosch H, et al, the CNS LCH Cooperative Group. Neuropathology of CNS disease in Langerhans cell histiocytosis. Brain 2005;128(4): 829–38.

63. Shields CL, Husson M, Shields JA, et al. Solitary Intraosseous Infantile Myofibroma of the Orbital Roof. Arch Ophthalmol 1998;116(11):1528–30.

64. Rodrigues EB, Shields CL, Eagle RCJ, et al. Solitary Intraosseous Orbital Myofibroma in Four Cases. Ophthalmic Plast Reconstr Surg 2006;22(4):292.

65. Madhuri BK, Tripathy D, Mittal R. Solitary orbital myofibroma in a child: A rare case report with literature review. Indian J Ophthalmol 2019;67(7):1240–5.

Common Neck and Otomastoid Infections in Children

William T. O'Brien Sr, DO

KEYWORDS

- Neck infection • Tonsillitis • Retropharyngeal infection • Abscess • Suppurative adenopathy
- Otomastoiditis • Lemierre syndrome • Infected congenital cyst

KEY POINTS

- Imaging is key in the workup of pediatric neck infections, as they may be difficult to localize based upon clinical presentation and physical exam findings alone.
- Primary roles of imaging in neck infections include identifying location and extent of infections, evaluating for potentially drainable collections, and assessing for airway and vascular complications.
- With temporal bone infections, it is critical to identify extratemporal spread, especially intracranial extension with associated complications.

INTRODUCTION

Neck infections are common in children and may be challenging to localize clinically, given overlapping clinical presentations and often nonspecific physical examination findings. Therefore, imaging plays an essential role in localizing the primary site of infection, identifying potentially drainable collections, and assessing for airway and vascular complications.[1] Knowledge of the characteristic imaging features of common pediatric neck infections is, therefore, paramount when interpreting imaging studies in children. This illustrative review focuses on characteristic imaging features and potential complications associated with common neck infections in children to include tonsillar, retropharyngeal, and otomastoid infections; suppurative adenopathy; superimposed inflammation or infection of congenital cystic lesions; and Lemierre syndrome.

TONSILLAR REGION INFECTIONS

Tonsillar region infections represent the most common neck infections in children and adolescents. Infections begin as tonsillitis, which may resolve or progress to more advanced phlegmon and eventually a tonsillar region abscess. Imaging findings in uncomplicated tonsillitis include tonsillar edema and enlargement with a characteristic striated or "tigroid" enhancement pattern (Fig. 1A).

If the infection progresses, a tonsillar region abscess may occur. Tonsillar region abscesses are characterized as peritonsillar in the vast majority of cases, with intratonsillar abscesses being far less common. The distinction may have clinical significance, because peritonsillar abscesses are typically drained, whereas patients with a suspected intratonsillar abscess may initially undergo a trial of medical therapy. Intratonsillar abscesses occur within the tonsillar capsule, most commonly within tonsillar crypts followed by the tonsillar parenchyma. On imaging, an intratonsillar abscess may be suggested when an abscess appears centered within the tonsil (Fig. 1B).

Peritonsillar abscesses present as rim-enhancing collections often located eccentrically in the tonsillar region between the tonsillar capsule and pharyngeal constrictor muscle. Because of the location, peritonsillar abscesses may extend into adjacent spaces of the neck, including the parapharyngeal, masticator, and submandibular spaces[2,3] (Fig. 1C). Although clinical presentations overlap, patients with

Division of Pediatric Neuroradiology, Orlando Health – Arnold Palmer Hospital for Children, 92 West Miller Street, Orlando, FL 32806, USA
E-mail address: William.obrien@orlandohealth.com

Neuroimag Clin N Am 33 (2023) 661–671
https://doi.org/10.1016/j.nic.2023.05.013

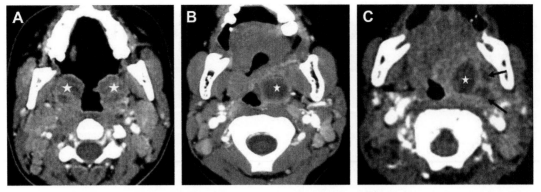

Fig. 1. Tonsillar regions infections. Contrast-enhanced CT images in three different patients demonstrate characteristic imaging features of tonsillitis (A) with symmetric enlargement of the palatine tonsils and a striated or "tigroid" enhancement pattern (*), an intratonsillar abscess (B) with a rim-enhancing collection centered within the left palatine tonsil (*), and a peritonsillar abscess (C) located eccentrically on the left (*) with extension into adjacent spaces of the neck (arrows). All three cases show varying degrees of reactive lymphadenopathy.

peritonsillar abscesses tend to have a higher incidence of dysphonia, trismus, and otalgia on presentation compared with patients with uncomplicated tonsillitis or intratonsillar abscesses.[4,5]

RETROPHARYNGEAL INFECTIONS

Retropharyngeal infectious and inflammatory processes in children include reactive retropharyngeal edema, suppurative adenopathy, and retropharyngeal abscesses.

Retropharyngeal edema refers to reactive, non-suppurative fluid within the retropharyngeal space secondary to a head and neck infection, most commonly pharyngitis in a child. Retropharyngeal edema can be recognized by its morphology, absence of rim enhancement, and relatively mild mass effect. In terms of morphology, reactive edema fills the retropharyngeal space from side to side with a midline waist as it crosses over the cervical vertebral bodies and flaring laterally, resulting in a "bowtie" configuration on axial images. Tapering of the fluid collection is noted at its cranial and caudal ends (Fig. 2). Surrounding inflammatory changes are typically absent.[6]

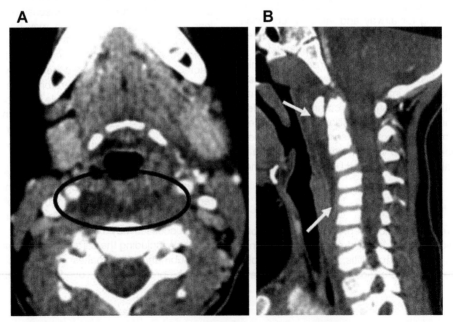

Fig. 2. Retropharyngeal edema. Contrast-enhanced axial CT image (A) shows a non-enhancing retropharyngeal fluid collection with a "bowtie" configuration, characterized by a midline waist and lateral flaring (o). "o" refers to the oval annotation encircling the fluid in the retropharyngealk space in image A. Sagittal reformatted image (B) demonstrates tapering of the retropharyngeal fluid at its cranial and caudal ends (arrows).

In the setting of suppurative adenopathy, an infection is contained within a lateral retropharyngeal lymph node, typically due to spread of a pharyngeal, otomastoid, or paranasal sinus infection. On cross-sectional imaging, a centrally necrotic lymph node is identified in the lateral retropharyngeal space, with variable peripheral solid nodal enhancement and a varying degree of surrounding inflammatory changes. The collection is round or ovoid, relatively small, and contained within the lymph node capsule. The adjacent vasculature needs to be closely evaluated for inflammatory complications, such as thrombosis or pseudoaneurysm formation. Vasospasm is commonly seen and typically transient and incidental with appropriate medical management of the underlying infection[6] (Fig. 3).

A retropharyngeal abscess most often results from rupture of a suppurative lymph node into the retropharyngeal space. Imaging findings show a larger retropharyngeal fluid collection that unlike a suppurative lymph node may cross midline and occasionally have intralesional foci of gas. Rim enhancement is often, but not always, present.[1] The abscess and surrounding inflammatory changes result in the regional mass effect; therefore, it is important to evaluate the airway for compression as well as any complications involving adjacent vasculature (Fig. 4).

An uncommon but important complication to identify is spread of a retropharyngeal abscess

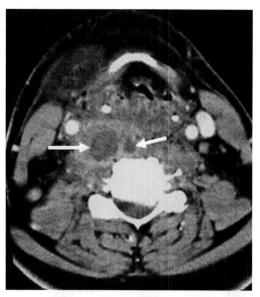

Fig. 4. Retropharyngeal abscess. Axial contrast-enhanced CT image shows a large, rim-enhancing right-sided retropharyngeal abscess (*arrows*), which crosses midline and causes mass effect on adjacent structures, including the aerodigestive tract and vasculature of the neck.

into the danger space, resulting in mediastinitis, along with potential pulmonary or cardiac infections.[6] The retropharyngeal and danger spaces cannot be directly differentiated on imaging, aside from their inferior extent. Inferiorly, the retropharyngeal space commonly extends to the T1–T3 levels, whereas the danger space can extend throughout the thoracic region to the level of the diaphragm (Fig. 5).

The question of drainability of a retropharyngeal collection comes up frequently and is often difficult to predict with a high degree of accuracy based on imaging findings. One study looked at volumes of retropharyngeal collections that were drainable versus those that were not. The average volume of drainable collections was 4.4 cm^3 and the average volume of those that were not drainable was 2.2 cm^3.[7]

OTOMASTOID INFECTIONS

Children are especially prone to otomastoid infections due to relatively horizontal orientation of their eustachian tubes and prominence of nasopharyngeal adenoidal tissue, both of which impair drainage from the middle ear cavity. Most cases are self-limited, diagnosed clinically, and treated medically. In the setting of mastoid and middle ear opacification with preservation of bony structures, the imaging findings themselves are

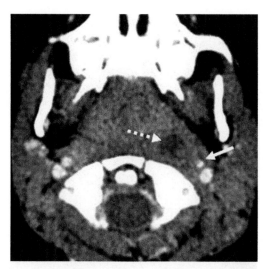

Fig. 3. Retropharyngeal suppurative adenopathy. Axial contrast-enhanced CT image demonstrates a small, round hypodense collection in a left lateral retropharyngeal lymph node (*dashed arrow*) with narrowing of the adjacent cervical internal carotid artery, consistent with vasospasm (*arrow*). Prominent adenoids are common in children.

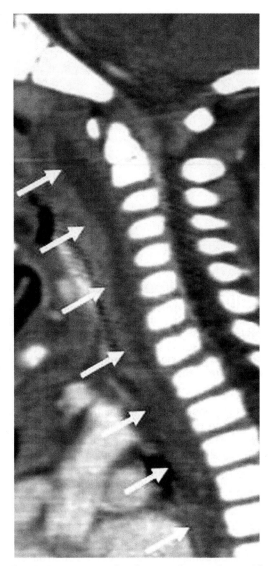

Fig. 5. Danger space involvement in a patient with mediastinitis as a complication of a retropharyngeal abscess. Sagittal contrast-enhanced CT image demonstrates a large retropharyngeal collection and adjacent inflammatory changes extending below the mid-thoracic region (*arrows*), compatible with danger space involvement.

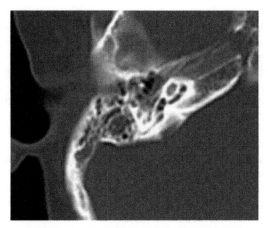

Fig. 6. Nonspecific otomastoid opacification. Axial CT image in bone algorithm demonstrates nonspecific opacification of the mastoid air cells and middle ear cavity, with preservation of bony structures.

mastoid walls may result in extratemporal spread of the infection. With lateral wall dehiscence, abscess formation occurs in the overlying postauricular soft tissues, and with dehiscence at the inferior mastoid tip, abscess formation and inflammatory changes may spread along the sternocleidomastoid muscle, which is referred to as a mastoid tip or Bezold abscess (Fig. 8). Not all cases of extratemporal abscesses, however, have frank bony dehiscence on imaging, as transvenous spread of infections may occur in children with intact bony margins.[8,9]

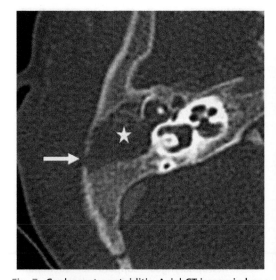

Fig. 7. Coalescent mastoiditis. Axial CT image in bone algorithm shows opacification throughout the mastoid air cells and epitympanum with erosion of mastoid septa (*) and dehiscence of the lateral mastoid wall (*arrow*) with overlying extratemporal soft tissue swelling.

nonspecific and should not be presumed to represent otomastoiditis, which remains a clinical diagnosis (Fig. 6).

Coalescent mastoiditis is a complication of otomastoiditis due to failed or untreated infections that result in obstruction of the aditus ad antrum with purulent debris accumulating in the mastoid air cells. The diagnosis is suggested on imaging when there is erosion of mastoid septa, resulting in coalescence of the mastoid cavity with suppurative debris (Fig. 7). Erosion of the

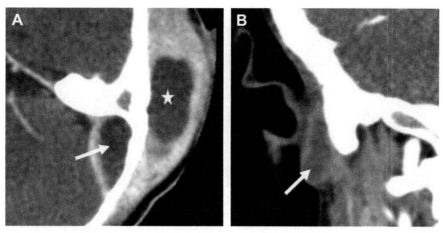

Fig. 8. Lateral and mastoid tip abscesses. Contrast-enhanced axial (A) and reformatted coronal (B) CT images in different patients demonstrates extratemporal abscesses superficial (*, A) and deep (epidural, arrow, A) to the lateral mastoid wall and extending along the mastoid tip (Bezold abscess, arrow, B).

Additional uncommon temporal bone complications of otomastoiditis include labyrinthitis and petrous apicitis. Labyrinthitis refers to inflammation within the inner ear structures and may occur due to direct or hematogenous spread of an infection. When due to an underlying otomastoid infections, there is direct spread through the oval or round window into the labyrinthine structures, so the associated labyrinthitis is unilateral.

There are three phases of labyrinthitis—acute, fibrous, and chronic, each of which has characteristic imaging features. In the acute phase, abnormal

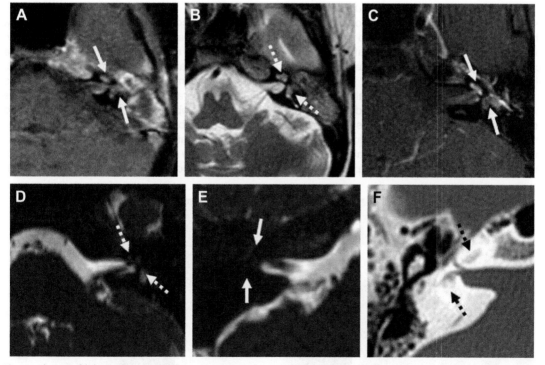

Fig. 9. Phases of labyrinthitis. Axial fat-suppressed T1 post-contrast (A) and high-resolution T2 (B) images in a patient with acute phase labyrinthitis show abnormal enhancement throughout the inner ear structures (arrows, A) with relative preservation of T2 signal intensity (dashed arrows, B). The same sequences (C, D) in a patient with fibrous phase labyrinthitis demonstrate persistent inner ear enhancement (arrows, C) with loss of the normal T2 signal intensity (dashed arrows, D). A follow-up CT examination (not show) did not show abnormal mineralization. Axial high-resolution T2 (E) and CT (F) images in a patient with chronic phase labyrinthitis show complete loss of T2 signal intensity within the inner ear structures (arrows, E) with abnormal mineralization on CT (dashed arrows, F).

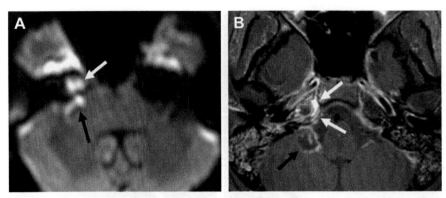

Fig. 10. Petrous apicitis. Axial diffusion-weighted (DWI, *A*) and fat-suppressed T1 post-contrast (*B*) images show central restricted diffusion (ADC map not shown) centered in the right petrous apex (*white arrow*, A) with surrounding inflammatory enhancement (*white arrows*, B). Mastoid enhancement and a small cerebellar abscess (*black arrows*, A and B) are also noted.

enhancement is seen within the inner ear structures, with relative preservation of T2 signal intensity and lack of ossification. In the fibrous phase, there is a loss of normal T2 signal intensity within the inner ear structures, with or without residual enhancement and a lack of ossification. In the chronic phase, there is essentially complete loss of T2 signal intensity and ossification throughout involved portions of inner structures, with no enhancement. It is important to recognize labyrinthitis in the acute or fibrous phase to help preserve or restore hearing, as once ossification occurs, it can be difficult or impossible to restore hearing through cochlear implantation.[10] (**Fig. 9**).

Petrous apicitis is a rare potential complication of otomastoiditis. Although debated, it is thought to preferentially occur in individuals with a pneumatized petrous apex. On imaging, there are bony erosive changes and signal abnormality centered in the petrous apex with peripheral and

surrounding inflammatory enhancement (**Fig. 10**). Gradenigo syndrome describes the classic clinical presentation where patients experience deep facial pain due to inflammation of the trigeminal or gasserian ganglion in Meckel cave and abducens nerve cranial nerve VI (CNVI) palsy due to inflammation along the dural reflection demarcating Dorello canal at the level of the petrous apex.[9,11]

Intracranial complications of otomastoiditis are common and an important cause of morbidity; therefore, early recognition and treatment of these complications are the key to improved outcomes. The most common intracranial complications include epidural abscesses and venous sinus thrombosis. Subdural empyemas, cerebritis, and parenchymal abscesses are less common complications associated with otomastoiditis.

As previously mentioned, coalescent mastoiditis may lead to bony erosion with formation of an

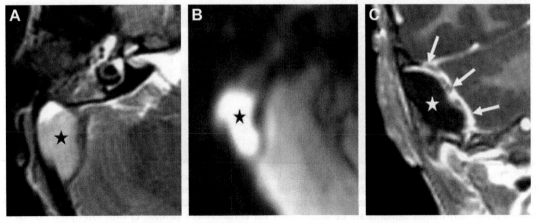

Fig. 11. Epidural abscess. Axial T2 (*A*), axial DWI (*B*), and coronal fat-suppressed T1 post-contrast (*C*) images show an epidural fluid collection (*, *A–C*) with restricted diffusion (*, *B*) as well as peripheral capsular and meningeal enhancement (*arrows*, *C*).

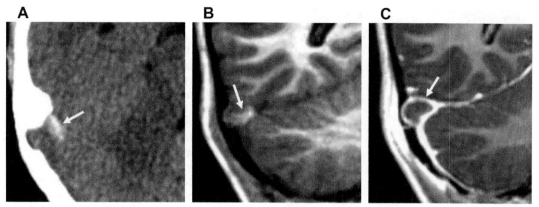

Fig. 12. Venous sinus thrombosis. Axial CT image demonstrates inward displacement and hyperdense thrombus within the right sigmoid sinus (*arrow, A*). Coronal T1 pre- (*B*) and post-contrast (*C*) sequences show that the thrombus is T1 hyperintense (*arrow, B*) with a characteristic "empty delta" sign (*arrow, C*) due to central nonenhancing thrombus on the post-contrast sequence.

extratemporal abscess. When the bony erosion occurs along the medial mastoid wall, an epidural abscess commonly forms and represents the most common intracranial complication of otomastoiditis. On imaging, an epidural abscess most often presents as a localized fluid collection along the inner margin of the mastoids with regional mass effect to include inward displacement of the adjacent dural venous sinus. Less commonly, an abscess may occur in the middle cranial fossa secondary to anterior mastoid wall dehiscence.

Smooth peripheral capsular and often adjacent meningeal enhancement is seen on both CT and MR imaging. MR imaging will also show characteristic restricted diffusion associated with the epidural abscess (**Fig. 11**).

Dural venous sinus thrombosis as a complication of otomastoiditis typically occurs in the setting of an overlying epidural abscess. On non-contrast CT, the thrombus can commonly be seen as area of hyperattenuation within the involved sigmoid

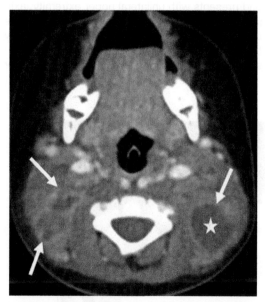

Fig. 13. Suppurative adenopathy, *S aureus*. Contrast-enhanced axial CT image shows bilateral conglomerate suppurative adenopathy (*arrows*) with surrounding inflammatory changes. The large left-sided suppurative lymph node (*) was drainable.

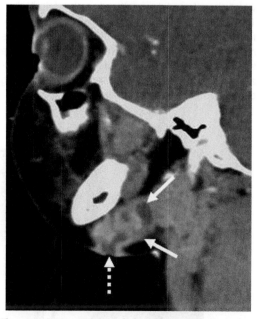

Fig. 14. Suppurative adenopathy, nontuberculous mycobacterium. Contrast-enhanced sagittal CT image demonstrates conglomerate suppurative adenopathy within the submandibular region (*arrows*) with a draining sinus to the skin surface (*dashed arrow*). Minimal surrounding inflammatory changes are present.

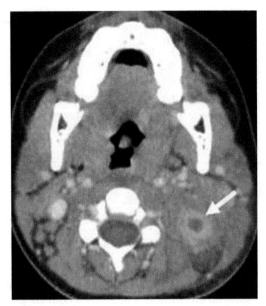

Fig. 15. Suppurative adenopathy, *B henselae.* Contrast-enhanced axial CT image shows unilateral conglomerate suppurative adenopathy (*arrow*) with surrounding inflammatory changes.

or distal transverse sinus. Thrombus can be confirmed on contrast-enhanced CT venogram or MR imaging, showing lack of venous sinus opacification in the region of intraluminal thrombus, which is referred to as the "empty delta" sign. Time-of-flight MR venogram will show absent flow-related signal intensity corresponding to the region of dural venous sinus thrombosis. The signal intensity of the thrombus will vary on MR imaging but is often T1 hyperintense with blooming on susceptibility-weighted imaging (Fig. 12).[9]

SUPPURATIVE ADENITIS

Suppurative adenitis in children may result from common or typical bacterial infections, such as *Staphylococcus aureus* or *Streptococcus pyogenes*, or atypical bacterial infections, such as *Mycobacterium* subspecies and *Bartonella henselae*. Infected lymph nodes are enlarged, may be conglomerate, and typically have surrounding inflammatory fat stranding. Central necrosis is a common feature of suppurative adenitis, and when large enough, may be drainable.[12]

Staphylococcus and *Streptococcus* are the most common etiologies of suppurative adenopathy in children and may be unilateral or bilateral. On CT, involved lymph nodes demonstrate peripheral solid enhancement and central hypoattenuation, with surrounding inflammatory changes (Fig. 13).

Nontuberculous mycobacterium infections are far more common than tuberculous (TB) infections in children in the United States. Both infections may calcify in the chronic stages, more commonly with TB, and both may cause skin discoloration as well as a sinus tract to the skin surface (Fig. 14). The degree of surrounding inflammatory changes is variable and often depends on the stage of infection, with decreased or a lack of perinodal inflammatory changes in the subacute and chronic stages.[12,13]

B henselae infection results from a cat bite or scratch, hence the term "cat scratch disease." It commonly occurs in children and young adults and presents with unilateral upper extremity, axillary, or neck adenopathy that may demonstrate central necrosis (Fig. 15). Clinical diagnosis may be challenging initially because patients often present in the subacute phase, so the initial cat bite or

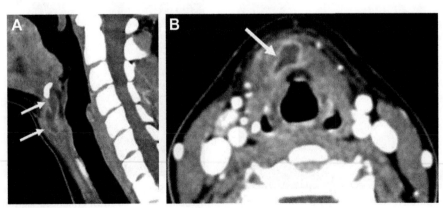

Fig. 16. Inflamed or infected thyroglossal duct cyst. Contrast-enhanced sagittal (*A*) and axial (*B*) CT images demonstrate a thin rim-enhancing fluid collection with surrounding inflammatory changes at and below the level of the hyoid bone (*arrows, A*). The collection is slightly off-midline and embedded within the strap muscles (*arrow, B*).

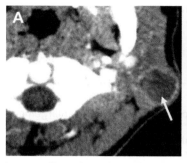
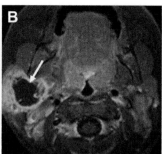
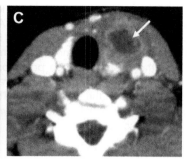

Fig. 17. Inflamed or infected branchial apparatus anomalies (BAAs). Contrast-enhanced axial CT image (*A*) shows a focal fluid collection centered in the left parotid gland (*arrow*) with slightly heterogeneous attenuation and mild surrounding inflammatory changes, compatible with the first BAA. Axial fat-suppressed T1 post-contrast image (*B*) demonstrates a slightly irregular fluid collection with peripheral inflammatory enhancement (*arrow*) centered at the level of the angle of the mandible, compatible with a second BAA. Contrast-enhanced axial CT image (*C*) shows a left thyroid abscess (*arrow*) with surrounding inflammatory changes, compatible with complication related to a third or fourth BAA sinus.

scratch may not be immediately recalled by the child or caregiver.[12,14]

INFLAMED OR INFECTED CONGENITAL LESIONS

The most common congenital cystic lesions of the neck include thyroglossal duct cysts (TGDCs) and branchial apparatus anomalies (BAAs). These congenital lesions are identified based on their characteristic locations and are relatively simple appearing when uncomplicated.[15] With superimposed inflammation or infection, imaging findings become more complex and include more pronounced peripheral enhancement, surrounding inflammatory changes and edema, and varying degrees of altered internal attenuation (CT) or signal intensity (MR imaging) due to internal debris.[1]

TGDCs may occur anywhere from the foramen cecum at the base of the tongue to the thyroid bed. Approximately 85% are midline and 75% occur at or below the level of the hyoid bone. When at or below the hyoid bone, they are characteristically embedded within the strap muscles. The more inferior the lesion is located in the neck, the more likely it is to be slightly off midline in location (Fig. 16). The most common suprahyoid location is at the foramen cecum at the base of the tongue.[16]

BAAs are characterized based on their embryologic origin and classified as first through fourth BAAs. The most common BAA is a cyst, followed by a sinus that may drain externally or internally, and rarely a fistula that extends from the mucosal surface of the pharynx to the skin surface. First BAAs occur anywhere from the external auditory canal to the submandibular region and are most

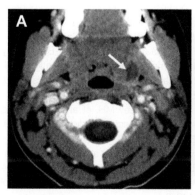
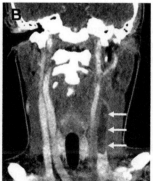
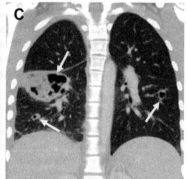

Fig. 18. Lemierre syndrome. Contrast-enhanced axial (*A*) and coronal (*B*) CT images through the neck demonstrate a left-sided peritonsillar abscess (*arrow*, *A*) and long-segment internal jugular venous sinus thrombosis (*arrows*, *B*). Coronal CT image through the chest (*C*) shows multiple septic pulmonary emboli with varying degrees of cavitation (*arrows*).

often intraparotid or periauricular in location. Second BAAs are the most common BAAs and classically occur at the level of the angle of the mandible. Third BAAs are uncommon and may be seen within the deep and often posterior neck. Third and fourth BAAs may form a sinus tract to the thyroid, typically on the left, or larynx. These patients commonly present with recurrent thyroiditis or thyroid abscess[17] (Fig. 17).

LEMIERRE SYNDROME

Lemierre syndrome refers to a head and neck infection that is complicated by thrombophlebitis and distant septic emboli. It preferentially occurs in children, adolescents, and young adults who are often otherwise healthy. The most common inciting infection is oropharyngeal, typically a tonsillar region infection, and the thrombophlebitis characteristically involves the internal jugular vein. Distant septic emboli may involve nearly any organ system; however, the lungs are essentially always involved, demonstrating peripheral pulmonary opacities with varying degrees of cavitation (Fig. 18).

Fusobacterium necrophorum, an anaerobe that is part of the normal oropharyngeal flora, is the classic organism associated with Lemierre syndrome, though many of these infections are polymicrobial. Treatment includes prolonged antibiotic therapy and drainage of any neck abscesses. The use of anticoagulation is still under discussion and debated in the literature. The risks of anticoagulation in the setting of Lemierre syndrome are low in the absence of underlying contraindications; however, most patients recover similarly with or without anticoagulation therapy. [18,19]

CT is the modality of choice in a patient with an acute presentation and is useful in identifying the primary site of neck infection, extent of venous thrombosis, and presence of pulmonary septic emboli. It is important for radiologists to be aware of this entity and its characteristic imaging features because imaging typically precedes the clinical diagnosis with confirmatory blood cultures. [20]

SUMMARY

Imaging is integral in the workup and management of neck infections in children, especially in the setting of a limited clinical history and non-localizing physical examination. Therefore, it is important to have a working knowledge of classic imaging features and potential complications of pediatric neck infections when interpreting pediatric imaging studies. This will help ensure appropriate treatment, prevent subsequent complications, and maximize clinical outcomes.

CLINICS CARE POINTS

- Tonsillitis presents with tonsillar enlargement and a "tigroid" enhancement pattern, whereas abscesses present as rim-enhancing collections.
- Retropharyngeal abscesses most often result from rupture of suppurative lateral retropharyngeal lymph nodes, exert mass effect, and often cross midline.
- The primary role of imaging in the clinical setting of otomastoiditis is to look for associated temporal and extra-temporal complications.
- Suppurative adenitis may result from typical or atypical infectious processes and often presents with conglomerate lymphadenopathy and varying degrees of surrounding inflammation.
- Superimposed inflammation or infection of an underlying congenital cystic lesion is suggested when an inflammatory process is centered in a characteristic location for a congenital lesion.
- Lemierre syndrome refers to a neck infection that is complicated by thrombophlebitis and distant septic pulmonary emboli.

DISCLOSURE

None.

REFERENCES

1. Ho ML, Courtier J, Glastonbury CM. The ABCs (airway, blood vessels, and compartments) of pediatric neck infections and masses. Am J Roentgenol 2016;206:963–72.
2. Capps EF, Kinsella JJ, Gupta M, et al. Emergency imaging assessment of acute, nontraumatic conditions of the head and neck. Radiographics 2010; 30(5):1335–52.
3. Kamalian S, Avery L, Lev MH, et al. Nontraumatic head and neck emergencies. Radiographics 2019; 39:1808–23.
4. Ali SA, Kovatch KJ, Smith J, et al. Predictors of intratonsillar abscess versus peritonsillar abscess in the pediatric patient. Int J Pediatr Otorhinolaryngol 2018;114:143–6.
5. Ali SA, Kovatch KJ, Smith J, et al. Predictors of intratonsillar versus peritonsillar abscess - a case-control series. Laryngoscope 2019;129(6):1354–9.

6. Hoang JK, Branstetter BF, Eastwood JD, et al. Multi-planar CT and MRI of collections in the retropharyngeal space: is it an abscess? Am J Roentgenol 2011;196(4):W426–32.

7. Shefelbine SE, Mancuso AA, Gajewski BJ, et al. Pediatric retropharyngeal lymphadenitis: differentiation from retropharyngeal abscess and treatment implications. Otolaryngol Head Neck Surg 2007;136(2):182–8.

8. Mansour S, Magnan J, Nicolas K, et al. Acute otitis media and acute coalescent mastoiditis. In: Middle ear diseases. Springer; 2018. p. 85–113.

9. Vazquez E, Castellote A, Piqueras J, et al. Imaging of complications of acute mastoiditis in children. Radiographics 2003;23:359–72.

10. Benson JC, Carlson ML, Lane JI. MRI of the internal auditory canal, labyrinth, and middle ear: how we do it. Radiology 2020;297:252–65.

11. Chapman PR, Shah R, Cure JK, et al. Petrous apex lesions: pictorial review. Am J Roentgenol 2011;196:WS26–37.

12. Ludwig BJ, Wang J, Nadgir RN, et al. Imaging of cervical lymphadenopathy in children and young adults. Am J Roentgenol 2012;199:1105–13.

13. Robson CD, Hazra R, Barnes PD, et al. Nontuberculous mycobacterial infection of the head and neck in immunocompetent children: CT and MR findings. Am J Neuroradiol 1999;20(10):1829–35.

14. Hopkins KL, Simoneaux SF, Patrick LE, et al. Imaging manifestations of cat-scratch disease. Am J Roentgenol 1996;166(2):435–8.

15. Ibrahim M, Hammoud K, Maheshwari M, et al. Congenital cystic lesions of the head and neck. Neuroimaging Clin N Am 2011;21(3):621–39.

16. Patel S, Bhatt AA. Thyroglossal duct pathology and mimics. Insights Imaging 2019;10(12):1–12.

17. Bagchi A, Hira P, Priyamvara A, et al. Branchial cleft cysts: a pictorial review. Pol J Radiol 2018;83:e204–9.

18. Nygren D, Elf J, Torisson G, et al. Jugular vein thrombosis and anticoagulation therapy in Lemierre's syndrome - a post hoc observational and population-based study of 82 patients. Open Forum Infect Dis 2020;8(1):1–7. ofaa585.

19. Campo F, Fusconi M, Ciotti M, et al. Antibiotic and anticoagulation therapy in Lemierre's syndrome: case report and review. J Chemother 2019;31(1):42–8.

20. O'Brien WT, Lattin GE, Thompson AK. Lemierre syndrome: an all-but-forgotten disease. Am J Roentgenol 2006;187:W324.

Pediatric Odontogenic and Paranasal Sinus Infections

Rebekah Clarke, MD

KEYWORDS

• Infection • Odontogenic • Paranasal sinus • Fungal

KEY POINTS

- Odontogenic and sinogenic infection is often suspected clinically, and the role of imaging is primarily to localize the infection and identify evidence of complications.
- Because of the proximity of the oral cavity and paranasal sinuses to the deep neck spaces, orbits, and skull base, there is a significant risk of potentially life-threatening spread of infection to these spaces.
- Computed tomography is typically the initial imaging modality; however, MR imaging can provide important information in select cases where there is concern for intracranial spread.

INTRODUCTION

In the setting of odontogenic or sinogenic facial infection, imaging appearances depend on the etiology and duration of the infectious process as well as the host immune response. Proximity of multiple soft tissue spaces within the head and neck contributes to the propensity for transcranial spread of infection. An understanding of this complex interplay of factors is essential for the radiologist to provide the most accurate and useful information to clinicians.

DISCUSSION

Odontogenic Infection

General imaging considerations

The role of imaging in odontogenic infection is to localize the source of infection and evaluate for complications such as abscess and spread of infection to surrounding spaces.[1] Plain radiography is still widely used for detection of dental caries or periodontal disease but is of little utility in evaluation of regional soft tissues. Contrast-enhanced computed tomography (ceCT) is ideal for evaluation of bony structures and provides additional information about the surrounding soft tissues. CT is the modality of choice for imaging in the emergent setting, given its acquisition speed and availability. MR imaging provides superior contrast resolution; however, scan time and availability limit its usefulness in the emergent setting.

Relevant Anatomy

Odontogenic infection may involve the tooth itself or any of the supporting structures. An understanding of dental anatomy provides a framework for understanding the various etiologies and imaging appearances of odontogenic infections. A challenge unique to pediatric odontogenic imaging is that one must be familiar with tooth classification systems for both primary and permanent teeth. There are two widely recognized classification systems: the universal system, used in the United States, and the Fédération Dentaire Internationale system, more widely used outside the United States. For the purposes of this article, only the universal system will be described. In this system, teeth are assigned a number, in the case of permanent teeth, or letter, in the case of primary teeth. Numbering of permanent teeth begins with the right maxillary third molar, assigning a number (1–16) to each tooth along the maxillary arch, and then continues with the left third mandibular molar, assigning a number (17–32) to each mandibular tooth. Similarly, primary teeth are designated

Department. of Pediatric Radiology, University of Texas Southwestern and Children's Health Dallas, 1935 Medical District Drive, Mail Code F1.02, Dallas, TX 75235, USA
E-mail address: Rebekah.Clarke@UTSouthwestern.edu

Neuroimag Clin N Am 33 (2023) 673–684
https://doi.org/10.1016/j.nic.2023.05.014

letters (A–T) beginning with the right maxillary second molar and ending with the right mandibular second molar (Fig. 1). The teeth may also be referred to by name, as shown in Fig. 1.

Each tooth is composed of a crown, the portion visible above the alveolar bone socket, and a root, which is seated within and attached to alveolar bone via the periodontal ligament (PDL). The root is divided into cervical, middle, and apical thirds, the latter containing the root terminus.[2] The crown is covered by an intensely radiopaque layer of enamel, and the root is covered by a layer of cementum, both of which serve as protective barriers for the underlying dentin which comprises the bulk of the tooth[3] (Fig. 2). The cementoenamel junction refers to the transition between the enamel and cementum. Within the center of the tooth is the root canal and pulp, which appear relatively radiolucent and contain abundant neurovascular tissue.[2,3]

Pathology

Caries

Dental caries is common in the pediatric population, with a prevalence of 45.8% among children aged 2 to 19 years according to one study.[4] Byproducts of the cariogenic bacteria that reside in the oral cavity promote demineralization of the enamel, resulting in defects in the tooth surface.[1,5] These defects appear as rounded lucencies, with predilection for the interproximal surfaces, but may also occur along the occlusive surfaces[5] (Fig. 3). Infection may then spread into the root canal, resulting in pulpitis, at which point root canal therapy is necessary to prevent tooth loss.

Periodontal and Endodontic Disease

Periodontal disease is infection and inflammation of the supporting structures around the teeth, leading to the loss of alveolar bone.[1] It is the result of chronic gingivitis, an inflammation of the gums, which leads to exposure of the underlying bone and PDL, and accumulation of infectious material within the PDL space.[1,5] On imaging, this appears as widening of the PDL space (Fig. 4). Apical periodontitis is involvement of the supporting structures around the root apex. Left untreated, apical periodontal disease may progress to endodontic disease involving pulpal structures, manifesting in the acute setting as periapical abscess. This

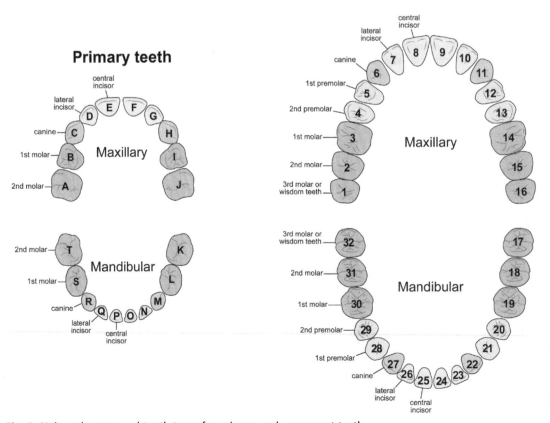

Fig. 1. Universal system and tooth types for primary and permanent teeth.

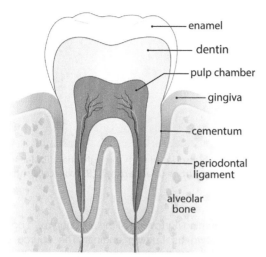

Fig. 2. Anatomy of a tooth, showing the structure of the root, crown, and periodontal tissues (gingiva, alveolar bone, periodontal ligament).

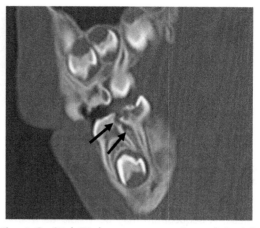

Fig. 4. Sagittal CT shows crown erosions of the left mandibular first and second molars with widening of the upper PDL space (*black arrows*).

Complications of Odontogenic Infection

Periodontal and endodontic disease may both lead to regional osteomyelitis. The mandible is more commonly involved, as the maxilla has more robust collateral blood supply.[7] CT in the acute phase typically shows areas of lucency surrounded by sclerotic marrow, representing areas of osteonecrosis and accumulation of purulent debris. This may be accompanied by overlying cortical breakthrough, periosteal new bone formation, and subperiosteal or soft tissue abscess (Figs. 7 and 8). There is a more mixed pattern of sclerotic trabeculation and lucency in the chronic

can be visualized on radiograph and CT as periapical lucency, with or without root resorption. Sclerosis of the surrounding bone, condensing osteitis, may be seen if there has been long-standing inflammation.[1,5] Eventually, cortical breakthrough may occur, with formation of subperiosteal abscess or extension into deep neck spaces[6,7] (Figs. 5 and 6).

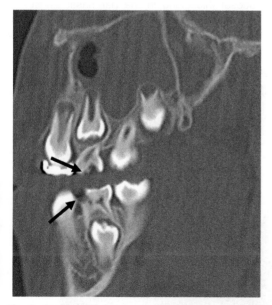

Fig. 3. Sagittal CT shows crown erosions of the left maxillary first molar and left mandibular first molar (*black arrows*).

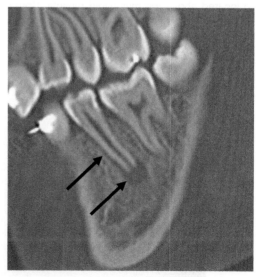

Fig. 5. Sagittal CT shows the evidence of apical periodontitis with periapical lucency, mild resorption of the root apex, and widening of the PDL space (*black arrows*).

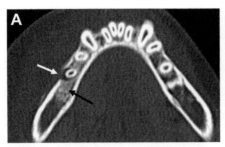
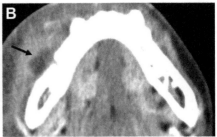

Fig. 6. (A) Axial CT shows periapical lucency and cortical breakthrough associated with the right mandibular second premolar (*white arrow*), with condensing osteitis of the surrounding bone (*black arrow*). (B) Axial ceCT shows adjacent subperiosteal abscess (*black arrow*).

phase. A sequestrum may be visible as a small fragment of bone surrounded by lucency.[8] MR imaging is useful for detecting osteomyelitis in its earliest stage, when T2 hyperintense marrow edema may be the only finding. In the setting of chronic osteomyelitis, marrow signal can be variable on T2-weighted images depending on the degree of sclerosis (Fig. 9). A sequestrum appears as focal low signal surrounded by high-signal tissue that enhances with gadolinium administration.[1,8] Both CT and MR imaging are useful for detection of soft tissue changes, including abscess and sinus tracts.[1,7,8]

Involvement of the mandibular molars is more likely to result in spread to the submandibular space due to the location of the root apices of these teeth below the mylohyoid muscle. Infection originating from the mandibular premolars and more anterior teeth is more likely to spread to the sublingual space due to the root apices of these teeth being located above the mylohyoid muscle. Spread of infection to the floor of the mouth may lead to

life-threatening narrowing of the oropharynx, a condition known as Ludwig angina. The source of infection is most often the second and third mandibular molars, with cellulitis spreading rapidly into the sublingual, submandibular, and submental spaces bilaterally. ceCT is most helpful in the acute setting to evaluate degree of airway compromise, presence of a drainable abscess, and to identify the source of infection.[7]

Paranasal Sinus Infection

General imaging considerations
There is no imaging modality sensitive and specific enough to diagnose acute sinusitis or differentiate between viral and bacterial causes.[9,10] The diagnosis is typically based on clinical signs and symptoms, and imaging is usually not appropriate in the setting of acute uncomplicated sinusitis.[10] Mucosal thickening in the paranasal sinuses is commonly seen on imaging in both symptomatic and asymptomatic individuals, especially in the

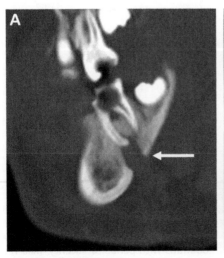
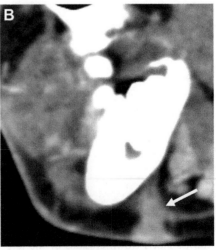

Fig. 7. Chronic osteomyelitis. (A) Sagittal CT shows periapical lucency and surrounding sclerosis with cortical breakthrough (*white arrow*). (B) Sagittal ceCT shows orocutaneous sinus tract (*white arrow*).

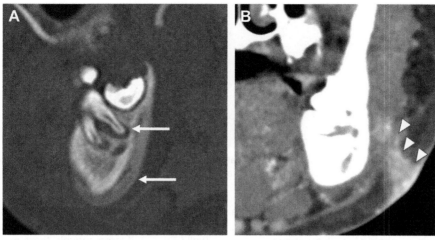

Fig. 8. Chronic osteomyelitis. (*A*) Sagittal CT shows periapical lucency with surrounding sclerosis and periosteal new bone formation (*white arrows*). (*B*) Coronal ceCT shows associated orocutaneous sinus tract (*arrowheads*).

pediatric population, and is therefore not helpful for distinguishing acute bacterial sinusitis from simple viral upper respiratory infection.[11] However, if complications of acute bacterial sinusitis are suspected, or if acute invasive fungal sinusitis (AIFS) is suspected, ceCT and/or MR imaging of the head and sinuses should be performed.[10,11] In both cases, it may also be appropriate to obtain CT arteriogram (CTA) or Magnetic resonance angiogram/magnetic resonance venogram (MRA/MRV) head to evaluate for vascular complications.[10] CT is typically obtained first and has several advantages over MR imaging, including speed of acquisition, availability, high spatial resolution, and ability to perform without sedation. Osseous anatomy of the sinuses is well depicted on CT; however, the effects of exposure to ionizing radiation must be considered in the pediatric population. MR imaging often requires the use of sedation in children and is not as widely available in the acute setting but avoids ionizing radiation and is superior to ceCT for delineation of intracranial involvement.[11]

Relevant Anatomy

The paranasal sinuses consist of the paired maxillary, ethmoid, frontal, and sphenoid sinuses. They are lined by ciliated columnar epithelium which plays a key role in both production and clearance of mucus. Impaired mucociliary clearance, most often a result of sinus outflow obstruction and/or viral upper respiratory infection, leads to accumulation of secretions and predisposes to secondary bacterial infection and sinusitis.[12]

Pathology

Bacterial sinusitis

Sinusitis is categorized as acute, subacute, chronic, and recurrent depending on the duration of illness. Acute bacterial sinusitis typically arises in the setting of a preexisting viral upper respiratory tract infection (URI). The viral infection sets off an inflammatory cascade within the sinus epithelium, resulting in impaired macrophage and lymphocyte function and increased susceptibility to secondary bacterial infection.[9] In addition to

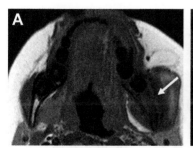
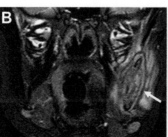
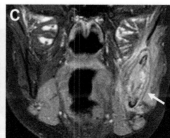

Fig. 9. Chronic osteomyelitis. (*A*) Axial T1-weighted image shows hypointense marrow in the left mandibular ramus (*arrow*). (*B*) Coronal Short Tau inversion recovery (STIR) and (*C*) post-contrast T1 fat-saturated sequences show corresponding mixed T2 signal and enhancement and periostitis (*white arrows*).

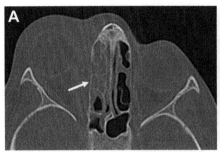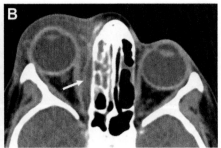

Fig. 10. Complicated sinusitis. Axial ceCT in bone (*A*) and soft tissue window (*B*) shows opacified ethmoid sinuses (*arrow, A*) with subperiosteal abscess along the medial orbital wall (*arrow, B*).

viral URI, other predisposing factors may include allergic rhinitis, asthma, gastroesophageal reflux, cystic fibrosis, or obstructive sleep apnea.[10]

Regardless of symptom duration, imaging findings are nonspecific and cannot distinguish between inflammation caused by viral, bacterial, allergic, and chemical etiology.[13] Mucosal thickening, air–fluid levels, and bubbly secretions may be seen in the setting of sinusitis; however, these same findings are frequently observed in patients being imaged for unrelated reasons and without clinical symptoms of sinusitis.[14] Therefore, imaging should be reserved for patients with recurrent or chronic sinusitis in whom surgery is being considered, or when complications of bacterial sinusitis are suspected.[10,15]

Complications of bacterial sinusitis are infrequent but may result in substantial morbidity and mortality if not recognized and treated in a timely manner.[9,14] The most common complications are related to spread of infection to the adjacent orbital or intracranial compartments. Orbital spread may be a result of osteitis of the very thin lamina papyracea separating the ethmoid air cells from the orbital contents and/or thrombophlebitis of the multiple small veins perforating the lamina papyracea.[9,11] Early ceCT may show findings of orbital cellulitis with or without preseptal cellulitis. The spread of infection is initially limited by the periosteum on the orbital side of the lamina papyracea, resulting in formation of a subperiosteal abscess along the medial or superior orbital wall (Fig. 10). If large enough, there may be mass effect resulting in proptosis and compromised extraocular muscle movement. The progression of orbital cellulitis or rupture of a subperiosteal abscess may lead to frank orbital abscess, typically in the extraconal space, and this is associated with more severe proptosis, extraocular muscle dysfunction, and potential vision loss.[11]

Intracranial complications include cavernous sinus thrombosis, epidural empyema, subdural empyema, meningitis, cerebritis, and cerebral abscess. Cavernous sinus thrombosis may occur as a result of retrograde thrombophlebitis of the multiple valveless veins that eventually drain into the cavernous sinus, including the superior ophthalmic vein (SOV)[11] (Figs. 11 and 12). On imaging, bulging of the lateral wall of the cavernous sinus is the most frequent finding.[16] Internal filling defects, the presence of susceptibility artifact or restricted diffusion in the cavernous sinus, and increased dural enhancement along the lateral borders of the cavernous sinus and ipsilateral tentorium can be additional clues to the diagnosis.[11,16]

Other intracranial complications can occur by either direct or indirect spread of infection, typically involving the frontal, ethmoid, or sphenoid sinuses given their proximity to the skull base.

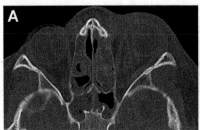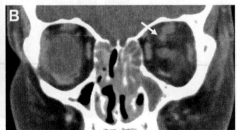

Fig. 11. Complicated sinusitis. Axial (*A*) and coronal (*B*) ceCT shows opacified ethmoid and sphenoid sinuses with and enlarged non-enhancing SOV (*arrow*).

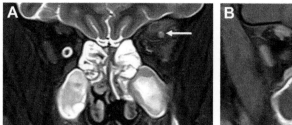
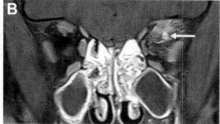

Fig. 12. Complicated sinusitis with SOV thrombosis. (A) Coronal STIR and (B) coronal post-contrast T1-weighted fat-saturated images show the enlarged SOV (*arrow, A*) with surrounding edema and enhancement and central non-enhancement (*arrow, B*).

Indirect spread via multiple valveless veins that traverse the sinus walls and skull base results in intracranial transmission often without frank bony destruction on imaging. Direct spread involves bony destruction of the skull base in the setting of osteomyelitis. Frontal sinusitis with osteomyelitis of the adjacent frontal bone and overlying subgaleal abscess is known as Pott puffy tumor, so named for the prominent forehead swelling associated with the abscess.[11,17] Involvement of the inner table of the skull typically leads to the development of an epidural abscess (Fig. 13). Further intracranial spread may lead to subdural empyema, meningitis, cerebritis, and cerebral abscess. In the acute setting, ceCT is often the initial imaging modality and demonstrates frank bony

destruction well, but may underestimate the extent of marrow involvement.[18] If large enough, epidural or subdural empyema may be visible on ceCT; however, MR imaging is considered the gold standard for imaging of intracranial complications of bacterial sinusitis because of its superior contrast resolution and ability to better detect early disease.[17,18] MR imaging protocols should include a fluid-sensitive fat-saturated sequence to assess extent of marrow involvement and presence of fluid collections, a post-gad T1 fat-saturated sequence, for detection of fluid collections, and diffusion-weighted images for detection of purulent material. Post-gadolinium T2 FLAIR images should be included for their sensitivity to leptomeningeal enhancement and parenchymal

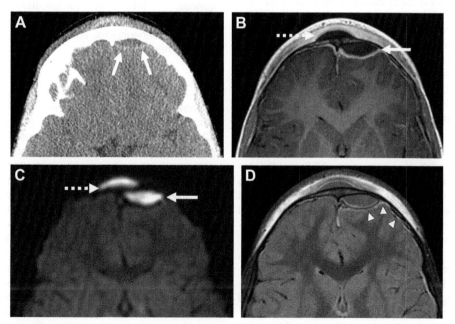

Fig. 13. Pott puffy tumor. (A) Axial unenhanced CT shows frontal scalp swelling and lentiform extra-axial collection over the left frontal lobe (*white arrows*). Axial post-contrast T1 (B), diffusion (C), and post-contrast T2-FLAIR (D) show subgaleal scalp abscess (dotted *arrows B, C*), epidural abscess (solid *arrows B, C*), and leptomeningeal enhancement (*arrowheads in D*).

edema.[11,19] In the setting of sphenoid involvement with the potential for cavernous sinus spread, MRA should be considered to evaluate for narrowing of the cavernous internal carotid arteries.[20] Gadolinium-enhanced MRV together with a post-contrast 3D T1 gradient echo sequence is helpful for detecting venous sinus thrombosis.[21]

Fungal sinusitis

The term fungal sinusitis comprises a spectrum of invasive and noninvasive forms of fungal infection of the paranasal sinuses. Invasive forms are characterized by the presence of fungal elements beyond the confines of the paranasal sinuses. These include acute and chronic invasive and chronic granulomatous fungal sinusitis. Noninvasive forms include allergic fungal sinusitis and mycetoma.[22] Inhalation of the spores of mycotic organisms within the environment leads to fungal colonization of the upper respiratory tract. In the immune competent individual, fungal proliferation is better controlled, and invasive infection prevented. However, in the immune compromised individual, there is greater potential for mucosal invasion and spread of infection.[22] Both invasive and noninvasive fungal sinusitis may be clinically indistinguishable from acute or chronic bacterial sinusitis, and histopathologic confirmation may be necessary; however, there are some important imaging characteristics that may suggest fungal etiology.[22] Non-contrast CT is typically sufficient for suspected noninvasive fungal sinusitis and may also be useful as a screening test for acute invasive fungal sinusitis if there is not yet clinical concern for orbital or intracranial involvement.[10,23] If there is clinical concern for complicated invasive fungal disease, initial imaging should include ceCT of the sinuses, orbits, and brain. Further evaluation with ceMR imaging may be warranted to better assess intracranial complications.[10]

Acute Invasive Fungal Sinusitis

Although relatively uncommon, AIFS rapidly progressive and can lead to serious complications or death within hours to weeks if not recognized and treated.[22] Clinicians must maintain a high level of suspicion for this disease, especially in immunocompromised or immunosuppressed patients, such as those with hematologic malignancies, poorly controlled diabetes, or organ transplant recipients. Effective treatment involves early diagnosis, aggressive surgical debridement, and timely administration of antifungal therapy.[24]

Most cases involve *Aspergillus* sp or *Mucor* sp, which rapidly invade the paranasal sinus and/or nasal cavity mucosa, causing inflammation and eventual tissue necrosis.[22] Spread beyond the paranasal sinuses may occur either directly or hematogenously via multiple valveless veins that permeate the sinus walls and may lead to orbital and intracranial complications.[25] The angioinvasive nature of both aspergillosis and mucormycosis can result in thrombosis with cerebral infarct, hemorrhage, or mycotic aneurysm.[24,25]

Although definitive diagnosis requires biopsy of infected tissue showing the presence of fungal invasion, imaging may provide clues that would support a diagnosis. On CT or MR imaging, one of the most reported findings is severe unilateral nasal cavity mucosal thickening, although this is not a highly specific finding.[23] Mucosal thickening and opacification of the paranasal sinuses may also be seen. The most common sites of involvement are the middle nasal turbinate, maxillary sinus, ethmoid, and sphenoid sinuses.[23] Areas of necrosis may appear as non-enhancing tissue on either ceCT or MR imaging[22] (**Fig. 14**). Bone dehiscence is best seen on CT and has been shown to be a specific indicator but is uncommon early in the disease process.[23,26] Extrasinus spread may occur in the absence of bone destruction because of its ability to spread along microvascular channels or nerves.[23] Infiltration of the maxillary periantral fat, pterygopalatine fossa, nasolacrimal duct, or sac are some of the best early predictors of acute invasive fungal sinusitis.[23,26] MR imaging has been shown to be more sensitive than CT, showing edema and enhancement in the involved tissue spaces.[22,26] Intracranial complications, such as meningitis, cerebritis, fungal granulomas, infarcts, and pseudoaneurysms, are also better visualized on MR imaging.[10,25]

Chronic Invasive Fungal Sinusitis

Compared with AIFS, chronic invasive fungal sinusitis is more indolent, lasting longer than 12 weeks, and is more likely to be seen in immune competent patients, though the subtly immunocompromised, such as poorly controlled diabetics or patients on chronic corticosteroid treatment, are still at risk.[25] *Aspergillus fumigatus* is the most common causative agent. Patients present with chronic sinusitis that is refractory to antibiotic treatment. Orbital apex syndrome may be seen if there is invasion into the orbital apex.[22,27] Fungal material within the involved sinus may have slightly greater density on CT compared with that seen in AIFS due to the increased deposition of calcium metabolites over time.[22,25] On MR imaging, the fungal mass is hypointense on T1-weighted images and markedly hypointense on T2-weighted images.[25] As with AIFS, bone erosion, invasion of the periantral soft tissues, and spread to the orbits

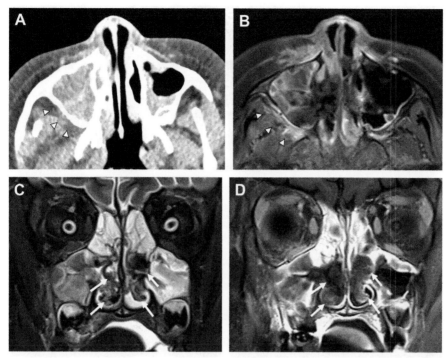

Fig. 14. AIFS. (*A*) Axial CT shows opacified right maxillary sinus with inflammatory stranding (white *arrowheads*) in the periantral fat. (*B*) Axial post-contrast T1 fat-saturated image shows corresponding periantral enhancement (white *arrowheads*). Coronal T2-DIXON (*C*) and post-contrast T1 fat-saturated (*D*) show areas of T2 hypointensity and non-enhancement within the turbinates indicating areas of tissue necrosis (*white arrows*).

or intracranial compartment are also possible, and treatment involves surgical debridement and antifungal therapy.

Chronic Granulomatous Invasive Fungal Sinusitis

The granulomatous form of chronic fungal sinusitis is most often reported in immunocompetent individuals from North Africa or Southeast Asia, and is typically caused by *Aspergillus flavus*.[22,25] The clinical and imaging characteristics are similar to chronic invasive fungal sinusitis, and orbital proptosis is a frequent presenting feature.[22,27] CT and MR imaging may show soft tissue opacification of the involved sinus with extrasinus invasion and possible intraorbital or intracranial spread. Bone erosion may also be seen.[22,25] Treatment typically involves surgical debridement and antifungal therapy.

Allergic Fungal Sinusitis

Allergic fungal sinusitis is the most common manifestation of fungal sinusitis. It is typically seen in young, immunocompetent, atopic individuals who have a history of chronic hypertrophic sinusitis and may have already undergone sinus surgery.[22,28] Fungal allergens, which are ubiquitous

in the environment, colonize the sinonasal passages, setting off an immunoglobulin E (IgE)-mediated allergic hypersensitivity reaction. Thick allergic mucin and cellular debris accumulate, and together with thickened, inflamed mucosa obstruct the sinonasal drainage pathways.

Imaging typically shows the involvement of multiple sinuses, although there may be asymmetric or unilateral involvement. The nasal passages are commonly involved.[22] Inflammatory debris within the sinuses appears hyperdense on non-contrast CT, surrounded by hypodense thickened sinonasal mucosa. There is characteristic expansion and bony remodeling of the involved sinuses, and potentially bony erosion, which can lead to intraorbital or intracranial extension, and may be mistaken for a mass.[22,28] On MR imaging, sinus contents are typically iso to hypointense on T2 due to the low water content of the inspissated mucin and may even appear as signal void due to accumulation of heavy metals such as iron, magnesium, and manganese by fungal elements[25] (Fig. 15). T1 signal is variable and can be hypointense; however, mixed signal and high T1 signal are also frequently seen.[25,28] There should be no enhancement of the sinus contents following gadolinium administration, which helps differentiate it from neoplastic disease of the sinuses.[28]

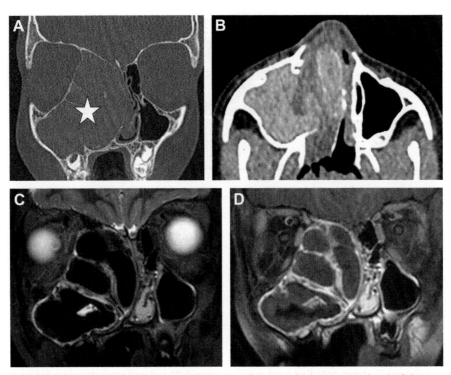

Fig. 15. Allergic fungal sinusitis. (*A*) Coronal and (*B*) axial CT shows marked expansion (star) of the opacified right maxillary and ethmoid sinuses and right nasal passage with hyperdense material. (*C*) Coronal STIR and (*D*) post-contrast T1 fat-saturated images show T2 signal void and non-enhancement of the sinus contents.

Sinonasal mucosa appears hyperintense on T2 and hypointense on T1-weighted images and enhances with contrast administration.

Treatment is surgical, aimed at removing the inspissated mucin and reestablishing normal sinonasal drainage pathways. Topical nasal steroids are useful for preventing recurrence by suppressing the underlying hypersensitivity reaction to fungal organisms.[28]

Fungus Ball

Fungus ball, or mycetoma, is an uncommon manifestation of fungal sinus disease, often occurring in older immunocompetent individuals, though any age may be affected, with a slight female predilection. It is thought to be a result of inadequate mucociliary clearance, leading to accumulation of fungal organisms, which then form a fungal mass as their hyphae become matted together.[28] *A fumigatus* is the most common organism involved.[22] Patients may present with mild sinus pressure, or the diagnosis may be made incidentally on imaging in asymptomatic individuals.[22]

Imaging shows the involvement of a single sinus, most often the maxillary sinus. Thickening, sclerosis, and remodeling of the sinus walls may occur due to chronic inflammation. On CT, the

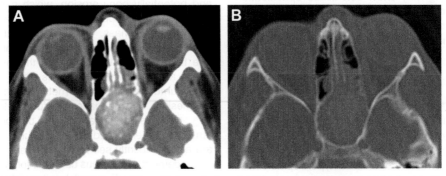

Fig. 16. Mycetoma. Axial soft-tissue (*A*) and bone window (*B*) CT shows opacified sphenoid sinus with mild bone remodeling and central hyperdensity.

affected sinus will be opacified with areas of central hyperdensity and calcifications surrounded by thickened hypodense inflamed mucosa[22,25] (Fig. 16). MR imaging typically shows a T1 hypointense mass with significant hypointensity on T2-weighted images due to the presence of calcifications and heavy metals. The fungal mass should not enhance following gadolinium administration, though there will be enhancement and thickening of the inflamed mucosa. Treatment is surgical to remove the fungus ball and create adequate sinus drainage pathways.

SUMMARY

Although the diagnosis of an odontogenic or sinus infection is often presumed clinically, imaging plays a key role not only in confirming the diagnosis but also alerting clinicians to the presence of drainable abscess or other potentially life-threatening complications such as intracranial spread of infection. The radiologist must be familiar with patient populations at risk, be able to recognize key imaging features, and understand the appropriate use of CT and/or MR imaging in each case.

CLINICS CARE POINTS

- The presence of a bony sequestrum on imaging in the setting of odontogenic osteomyelitis indicates chronic infection in which a central necrotic infectious focus has become walled off from vascularized bone and insusceptible to antibiotics.

- Odontogenic sinusitis is clinically indistinguishable from rhinosinusitis from other causes but is more often polymicrobial and requires different antibiotic regimen with anaerobe coverage. Imaging can therefore play an important role in identifying the source of infection.

- Spread of infection from the sinuses may occur in the absence of bone destruction due to the ability to spread along vascular channels.

- Infiltration of the maxillary periantral fat planes or pterygopalatine fossa has been shown to be one of the best early signs of acute invasive fungal sinusitis.

DISCLOSURE

The author has nothing to disclose.

REFERENCES

1. Mardini S, Gohel A. Imaging of Odontogenic Infections. Radiol Clin North Am 2018;56(1):31–44.
2. Husain MA. Dental Anatomy and Nomenclature for the Radiologist. Radiol Clin North Am 2018;56(1):1–11.
3. Chapman MN, Nadgir RN, Akman AS, et al. Periapical lucency around the tooth: radiologic evaluation and differential diagnosis. Radiographics 2013;33(1):E15–32.
4. National Center for Health Statistics. National Health and Nutrition Examination Survey (NHANES): Examination manuals, 2011–2012, 2013–2014, 2015–2016. Available from: https://wwwn.cdc.gov/nchs/nhanes/Default.aspx).
5. Steinklein J, Nguyen V. Dental anatomy and pathology encountered on routine CT of the head and neck. AJR Am J Roentgenol 2013;201(6):W843–53.
6. Gonzalez-Beicos A, Nunez D. Imaging of acute head and neck infections. Radiol Clin North Am 2012;50(1):73–83.
7. Loureiro RM, Naves EA, Zanello RF, et al. Dental Emergencies: A Practical Guide. Radiographics 2019;39(6):1782–95.
8. Lee YJ, Sadigh S, Mankad K, et al. The imaging of osteomyelitis. Quant Imaging Med Surg 2016;6(2):184–98.
9. Kölln KA, Senior BA. Diagnosis and Management of Acute Rhinosinusitis. In: Thaler EH, Kennedy DW, editors. Rhinosinusitis: a Guide for diagnosis and Management. New York: Springer; 2008. p. 1–11.
10. Expert Panel on Pediatric Imaging, Tekes A, Palasis S, et al. ACR Appropriateness Criteria® Sinusitis-Child. J Am Coll Radiol 2018;15(11S):S403–12.
11. Dankbaar JW, van Bemmel AJ, Pameijer FA. Imaging findings of the orbital and intracranial complications of acute bacterial rhinosinusitis. Insights Imaging 2015;6(5):509–18.
12. Joshi VM, Sansi R. Imaging in Sinonasal Inflammatory Disease. Neuroimaging Clin N Am 2015;25(4):549–68.
13. Wald ER, Applegate KE, Bordley C, et al. Clinical practice guideline for the diagnosis and management of acute bacterial sinusitis in children aged 1 to 18 years. Pediatrics 2013;132(1):e262–80.
14. Wald AAP 2001: American Academy of Pediatrics, Subcommittee on Management of Sinusitis and Committee on Quality Improvement. Clinical practice guideline: management of sinusitis. Pediatrics 2001;108(3):798–808.
15. Brook I. Acute sinusitis in children. Pediatr Clin North Am 2013;60(2):409–24.
16. Bhatia H, Kaur R, Bedi R. MR imaging of cavernous sinus thrombosis. Eur J Radiol Open 2020;7:100226.
17. Connor SE. The Skull Base in the Evaluation of Sinonasal Disease: Role of Computed Tomography and

MR Imaging. Neuroimaging Clin N Am 2015;25(4): 619–51.

18. Vaidyanathan S, Lingam RK. Imaging of Acute and Chronic Skull Base Infection. Neuroimaging Clin N Am 2021;31(4):571–98.

19. Younis RT, Anand VK, Davidson B. The role of computed tomography and magnetic resonance imaging in patients with sinusitis with complications. Laryngoscope 2002;112(2):224–9.

20. Wong AM, Bilaniuk LT, Zimmerman RA, et al. Magnetic resonance imaging of carotid artery abnormalities in patients with sphenoid sinusitis. Neuroradiology 2004;46(1):54–9.

21. Wetzel SG, Johnson G, Tan AG, et al. Three-dimensional, T1-weighted gradient-echo imaging of the brain with a volumetric interpolated examination. AJNR Am J Neuroradiol 2002;23(6):995–1002.

22. Raz E, Win W, Hagiwara M, et al. Fungal Sinusitis. Neuroimaging Clin N Am 2015;25(4):569–76.

23. Middlebrooks EH, Frost CJ, De Jesus RO, et al. Acute Invasive Fungal Rhinosinusitis: A Comprehensive Update of CT Findings and Design of an Effective Diagnostic Imaging Model. AJNR Am J Neuroradiol 2015;36(8):1529–35.

24. Shih RY, Koeller KK. Bacterial, Fungal, and Parasitic Infections of the Central Nervous System: Radiologic-Pathologic Correlation and Historical Perspectives. Radiographics 2015;35(4):1141–69.

25. Mossa-Basha M, Ilica AT, Maluf F, et al. The many faces of fungal disease of the paranasal sinuses: CT and MRI findings. Diagn Interv Radiol 2013; 19(3):195–200.

26. Groppo ER, El-Sayed IH, Aiken AH, et al. Computed tomography and magnetic resonance imaging characteristics of acute invasive fungal sinusitis. Arch Otolaryngol Head Neck Surg 2011;137(10): 1005–10.

27. Chakrabarti A, Denning DW, Ferguson BJ, et al. Fungal rhinosinusitis: a categorization and definitional schema addressing current controversies. Laryngoscope 2009;119(9):1809–18.

28. Aribandi M, McCoy VA, Bazan C 3rd. Imaging features of invasive and noninvasive fungal sinusitis: a review. Radiographics 2007;27(5):1283–96.

Infectious and Inflammatory Processes of the Orbits in Children

Julie B. Guerin, MD[a],*, Michael C. Brodsky, MD[b], V. Michelle Silvera, MD[a]

KEYWORDS

• Orbit • Infection • Inflammation • Abscess • Neuroimaging • Pediatric

KEY POINTS

- The most reliable clinical predictors of postseptal infection are proptosis, limited ocular motility, pain, and ophthalmoplegia; in these cases, imaging should be obtained to rule out postseptal infection and complications including abscess and venous thrombosis.
- Computed tomography of the orbits with IV contrast is the first-line modality for evaluating orbital inflammation with MR imaging typically reserved for cases in which intracranial extension is suspected.
- Noninfectious orbital inflammatory processes are rare in children; many have shared imaging features of mass-like, infiltrative orbital soft tissue, frequently involving the lacrimal gland and extraocular musculature.
- Neonates with congenital dacryocystocele and nasolacrimal duct cyst due to failed canalization of the distal nasolacrimal duct are susceptible to acute dacryocystitis.

INTRODUCTION

Primary orbital pathology in children is usually due to infection, with most cases being bacterial in nature. Preseptal cellulitis is common in young children and often does not require imaging. Postseptal cellulitis is usually a result of paranasal sinus infection. Radiologists typically encounter these cases when the clinician finds signs and symptoms indicating postseptal orbital involvement such as ophthalmoplegia, proptosis, or pain with eye movement. Performing timely and appropriate imaging is important for the detection and early management of subperiosteal/orbital abscess, venous thrombosis, and intracranial spread of infection. Noninfectious inflammatory processes are much rarer in the pediatric orbit, with the most common condition being idiopathic orbital inflammatory disease (formerly called orbital pseudotumor). Less common benign mass-like inflammatory processes involving the

pediatric orbit can have overlapping imaging features and must be distinguished from life-threatening malignancies such as rhabdomyosarcoma and lymphoma. Inflammation of the sclera is often a clinical diagnosis, though recognition of its imaging features is important.

DISCUSSION
Imaging Considerations

Computed tomography (CT) of the orbits with intravenous (IV) contrast is the first-line modality for evaluating orbital infection and inflammation. It offers rapid image acquisition and high spatial resolution. The American College of Radiology (ACR) 2018 Appropriateness Criteria for orbital imaging state that orbital CT with IV contrast is the appropriate initial imaging modality in the emergent setting for suspected orbital infection, including in children.[1] Advantages of CT include superior detection of foreign bodies, calcification,

[a] Department of Radiology, Mayo Clinic, 200 1st Street SW, Rochester MN 55905, USA; [b] Department of Ophthalmology, Mayo Clinic, 200 1st Street SW, Rochester MN 55905, USA
* Corresponding author.
E-mail address: guerin.julie@mayo.edu

Neuroimag Clin N Am 33 (2023) 685–697
https://doi.org/10.1016/j.nic.2023.05.015
1052-5149/23/© 2023 Elsevier Inc. All rights reserved.

and integrity of osseous structures. Multiplanar views and contrast administration allow for visualization of subperiosteal abscess (SPA), venous patency, and intracranial complications. Per the ACR, patients with orbital infectious and inflammatory conditions may be imaged with CT or MR imaging as they provide overlapping information.[1]

MR imaging provides superior soft tissue characterization compared with CT. For CT cases with suspected intracranial extension of orbital infection or inflammation, MR imaging of the head is the preferred next step. MR imaging is important for evaluation of cavernous and venous sinus thrombosis and for assessment of intracranial empyema, meningitis, septic emboli, cerebritis, and cerebral abscess.[1–3]

Orbital ultrasound has a limited role in the urgent workup of orbital pathology. In the setting of orbital infections, high-frequency (>10 MHz) linear array transducers can be used to assess for drainable superficial fluid collections.[2] However, the small field of view and artifact produced by the bony orbit make this imaging modality insufficient for assessing many intraorbital pathologies.[3]

ORBITAL INFECTION
Chandler Classification System

In 1970, before the widespread use of CT and MR imaging, Chandler and colleagues proposed a classification system for orbital complications of sinusitis which was based on clinical criteria.[4] This system is still in use today, though has been modified to include correlating imaging findings for each group.[5] The system is organized as follows: Group I, preseptal cellulitis; Group II, orbital cellulitis without abscess; Group III, SPA; Group IV, orbital abscess; and Group V, cavernous sinus thrombosis (CST).[4,5]

Preseptal Cellulitis (Group 1)

Preseptal, or periorbital, cellulitis is an acute infection, which is limited to the soft tissues anterior to the orbital septum. It is much more common than postseptal infection and inflammation and presents predominately in children between 2 and 6 years of age.[6–9] The most common causes are direct trauma, insect bites, and dental abscess with *Staphylococcus aureus* or group A *Streptococcus* as the most commonly associated pathogens.[2,7] These children present with soft tissue swelling, erythema, and marked tenderness of periorbital tissues. Imaging is often not obtained if there is no clinical concern for infection involving the postseptal orbit. However, if the degree of orbital soft tissue swelling prevents assessment of the globe or an adequate physical examination,

or is otherwise challenging in a young child, imaging may be requested to assess for deeper extent (Box 1).

Management
When clinical assessment or imaging is consistent with isolated preseptal infection, children are treated with oral antibiotics on an outpatient basis. Many advocate for close follow-up in 24 to 48 hours; if there is no improvement or if there is clinical deterioration, orbital CT should be repeated to reassess for postseptal involvement.[10]

Postseptal (Orbital) Cellulitis Without Abscess (Group 2)

Postseptal cellulitis is an acute infection involving tissues posterior to the orbital septum and within the bony orbit. Most cases result from the direct extension of rhinosinusitis, with the ethmoid sinus being the most common source.[6,7,9,11–13] Children presenting with postseptal orbital infection are older compared with those with preseptal cellulitis, ranging in age from 5 to 12 years at presentation and coinciding with further development of the paranasal sinuses.[2,7–9] Infection may also be introduced by penetrating trauma, dental infection, or hematogenous spread from a systemic infection, though these etiologies are less common. The most reliable clinical predictors of postseptal infection are proptosis, limited ocular motility, pain, and ophthalmoplegia.[8,9,13] Photophobia, fever, leukocytosis, and an elevated C-reactive protein (CRP) have also been reported as indicators of postseptal disease[8,9,11] (Box 2).

Management
Like preseptal cellulitis, medical management is the main treatment of orbital cellulitis without abscess, though children are typically admitted to the hospital for intravenous antibiotics.[14]

Subperiosteal and Orbital Abscess (Groups 3 and 4)

Subperiosteal and orbital abscesses are drainable, purulent collections which present in the setting of postseptal/orbital cellulitis, typically in children 5 to 12 years of age.[7–9] An SPA is the most common and occurs between the periorbita and the bony orbital wall, adjacent to infected paranasal sinuses. An orbital abscess is not contained within the periorbita, occurs within the intraconal or extraconal orbital tissues, and is relatively rare.[11] Focal phlegmon, unbounded soft tissue inflammation which does not have a liquid component, typically precedes formation of an abscess. Intraoperative cultures of SPAs most commonly demonstrate gram-positive bacteria.[11,12] Similar to postseptal

<table>
<tr><td>

Box 1

Imaging features of preseptal cellulitis (Chandler group 1)

- Periorbital soft tissue swelling and inflammatory fat stranding which does not extend deep to the orbital septum (**Fig. 1**).

- In the setting of acute infection, location of the orbital septum may be inferred by appreciating a sharp transition from hyperattenuating and enhancing preseptal soft tissues to clean postseptal orbital fat.

</td><td>

Box 2

Imaging features of postseptal (orbital) cellulitis without abscess (Chandler group 2)

- Edema and inflammatory stranding of the orbital fat, often initially in the medial extraconal space.

- Swelling and hyperenhancement of the extraocular muscles if associated myositis is present.

- Hyperenhancement of the optic nerve if concomitant optic neuritis is present.

- Concurrent paranasal sinus inflammation.

</td></tr>
</table>

cellulitis, SPAs and orbital abscesses present with proptosis, ophthalmoplegia, and painful eye movements with proptosis being the most significant predictor for surgical intervention.[6,8,9,13,15] Orbital abscess is more likely than phlegmon to cause complete ophthalmoplegia and lead to vision impairment[15] (**Box 3**).

An SPA can increase quickly in size over a few days with radiographic resolution requiring 1 to 3 weeks.[17] Associated findings of postseptal cellulitis described above are seen concurrently.

Management

Although orbital abscesses are typically managed surgically, there are no established guidelines for treatment of SPAs. Successful medical management has been reported for patients with low volume SPAs less than 3.8 mL, however, those with volumes greater than 3.8 mL have a significantly higher probability of requiring surgery.[15,18] Intracranial complications also increase the likelihood of surgical intervention.[18]

Cavernous Sinus Thrombosis (Group 5)

Septic CST is a severe phlebitic process that can be life-threatening. Orbital cellulitis is an uncommon source, and most cases arise from the paranasal sinuses.[19] The incidence has greatly

declined since the introduction of antibiotics though morbidity and mortality rates related to CST remain significant. In the context of orbital infection, spread is typically through the ophthalmic veins with propagation of phlebitis and/or thrombophlebitis. Infectious organisms are typically bacterial with S aureus the most common pathogen.[19] Children can present with ophthalmoplegia, proptosis, and chemosis. Cranial nerve palsy affecting cranial nerves II, III, IV, VI, and the ophthalmic division of Vth nerve can be seen with CST but can also be seen with phlegmonous involvement of the orbital apex and superior orbital fissure.[20] Both contrast-enhanced head CT and contrast-enhanced head MR imaging are highly sensitive for detecting CST,[21] though MR imaging is superior for identifying further intracranial spread. Importantly, imaging may be normal early in the course of CST; therefore, high clinical suspicion is crucial (**Box 4**).

Management

Treatment mainstay is systemic antibiotic therapy with some patients requiring paranasal sinus debridement or orbital decompression. Anticoagulation therapy may be considered for superior

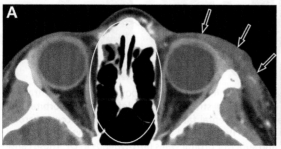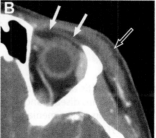

Fig. 1. Preseptal cellulitis in a 10-year-old boy. Axial CT images with IV contrast (*A, B*) show left periorbital soft tissue swelling (*open arrows*) with normal-appearing left postseptal orbital fat. The orbital septum extends across the bony orbit (*white arrows*). The ethmoid sinuses are clear (*oval* in *A*).

ophthalmic and CST, though prospective data are limited.[2,22]

Other Intracranial Spread of Infection

MR imaging should be obtained for any concern of intracranial involvement, including cavernous and dural venous sinus thrombosis, meningitis, empyema, cerebritis, and cerebral abscess.[3] Intracranial spread of sinusitis typically occurs via the propagation of septic thrombi through the valveless diploic venous system that connects sinus mucosal veins to meninges intracranially; intracranial spread of infection is less commonly a direct extension of osteomyelitis.[23,24]

DACRYOCYSTITIS

Dacryocystitis is inflammation of the lacrimal sac which usually results from obstruction of the nasolacrimal duct. Subsequent backup and stasis of fluid in the lacrimal system can lead to infection. Nasolacrimal duct obstruction without dacryocystitis is common in infants, and superimposed infection is most often chronic and low grade. As such, it is usually treatable with simple probing and irrigation and does not require cross-

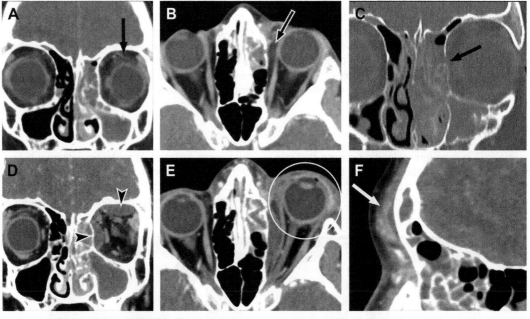

Fig. 2. Postseptal cellulitis and subperiosteal abscesses in a 12-year-old boy. CT with IV contrast (A–C) demonstrates left paranasal sinus disease and mild inflammatory stranding of the left postseptal orbital fat (*black arrow* in A). Subtle infiltration of the medial extraconal postseptal fat (*open arrow* in B) adjacent to erosive change of the left lamina papyracea (*black arrow* in C). CT with IV contrast 1 day later (D–F) shows subsequent development of subperiosteal abscesses along the medial and superior orbital walls (*arrowheads* in D). These cause mass effect on the medial and superior rectus muscles, left-sided proptosis with posterior tenting of the globe (circle in E), and straightening of the optic nerve. An additional subperiosteal abscess overlies the opacified frontal sinus (*white arrow* in F). (*Courtesy of* C Carr, MD, Rochester, MN.)

<table>
<tr><td>

Box 4

Imaging features of cavernous sinus thrombosis (Chandler group 5)

Direct signs

- Loss of concavity with lateral bulging (ie, convexity) of the cavernous sinus margins (often best appreciated in the coronal plane) and heterogeneous filling defects within the cavernous sinus[19] (Fig. 3).

Indirect signs

- Thickened dural enhancement along the sinus margins, orbital apex inflammation, and exophthalmos.

Careful attention to the orbital and intracranial vessels is advised.

- Narrowing or occlusion of the ipsilateral cavernous internal carotid artery can lead to arterial ischemic stroke.

- Thrombosis of the superior and inferior ophthalmic veins, the inferior petrosal sinus, and sphenoparietal sinus may be identified with luminal filling defects, venous expansion, wall thickening with hyperenhancement, and magnetic susceptibility on gradient sequences (Fig. 4).

- Associated intraluminal diffusion restriction can be due to purulent material or evolving thrombus.[19,22]

</td></tr>
</table>

sectional imaging. A small percentage of neonates will have a congenital dacryocystocele and a nasolacrimal duct cyst due to failure of

canalization of the distal nasolacrimal duct at the valve of Hasner. These infants are more susceptible to acute dacryocystitis and typically present in the first 2 weeks of life with pronounced swelling and erythema over the lacrimal sac. More severe infections can be accompanied by progressive cellulitis and formation of an abscess in the lacrimal sac. This can lead to breathing difficulties and cyanosis[2,25] (Box 5).

Management

Management of dacryocystitis is done in consultation with an ophthalmologist and typically involves endoscopic decompression and antibiotics.

Orbital Inflammatory Processes

Noninfectious orbital inflammatory processes are rare in children; many have shared imaging features of mass-like, infiltrative soft tissue within the pediatric orbit.

Idiopathic Orbital Inflammation

Idiopathic orbital inflammation (IOI), formerly known as orbital pseudotumor, is a noninfectious and nonneoplastic space-occupying inflammatory process of the orbit that is typically a diagnosis of exclusion.[27] It is relatively uncommon in the pediatric population with larger cohort studies reporting 11% to 17% of affected patients being less than 18 to 20 years of age.[28,29] The most common presenting symptoms are periorbital edema and blepharoptosis, a palpable mass, limited ocular motility, and ocular or orbital pain.[28,30–32] IOI may present with orbital myositis, dacryoadenitis, optic

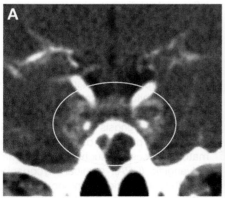
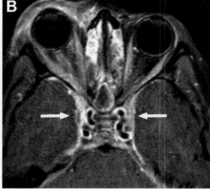

Fig. 3. Cavernous sinus thrombosis in an adolescent. Coronal CT angiogram (*A*) shows outward bulging of cavernous sinus margins and patchy hypoenhancement (*circle*). Axial post-gadolinium T1W image (*B*) shows heterogenous filling defects in the cavernous sinus, carotid artery wall enhancement, and abnormal dural enhancement in the middle cranial fossae (*white arrows*). Within the right orbit, there are signs of preseptal and postseptal cellulitis, perineural optic nerve enhancement, shading of the orbital fat, and enlargement of the extraocular muscles with crowding of the right orbital apex and right-sided proptosis. (*Courtesy of* W O'Brien Sr., DO, Orlando, FL.)

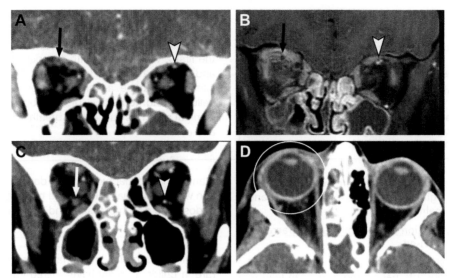

Fig. 4. Two cases of venous thrombosis in the setting of orbital infection. Coronal contrast-enhanced CT and MR imaging (*A, B*) in an adolescent with congestion and visual impairment show a luminal filling defect in the right superior ophthalmic vein (*black arrows*) with slight venous expansion and peripheral hyperenhancement. The left superior ophthalmic vein is normal (*arrowheads*). Enhancing fat stranding in the right orbit represents postseptal orbital cellulitis. Coronal and axial contrast-enhanced CT images (*C, D*) in a child with right-sided sinusitis show a luminal filling defect in the right inferior ophthalmic vein with slight venous expansion (*white arrow* in *C*). The left inferior ophthalmic vein is normal (*arrowhead* in *C*). There is right-sided proptosis from the orbital infection (*circle* in *D*). (*Courtesy of* W O'Brien Sr., DO, Orlando, FL.)

perineuritis, posterior scleritis, or any combination thereof, with each component producing enlargement and/or enhancement of their respective structures. Although any area of the orbit can be involved, the lacrimal gland and extraocular musculature are the most commonly involved structures in both adults and children.[30] A focal orbital mass is a typical finding in children, potentially resulting in orbital apex syndrome. Ptosis,

uveitis, and disc edema have been reported as more common in children with IOI compared with adults[31–34]; in contrast, proptosis and pain are reported as less common in children compared with adults.[30] Although IOI is typically unilateral, a larger cohort of pediatric IOI reported 13% of children with bilateral disease.[30] Pediatric IOI may be accompanied by constitutional symptoms[30] or may precede the later development of a systemic inflammatory disease.[35]

Imaging

Imaging features of IOI are described in **Table 1**. An example of IOI is shown in **Fig. 6**. Tolosa–Hunt syndrome is a variant form of IOI extending from the orbital apex to the cavernous sinus and is characterized by painful ophthalmoplegia. The differential diagnosis for mass-like, infiltrative lesions in the pediatric orbit includes other inflammatory processes such as granulomatosis with polyangiitis (GPA), atypical mycobacterial infection, fungal infection, immunoglobulin G4-related ophthalmic disease (IgG4-ROD), thyroid orbitopathy, and sarcoidosis,[31] though collectively, these are also rare in children. Malignant lesions including ocular adnexal lymphoma and rhabdomyosarcoma are important to differentiate from IOI as all may manifest as pliant enhancing soft tissue that molds to the orbital contour. The highly

---

Box 5
Imaging features of dacryocystitis

- On ultrasound: heterogeneously echogenic material in the region of the medial canthus and lacrimal sac.

- On CT: tubular low-attenuating soft tissue in the lacrimal sac and duct with peripheral enhancement.

- On MR imaging: purulent contents demonstrate intermediate to hypointense signal on T2-weighted imaging and diffusion restriction (**Fig. 5**).

- Congenital dacryocystoceles and nasolacrimal duct cysts can appear as mass-like expansion extending to the inferior meatus with asymmetric enlargement of the ipsilateral bony nasolacrimal canal.[26]

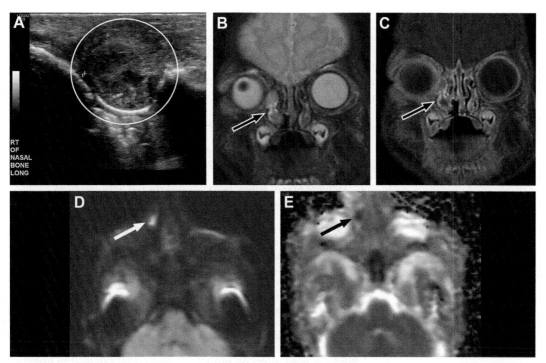

Fig. 5. Acute dacryocystitis in a 4-day-old term infant. Targeted ultrasound (*A*) demonstrates heterogeneously echogenic material in the lacrimal sac. Coronal fat-saturated, T2W (*B*) and post-gadolinium T1W MR images (*C*) show T2 hyperintense and peripherally enhancing lobular expansion of the lacrimal sac and nasolacrimal duct (*open arrows*). Axial DWI MR image (*D*) and corresponding ADC map (*E*) demonstrate focal diffusion restriction indicating purulent material (*white* and *black arrows*).

cellular and hypermetabolic content of malignant mimics may be identified on imaging with quantifiable decreased signal on apparent diffusion coefficient (ADC) maps (<0.84 10^{-3} mm^2/s to $<1.14 \times 10^{-3}$ mm^2/s[16,36,37]), increased perfusion, and substantial F-fluorodeoxyglucose avidity on PET/CT images.[16,36,37]

Management

High-dose corticosteroid therapy is the typical treatment of acute and subacute IOI disease. Orbital biopsy may be necessary in cases that are unresponsive, progressive, or demonstrate recurrence following corticosteroid treatment, although identifiable causes are common.[38]Local radiation therapy is also sometimes used. Full recovery rates are low in both adults and children with post-treatment recurrence in children reported in the range of 37% to 71%.[30,33]

Immunoglobulin G4-Related Ophthalmic Disease

IgG4-ROD is a systemic fibroinflammatory condition with an undetermined pathophysiological mechanism. It is exceedingly rare in children with

fewer than 20 reported cases in the literature.[39] Of those few cases, most of the children have presented with unilateral orbital swelling.

Imaging

Imaging features of IgG4-ROD in children, based on limited reports in the literature,[39–41] are described in **Table 1**.

Management

In larger adult series, cases are typically responsive to prednisone therapy, though maintenance therapy with disease-modifying antirheumatic drugs is sometimes required.[42,43] It is important to treat this disease in its active stage before fibrotic changes predominate.

ORBITAL GRANULOMATOSIS WITH POLYANGIITIS (PREVIOUSLY KNOWN AS WEGENER GRANULOMATOSIS)

GPA is an autoimmune granulomatous disease causing a small-vessel vasculitis that typically affects the orbit, paranasal sinuses, nose, throat, lungs, and kidneys. It usually presents in the fourth to fifth decade of life and is rare in children.[44–46]

Table 1
Shared and differentiating features of idiopathic orbital inflammation, immunoglobulin G4-related ophthalmic disease, and orbital granulomatosis with polyangiitis

Disease Entity	Shared Imaging Features	Distinctive Features
Idiopathic orbital inflammation	Unilateral disease is most common Infiltrative, trans-spatial, and often mass-like soft tissue process which can involve any part of the orbit (including optic nerve/sheath, orbital fat, lacrimal gland, sclera, uvea, and extraocular muscles without sparing of the myotendinous junctions) Infiltrates are usually isointense to hypointense on T1-weighted MR images and show moderate diffuse enhancement Variable signal intensity on T2-weighted images becomes more T2 hypointense with greater fibrosis No diffusion restriction Produces mass effect on orbital contents	Most common noninfectious inflammatory lesion involving the pediatric orbit Although any area of the orbit can be involved, extraocular musculature and lacrimal glands are most commonly affected with resulting enlargement of structures Though unilateral disease is most common, children may have bilateral involvement
Immunoglobulin G4-related ophthalmic disease		Rare in children; available reports describe common features in middle column in addition to involvement of optic nerve and trigeminal nerve branches, sclera, and choroid[40]
Orbital granulomatosis with polyangiitis (GPA)		Rare in children Extension of the mass into the bony orbit can lead to osseous destruction or neo-ossification[45,48,49,51,52] More likely to have T2 hypointense signal and diffusion restriction from fibrotic tissue Mass effect from an orbital mass may lead to proptosis and optic nerve compression with potential for optic neuropathy and vision loss[44,45,47–49] Later stages of fibrosis can show globe retraction and enophthalmos[51,52]

Ophthalmologic features of GPA can occur in approximately half of patients and can affect nearly every structure of the eye. This can result as extension from paranasal sinus disease, or the disease may arise primarily within the orbit. The most common manifestation is an orbital mass, which represents the granulomatous inflammatory component of GPA.[44,45,47–49] Associated dacryoadenitis or extraocular myositis coexists in a smaller percentage of patients.[47] The small vessel vasculitis component of GPA may contribute to episcleritis/conjunctivitis, scleritis, optic neuritis, and retinitis.[44]

Imaging

Imaging features of orbital GPA are described in Table 1. A case example is shown in Fig. 7.

Management

Owing to nonspecific imaging features, biopsy is usually necessary. GPA is very responsive to corticosteroid therapy combined with cyclophosphamide or rituximab.[46,50]

POSTERIOR SCLERITIS

The outer sheath of the globe is trilaminar in design and consists of sclera, choroid, and retina, listed from superficial to deep. Scleritis is inflammation of the sclera, the superficial layer of the globe, which extends from the margin of the cornea anteriorly to the optic nerve posteriorly where it is contiguous with the optic nerve sheath. Most of the cases are noninfectious or idiopathic in nature.[53,54] Uveitis, inflammation of the choroid,

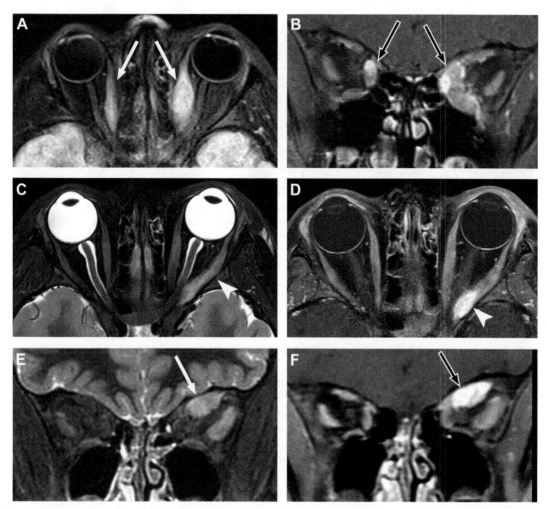

Fig. 6. Bilateral idiopathic orbital inflammation in an 8-year-old girl. Axial fat-saturated T2 FLAIR (*A*) and coronal post-gadolinium T1W images (*B*) from the initial MR imaging examination show signal prolongation and enlargement of the medial rectus muscles (*white arrows*) with corresponding enhancement (open *arrows*) and additional involvement of the left superior oblique and inferior rectus muscles. Axial fat-saturated T2W (*C*) and axial post-gadolinium T1W MR images (*D*) 4 months later show new abnormal T2 prolongation and enlargement of the left lateral rectus muscle with a focus of abnormal enhancement (*arrowheads*). Coronal fat-saturated T2W (*E*) and coronal post-gadolinium T1W MR images (*F*) 1 year from presentation demonstrate new T2 signal prolongation (*white arrow*) and enlargement of the left superior rectus muscle with associated enhancement (*open arrow*) as well as enlargement of the left superior oblique and lateral rectus muscles.

ciliary body and iris, and endophthalmitis, and inflammation of the vitreous and/or aqueous humor within the anterior chamber are beyond the scope of pediatric orbital disease and will not be further discussed.

Scleritis is classified clinically as anterior or posterior in location. Anterior scleritis is usually diagnosed clinically and is typically not considered an orbital disease. Posterior idiopathic scleritis is the most common type of scleritis observed, including in the context of IOI as mentioned previously. It is usually not readily evident on physical examination and it is widely underdiagnosed.[53,55,56] Posterior

scleritis is characterized by pain and redness of the eye, with choroidal folds, retinal striae, and optic disc edema.[57]

Prompt workup should be performed to exclude infectious and systemic causes.[56] The diagnosis and management of posterior scleritis is primarily achieved clinically by ophthalmologic examination. Orbital ophthalmologic imaging is particularly helpful in the diagnosis as B-scan ultrasonography shows retrobulbar edema producing a characteristic "T-sign."[57,58] CT and MR imaging are rarely indicated, though both imaging modalities may show findings that support the diagnosis (Box 6).

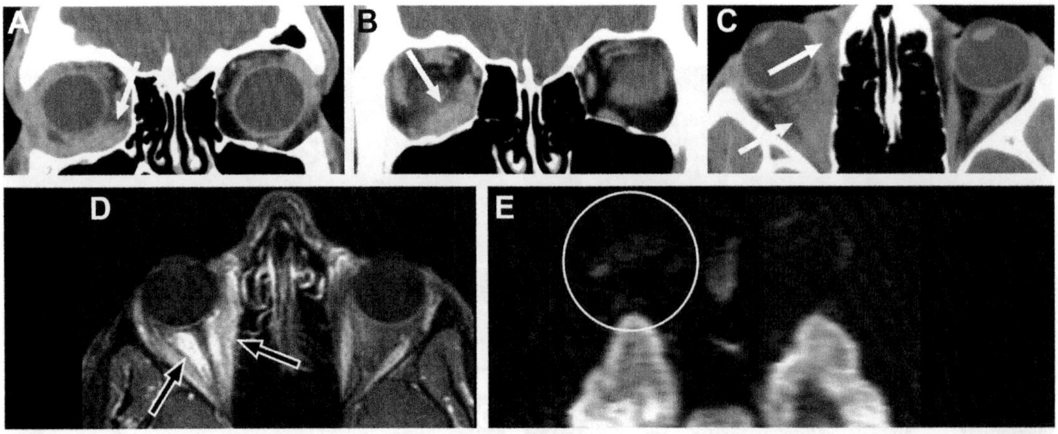

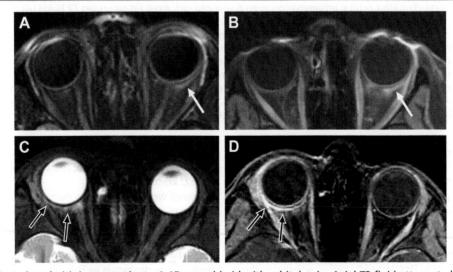

Fig. 7. Orbital granulomatosis with polyangiitis in a 16-year-old boy. Coronal (*A, B*) and axial (*C*) non-contrast CT images show an infiltrative soft tissue process in the right orbit, mostly concentrated inferiorly, with obscuration of the normal tissue planes with the adjacent extraocular musculature (*white arrows*). Axial post-gadolinium T1W MR image (*D*) demonstrates avid enhancement (*open arrows*) of this process. There is no associated restricted diffusion on the axial diffusion-weighted sequence (*circle* in *E*).

Box 6
Imaging features of posterior scleritis

- The normal sclera can be delineated as the outer hypointense rim of the globe.

- Posterior scleritis manifests with abnormal thickening and enhancement of the outer globe wall with adjacent periscleral cellulitis of the retrobulbar fat[2,55] (Fig. 8).

- Scleral enhancement is always abnormal and can be made more conspicuous on MR imaging using post-contrast T1-weighting imaging with fat saturation.

- Inflammation of the sclera may be diffuse or less commonly focal and nodular. Nodular scleritis may mimic malignancy; lack of diffusion restriction of the sclera is a differentiating feature from tumors such as retinoblastoma.

- May be accompanied by more extensive inflammation in the orbit, which can mimic infectious post-septal cellulitis.[55]

- MR imaging may show imaging features of scleritis even when ophthalmoscopic findings are absent.[59]

Fig. 8. Posterior scleritis in two patients. A 15-year-old girl with orbital pain: Axial T2 fluid-attenuated inversion recovery (FLAIR) image (*A*) and axial post-gadolinium T1W MR image (*B*) demonstrate thickening and enhancement of the posterolateral left sclera with adjacent retrobulbar cellulitis (*white arrows*). A 8-year-old girl with orbital pain: Axial T2W MR image with fat saturation (*C*) and axial post-gadolinium T1W MR image (*D*) show abnormal right-sided scleral thickening and enhancement with adjacent retrobulbar cellulitis (*open arrows*). ADC, apparent diffusion coefficient; DWI, diffusion-weighted imaging; T1W, T1-weighted; T2W, T2-weighted.

Management

Corticosteroid therapy is the standard initial treatment with disease-modifying antirheumatic drugs and immunomodulatory agents becoming a mainstay in long-term therapy.

SUMMARY

Contrast-enhanced cross-sectional imaging plays a vital role in characterizing suspected postseptal orbital infection and inflammation. Specifically, it assists in detecting involvement of orbital and intracranial structures and narrowing differential considerations. This information is necessary for clinicians to make management decisions and implement therapy to preserve vision and limit extension of disease and complications. Infectious conditions of the orbit may have overlapping imaging features with uncommon noninfectious inflammatory processes and orbital malignancies. Preseptal periorbital conditions usually do not require cross-sectional imaging. Radiologists should be aware of orbital pathology in children, the role of imaging, and differentiating imaging features to optimize patient care.

CLINICS CARE POINTS

- Orbital computed tomography with IV contrast is the appropriate initial imaging modality in the emergent setting for suspected orbital infection in children, per The American College of Radiology (ACR) 2018 Appropriateness Criteria.[1]
- Most cases of postseptal orbital infection result from the direct extension of rhinosinusitis, with the ethmoid sinus being the most common source.[6,7,9,11–13]
- Although there are no established treatment guidelines for subperiosteal abscess, successful medical management has been reported for patients with low volume subperiosteal abscess less than 3.8 mL.[15,18]
- Diffusion restriction can be a helpful for differentiating benign inflammatory processes in the pediatric orbit from malignancies such as rhabdomyosarcoma and lymphoma; suggested ADC cutoff values range from 0.84 10^{-3} to 1.14 $\times$ 10^{-3} mm^2/s.[16,36,37]
- Posterior idiopathic scleritis is the most common type of scleritis observed; it is not readily evident on physical examination and it is widely underdiagnosed.[53,55,56]

FUNDING AND CONFLICTS OF INTEREST

The authors have no funding or conflicts of interest to declare.

ACKNOWLEDGMENTS

The authors would like to thank the assistance of Sonia Watson, PhD, in preparation of the manuscript.

REFERENCES

1. Expert Panel on Neurologic Imaging, Kennedy TA, Corey AS, et al. ACR Appropriateness Criteria® Orbits Vision and Visual Loss. J Am Coll Radiol JACR 2018;15(5S):S116–31.
2. Nagaraj UD, Koch BL. Imaging of orbital infectious and inflammatory disease in children. Pediatr Radiol 2021;51(7):1149–61.
3. Burek AG, Melamed S, Liljestrom T, et al. Evaluation and Medical Management of the Pediatric Patient With Orbital Cellulitis/Abscess: A Systematic Review. J Hosp Med 2021;16(11):680–7.
4. Chandler JR, Langenbrunner DJ, Stevens ER. The pathogenesis of orbital complications in acute sinusitis. Laryngoscope 1970;80(9):1414–28.
5. Healy GB. Chandler et al.: "The pathogenesis of orbital complications in acute sinusitis." (Laryngoscope 1970;80:1414-1428). Laryngoscope 1997; 107(4):441–6.
6. Jabarin B, Eviatar E, Israel O, et al. Indicators for imaging in periorbital cellulitis secondary to rhinosinusitis. Eur Arch Oto-Rhino-Laryngol 2018;275(4): 943–8.
7. Santos JC, Pinto S, Ferreira S, et al. Pediatric preseptal and orbital cellulitis: A 10-year experience. Int J Pediatr Otorhinolaryngol 2019;120:82–8.
8. Murphy DC, Meghji S, Alfiky M, et al. Paediatric periorbital cellulitis: A 10-year retrospective case series review. J Paediatr Child Health 2021;57(2):227–33.
9. Miranda-Barrios J, Bravo-Queipo-de-Llano B, Baquero-Artigao F, et al. Preseptal Versus Orbital Cellulitis in Children: An Observational Study. Pediatr Infect Dis J 2021;40(11):969–74.
10. Najarian C, Brown AM. What Is the Best Treatment for a Subperiosteal Abscess? A Case Report in a Pediatric Patient. J Pediatr Health Care 2019;33(4): 489–93.
11. Martins M, Martins SP, Pinto-Moura C, et al. Management of post-septal complications of acute rhinosinusitis in children: A 14-year experience in a tertiary hospital. Int J Pediatr Otorhinolaryngol 2021;151:110925.
12. Coudert A, Ayari-Khalfallah S, Suy P, et al. Microbiology and antibiotic therapy of subperiosteal orbital abscess in children with acute ethmoiditis. Int J Pediatr Otorhinolaryngol 2018;106:91–5.

13. Singh M, Negi A, Zadeng Z, et al. Long-Term Ophthalmic Outcomes in Pediatric Orbital Cellulitis: A Prospective, Multidisciplinary Study From a Tertiary-Care Referral Institute. J Pediatr Ophthalmol Strabismus 2019;56(5):333–9.

14. Sciarretta V, Demattè M, Farneti P, et al. Management of orbital cellulitis and subperiosteal orbital abscess in pediatric patients: A ten-year review. Int J Pediatr Otorhinolaryngol 2017;96:72–6.

15. Le TD, Liu ES, Adatia FA, et al. The effect of adding orbital computed tomography findings to the Chandler criteria for classifying pediatric orbital cellulitis in predicting which patients will require surgical intervention. J Am Assoc Pediatr Ophthalmol Strabismus 2014;18(3):271–7.

16. Sepahdari AR, Politi LS, Aakalu VK, et al. Diffusion-weighted imaging of orbital masses: multi-institutional data support a 2-ADC threshold model to categorize lesions as benign, malignant, or indeterminate. AJNR Am J Neuroradiol 2014;35(1):170–5.

17. Cossack MT, Herretes SP, Cham A, et al. Radiographic Course of Medically Managed Pediatric Orbital Subperiosteal Abscesses. J Pediatr Ophthalmol Strabismus 2018;55(6):387–92.

18. Wong SJ, Levi J. Management of pediatric orbital cellulitis: A systematic review. Int J Pediatr Otorhinolaryngol 2018;110:123–9.

19. Caranfa JT, Yoon MK. Septic cavernous sinus thrombosis: A review. Surv Ophthalmol 2021;66(6):1021–30.

20. Saini L, Chakrabarty B, Kumar A, et al. Orbital Apex Syndrome: A Clinico-anatomical Diagnosis. J Pediatr Neurosci 2020;15(3):336–7.

21. Smith DM, Vossough A, Vorona GA, et al. Pediatric cavernous sinus thrombosis: A case series and review of the literature. Neurology 2015;85(9):763–9.

22. Press CA, Lindsay A, Stence NV, et al. Cavernous Sinus Thrombosis in Children: Imaging Characteristics and Clinical Outcomes. Stroke 2015;46(9):2657–60.

23. Masuoka S, Miyazaki O, Takahashi H, et al. Predisposing conditions for bacterial meningitis in children: what radiologists need to know. Jpn J Radiol 2022;40(1):1–18.

24. Patel NA, Garber D, Hu S, et al. Systematic review and case report: Intracranial complications of pediatric sinusitis. Int J Pediatr Otorhinolaryngol 2016;86:200–12.

25. Lueder GT. The association of neonatal dacryocystoceles and infantile dacryocystitis with nasolacrimal duct cysts (an American Ophthalmological Society thesis). Trans Am Ophthalmol Soc 2012;110:74–93.

26. Rand PK, Ball WS, Kulwin DR. Congenital nasolacrimal mucoceles: CT evaluation. Radiology 1989;173(3):691–4.

27. Boulter EL, Eleftheriou D, Sebire NJ, et al. Inflammatory lesions of the orbit: a single paediatric rheumatology centre experience. Rheumatol Oxf Engl 2012;51(6):1070–5.

28. Eshraghi B, Sonbolestan SA, Abtahi MA, et al. Clinical characteristics, histopathology, and treatment outcomes in adult and pediatric patients with nonspecific orbital inflammation. J Curr Ophthalmol 2019;31(3):327–34.

29. Blodi FC, Gas JD. Inflammatory pseudotumour of the orbit. Br J Ophthalmol 1968;52(2):79–93.

30. Spindle JMD, Tang SXMD, Davies BMD, et al. Pediatric Idiopathic Orbital Inflammation: Clinical Features of 30 Cases. Ophthal Plast Reconstr Surg 2016;32(4):270–4.

31. Belanger C, Zhang KS, Reddy AK, Yen MT, Yen KG. Inflammatory Disorders of the Orbit in Childhood: A Case Series. Am J Ophthalmol.

32. Berger JW, Rubin PA, Jakobiec FA. Pediatric orbital pseudotumor: case report and review of the literature. Int Ophthalmol Clin 1996;36(1):161–77.

33. Yan J, Qiu H, Wu Z, et al. Idiopathic orbital inflammatory pseudotumor in Chinese children. Orbit Amst Neth 2006;25(1):1–4.

34. Mottow-Lippa L, Jakobiec FA, Smith M. Idiopathic inflammatory orbital pseudotumor in childhood. II. Results of diagnostic tests and biopsies. Ophthalmology 1981;88(6):565–74.

35. Tsukikàwa M, Lally SE, Shields CL, et al. Idiopathic Orbital Pseudotumor Preceding Systemic Inflammatory Disease in Children. J Pediatr Ophthalmol Strabismus 2019;56(6):373–7.

36. Eissa L, Abdel Razek AAK, Helmy E. Arterial spin labeling and diffusion-weighted MR imaging: Utility in differentiating idiopathic orbital inflammatory pseudotumor from orbital lymphoma. Clin Imaging 2020;71:63–8.

37. Jaju A, Rychlik K, Ryan ME. MRI of Pediatric Orbital Masses: Role of Quantitative Diffusion-weighted Imaging in Differentiating Benign from Malignant Lesions. Clin Neuroradiol 2020;30(3):615–24.

38. Mombaerts I, Rose GE, Garrity JA. Orbital inflammation: Biopsy first. Surv Ophthalmol 2016;61(5):664–9.

39. Smerla RG, Rontogianni D, Fragoulis GE. Ocular manifestations of IgG4-related disease in children. More common than anticipated? Review of the literature and case report. Clin Rheumatol 2018;37(6):1721–7.

40. Derzko-Dzulynsky L. IgG4-related disease in the eye and ocular adnexa. Curr Opin Ophthalmol 2017;28(6):617–22.

41. Griepentrog GJ, Vickers RW, Karesh JW, et al. A clinicopathologic case study of two patients with pediatric orbital IgG4-related disease. Orbit Amst Neth 2013;32(6):389–91.

42. Karim F, Loeffen J, Bramer W, et al. IgG4-related disease: a systematic review of this unrecognized disease in pediatrics. Pediatr Rheumatol Online J

2016;14. https://doi.org/10.1186/s12969-016-0079-3.

43. Wallace ZS, Deshpande V, Stone JH. Ophthalmic manifestations of IgG4-related disease: single-center experience and literature review. Semin Arthritis Rheum 2014;43(6):806–17.

44. Davila-Camargo A, Tovilla-Canales JL, Olvera-Morales O, et al. Orbital manifestations of granulomatosis with polyangiitis: 12-year experience in Mexico City. Orbit Amst Neth 2020;39(5):357–64.

45. Sfiniadaki E, Tsiara I, Theodossiadis P, et al. Ocular Manifestations of Granulomatosis with Polyangiitis: A Review of the Literature. Ophthalmol Ther 2019; 8(2):227–34.

46. Durel CA, Hot A, Trefond L, et al. Orbital mass in ANCA-associated vasculitides: data on clinical, biological, radiological and histological presentation, therapeutic management, and outcome from 59 patients. Rheumatol Oxf Engl 2019;58(9):1565–73.

47. Ismailova DS, Abramova JV, Novikov PI, et al. Clinical features of different orbital manifestations of granulomatosis with polyangiitis. Graefes Arch Clin Exp Ophthalmol Albrecht Von Graefes Arch Klin Exp Ophthalmol 2018;256(9):1751–6.

48. Andrada-Elena M, Ioana TT, Mihaela FM, et al. Wegener's granulomatosis with orbital involvement: case report and literature review. Romanian J Ophthalmol 2021;65(1):93–7.

49. Ure E, Kayadibi Y, Sanli DT, et al. Orbital involvement as the initial presentation of Wegener granulomatosis in a 9-year-old girl: MR imaging findings. Diagn Interv Imaging 2016;97(11):1181–2.

50. Muller K, Lin JH. Orbital Granulomatosis With Polyangiitis (Wegener Granulomatosis). Arch Pathol Lab Med 2014;138(8):1110–4.

51. Guzman-Soto MI, Kimura Y, Romero-Sanchez G, et al. From Head to Toe: Granulomatosis with Polyangiitis. Radiographics 2021;41(7):1973–91.

52. Pakalniskis MG, Berg AD, Policeni BA, et al. The Many Faces of Granulomatosis With Polyangiitis: A Review of the Head and Neck Imaging Manifestations. Am J Roentgenol 2015;205(6):W619–29.

53. Waduthantri S, Chee SP. Pediatric Uveitis and Scleritis in a Multi-Ethnic Asian Population. Ocul Immunol Inflamm 2021;29(7–8):1304–11.

54. Sun N, Wang C, Linghu W, et al. Demographic and clinical features of pediatric uveitis and scleritis at a tertiary referral center in China. BMC Ophthalmol 2022;22(1):174.

55. Diogo MC, Jager MJ, Ferreira TA. CT and MR Imaging in the Diagnosis of Scleritis. AJNR Am J Neuroradiol 2016;37(12):2334–9.

56. Tarsia M, Gaggiano C, Gessaroli E, et al. Pediatric Scleritis: An Update. Ocul Immunol Inflamm 2022; 28:1–10.

57. Benson WE. Posterior scleritis. Surv Ophthalmol 1988;32(5):297–316.

58. Cheung CMG, Chee SP. Posterior scleritis in children: clinical features and treatment. Ophthalmology 2012;119(1):59–65.

59. Bang GM, Brodsky MC. Pediatric posterior scleritis. Ophthalmology 2012;119(7):1505. e1; author reply 1505.

UNITED STATES POSTAL SERVICE ® Statement of Ownership, Management, and Circulation
(All Periodicals Publications Except Requester Publications)

1. Publication Title	2. Publication Number	3. Filing Date
NEUROIMAGING CLINICS OF NORTH AMERICA	010 – 548	9/18/2023

4. Issue Frequency	5. Number of Issues Published Annually	6. Annual Subscription Price
FEB, MAY, AUG, NOV	4	$413.00

7. Complete Mailing Address of Known Office of Publication (Not printer) (Street, city, county, state, and ZIP+4®)

ELSEVIER INC.
230 Park Avenue, Suite 800
New York, NY 10169

Contact Person
Malathi Samayan

Telephone (Include area code)
91-44-4299-4507

8. Complete Mailing Address of Headquarters or General Business Office of Publisher (Not printer)

ELSEVIER INC.
230 Park Avenue, Suite 800
New York, NY 10169

9. Full Names and Complete Mailing Addresses of Publisher, Editor, and Managing Editor (Do not leave blank)

Publisher (Name and complete mailing address)

DOLORES MELONI, ELSEVIER INC.
1600 JOHN F KENNEDY BLVD. SUITE 1800
PHILADELPHIA, PA 19103-2899

Editor (Name and complete mailing address)

JOHN VASSALLO, ELSEVIER INC.
1600 JOHN F KENNEDY BLVD. SUITE 1800
PHILADELPHIA, PA 19103-2899

Managing Editor (Name and complete mailing address)

PATRICK MANLEY ELSEVIER INC.
1600 JOHN F KENNEDY BLVD. SUITE 1800
PHILADELPHIA, PA 19103-2899

10. Owner (Do not leave blank. If the publication is owned by a corporation, give the name and address of the corporation immediately followed by the names and addresses of all stockholders owning or holding 1 percent or more of the total amount of stock. If not owned by a corporation, give the names and addresses of the individual owners. If owned by a partnership or other unincorporated firm, give its name and address as well as those of each individual owner. If the publication is published by a nonprofit organization, give its name and address.)

Full Name	Complete Mailing Address
WHOLLY OWNED SUBSIDIARY OF REED/ELSEVIER, US HOLDINGS	1600 JOHN F KENNEDY BLVD, SUITE 1800 PHILADELPHIA, PA 19103-2899

11. Known Bondholders, Mortgagees, and Other Security Holders Owning or Holding 1 Percent or More of Total Amount of Bonds, Mortgages, or Other Securities. If none, check box. ▶ ☐ None

Full Name	Complete Mailing Address
N/A	

12. Tax Status (For completion by nonprofit organizations authorized to mail at nonprofit rates) (Check one)
The purpose, function, and nonprofit status of this organization and the exempt status for federal income tax purposes:

☒ Has Not Changed During Preceding 12 Months
☐ Has Changed During Preceding 12 Months (Publisher must submit explanation of change with this statement)

PS Form 3526, July 2014 [Page 1 of 4 (see instructions page 4)] PSN: 7530-01-000-9931   PRIVACY NOTICE: See our privacy policy on www.usps.com.

13. Publication Title	14. Issue Date for Circulation Data Below
NEUROIMAGING CLINICS OF NORTH AMERICA	MAY 2023

15. Extent and Nature of Circulation			Average No. Copies Each Issue During Preceding 12 Months	No. Copies of Single Issue Published Nearest to Filing Date
a. Total Number of Copies (Net press run)			394	371
b. Paid Circulation (By Mail and Outside the Mail)	(1)	Mailed Outside-County Paid Subscriptions Stated on PS Form 3541 (Include paid distribution above nominal rate, advertiser's proof copies, and exchange copies)	293	276
	(2)	Mailed In-County Paid Subscriptions Stated on PS Form 3541 (Include paid distribution above nominal rate, advertiser's proof copies, and exchange copies)	0	0
	(3)	Paid Distribution Outside the Mails Including Sales Through Dealers and Carriers, Street Vendors, Counter Sales, and Other Paid Distribution Outside USPS®	63	49
	(4)	Paid Distribution by Other Classes of Mail Through the USPS (e.g., First-Class Mail®)	0	0
c. Total Paid Distribution (Sum of 15b (1), (2), (3), and (4))		▶	356	325
d. Free or Nominal Rate Distribution (By Mail and Outside the Mail)	(1)	Free or Nominal Rate Outside-County Copies included on PS Form 3541	22	31
	(2)	Free or Nominal Rate In-County Copies Included on PS Form 3541	0	0
	(3)	Free or Nominal Rate Copies Mailed at Other Classes Through the USPS (e.g., First-Class Mail)	0	0
	(4)	Free or Nominal Rate Distribution Outside the Mail (Carriers or other means)	0	0
e. Total Free or Nominal Rate Distribution (Sum of 15d (1), (2), (3) and (4))		▶	22	31
f. Total Distribution (Sum of 15c and 15e)		▶	378	356
g. Copies not Distributed (See Instructions to Publishers #4 (page #3))		▶	16	15
h. Total (Sum of 15f and g)		▶	394	371
i. Percent Paid (15c divided by 15f times 100)			94.17%	91.29%

* If you are claiming electronic copies, go to line 16 on page 3. If you are not claiming electronic copies, skip to line 17 on page 3.

PS Form 3526, July 2014 (Page 2 of 4)

16. Electronic Copy Circulation	Average No. Copies Each Issue During Preceding 12 Months	No. Copies of Single Issue Published Nearest to Filing Date
a. Paid Electronic Copies ▶		
b. Total Paid Print Copies (Line 15c) + Paid Electronic Copies (Line 16a) ▶		
c. Total Print Distribution (Line 15f) + Paid Electronic Copies (Line 16a) ▶		
d. Percent Paid (Both Print & Electronic Copies) (16b divided by 16c × 100) ▶		

☒ I certify that 50% of all my distributed copies (electronic and print) are paid above a nominal price.

17. Publication of Statement of Ownership

☒ If the publication is a general publication, publication of this statement is required. Will be printed in the NOVEMBER 2023 issue of this publication. ☐ Publication not required.

18. Signature and Title of Editor, Publisher, Business Manager, or Owner

Malathi Samayan - Distribution Controller

Malathi Samayan   Date 9/18/2023

I certify that all information furnished on this form is true and complete. I understand that anyone who furnishes false or misleading information on this form or who omits material or information requested on the form may be subject to criminal sanctions (including fines and imprisonment) and/or civil sanctions (including civil penalties).

PS Form 3526, July 2014 (Page 3 of 4)   PRIVACY NOTICE: See our privacy policy on www.usps.com.

Moving?

Make sure your subscription moves with you!

To notify us of your new address, find your **Clinics Account Number** (located on your mailing label above your name), and contact customer service at:

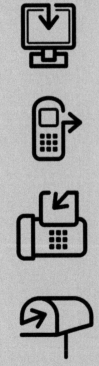

Email: journalscustomerservice-usa@elsevier.com

800-654-2452 (subscribers in the U.S. & Canada)
314-447-8871 (subscribers outside of the U.S. & Canada)

Fax number: 314-447-8029

Elsevier Health Sciences Division
Subscription Customer Service
3251 Riverport Lane
Maryland Heights, MO 63043

*To ensure uninterrupted delivery of your subscription, please notify us at least 4 weeks in advance of move.

Printed and bound by CPI Group (UK) Ltd, Croydon, CR0 4YY

03/10/2024

01040367-0017